D1068831

CRITICAL CARE MANAGEMENT OF
The Obese Patient

CRITICAL CARE MANAGEMENT OF
The Obese Patient

EDITED BY

Ali A. El Solh MD MPH

Associate Professor of Medicine, Anesthesiology, and Social and Preventive Medicine
Division of Pulmonary, Critical Care & Sleep Medicine
School of Medicine and Biomedical Sciences
University at Buffalo;
Chief, Critical Care
Western New York Healthcare System;
Director, Western New York Respiratory Research Center
Buffalo, NY, USA

WILEY-BLACKWELL

A John Wiley & Sons, Ltd., Publication

This edition first published 2012 © 2012 by John Wiley & Sons, Ltd

Wiley-Blackwell is an imprint of John Wiley & Sons, formed by the merger of Wiley's global Scientific, Technical and Medical business with Blackwell Publishing.

Registered Office
John Wiley & Sons, Ltd, The Atrium, Southern Gate, Chichester, West Sussex, PO19 8SQ, UK

Editorial Offices
9600 Garsington Road, Oxford, OX4 2DQ, UK
The Atrium, Southern Gate, Chichester, West Sussex, PO19 8SQ, UK
111 River Street, Hoboken, NJ 07030–5774, USA

For details of our global editorial offices, for customer services and for information about
how to apply for permission to reuse the copyright material in this book please see our website at
www.wiley.com/wiley-blackwell

The right of the author to be identified as the author of this work has been asserted in accordance with
the UK Copyright, Designs and Patents Act 1988.

Library of Congress Cataloging-in-Publication Data

Critical care management of the obese patient / edited by Ali A. El Solh.
     p. ; cm.
   Includes bibliographical references and index.
   ISBN-13: 978-0-470-65590-0 (hard cover : alk. paper)
   ISBN-10: 0-470-65590-9 (hard cover : alk. paper)   1. Critical care medicine.
2. Obesity–Complications.   I. El Solh, Ali A.
   [DNLM: 1. Critical Care–methods.   2. Comorbidity.   3. Critical Illness.   4. Obesity–complications.
5. Obesity–physiopathology. WX 218]
   RC86.C75 2012
   616.3′98028–dc23
                                            2011024782

A catalogue record for this book is available from the British Library.

Wiley also publishes its books in a variety of electronic formats. Some content that appears in print may
not be available in electronic books.

Set in 9.25/11.5pt Minion by SPi Publisher Services, Pondicherry, India
Printed and bound in Singapore by Markono Print Media Pte Ltd

1   2012

Contents

Part VII   Prognosis and Ethics

Contributors

Martin A. Alpert MD
Brent M. Parker Professor of Medicine
Division of Cardiovascular Medicine
University of Missouri-Columbia School of Medicine
Columbia, MO, USA

Paula Alvarez-Castro MD
Xeral Lugo Hospital
Lugo, Spain

Bikram S. Bal MD
Section of Gastroenterology
Washington Hospital Center and Georgetown
University School of Medicine
Washington, DC, USA

Robert L. Bell MD MA FACS
Director, Minimally Invasive Surgery
Director, Bariatric Surgery
Associate Professor
Department of Surgery
Yale University School of Medicine
New Haven, CT, USA

Eric J. Chan MD
Fellow in Cardiovascular Disease
University of Missouri-Columbia
School of Medicine
Columbia, MO, USA

Hui Sen Chong MD
Clinical Assistant Professor
Department of Surgery Gastrointestinal,
Minimally Invasive Surgery University of Iowa
Hospitals and Clinics
Iowa City, IA, USA

Fernando Cordido MD PhD
Professor of Endocrinology and Nutrition
Endocrine Department
University Hospital A Coruña
University of A Coruña
A Coruña, Spain

Jan J. De Waele MD PhD
Senior Lecturer
Department of Intensive Care Medicine
Ghent University Hospital
Ghent University
Ghent, Belgium

Thérèse M. Duane MD FACS
Associate Professor of Surgery
Department of General Surgery
Virginia Commonwealth University
Medical College of Virginia
Richmond, VA, USA

Brian L. Erstad PharmD FCCM
Professor
University of Arizona College of Pharmacy
Department of Pharmacy Practice & Science
Tucson, AZ, USA

Ilse M. Espina MS
Research Assistant
Dorrington Medical Associates
Houston, TX, USA;
Universidad Popular Autónoma del
Estado de Puebla
Puebla, Mexico

Frederick C. Finelli MD JD
Department of Surgery
Washington Hospital Center and Georgetown
University School of Medicine
Washington, DC, USA

Erin C. Hall MD MPH
Department of Surgery
Johns Hopkins School of Medicine
Baltimore, MD, USA;
Department of Surgery
Georgetown University
Washington, DC, USA

Hadley K. Herbert MD
General Surgery Resident
Department of General Surgery
Virginia Commonwealth University
Medical College of Virginia
Richmond, VA, USA

Eric A.J. Hoste MD PhD
Senior Lecturer
Department of Intensive Care Medicine
Ghent University Hospital, Ghent University
Ghent, Belgium;
Research Foundation
Flanders, Belgium

Tjasa Hranjec MD
Department of Surgery
University of Virginia Health System
Charlottesville, VA, USA

Christopher G. Hughes MD
Assistant Professor of Anesthesiology
Vanderbilt University School of Medicine
Nashville, TN, USA

Philippe Abou Jaoude MD
Pulmonary/Critical Care Fellow
Department of Medicine
Division of Pulmonary Care and Critical Care Medicine
State University of New York at Buffalo
Buffalo, NY, USA

David A. Johnson MD FACG FASGE
Professor of Medicine
Chief of Gastroenterology
Eastern Virginia Medical School
Norfolk, VA, USA

Venkata S. Katabathina MD
Assistant Professor
Section of Abdominal Imaging/Intervention,
Department of Radiology
University of Texas Health Science Center
San Antonio, TX, USA

Timothy R. Koch MD FACG
Professor of Medicine (Gastroenterology)
Georgetown University School of Medicine
Washington, DC, USA;
Washington Hospital Center
Washington, DC, USA

Wim K. Lagrand MD PhD
Cardiologist-Intensivist
Department of Intensive Care Adults
Academic Medical Center
Amsterdam, The Netherlands

Neeraj Lalwani MD
Department of Radiology
University of Texas Health Science Center
San Antonio, TX, USA

Carel W. le Roux MBChB MSc MRCP
MRCPath PhD
Reader and Honorary Consultant
in Metabolic Medicine
Imperial Weight Centre
Imperial College London
London, UK

Benjamin H. Levy III MD
Department of Internal Medicine
University of Arizona
Tucson, AZ, USA

M. Jeffrey Mador MD
Associate Professor of Medicine
Division of Pulmonary, Critical Care and Sleep Medicine
State University of New York at Buffalo
Buffalo, NY, USA;
Staff Physician
Western New York Veteran Affairs Healthcare System
Buffalo, NY, USA

Juliana Marques MD
Department of Anaesthesiology and Intensive Care
Friedrich Schiller University Hospital
Jena, Germany

Samer G. Mattar MD FACR FRCS (Edin) FASMBS
Associate Professor of Surgery
Indiana University
Indianapolis, IN, USA;
Director, IU Health Bariatics and Weight Loss
Indianapolis, IN, USA;
Indiana University Health Bariatics and Weight Loss,
Indiana University Health North,
Carmel, IN, USA

Richard A. Matthay MD
Boehringer Ingelheim Emeritus Professor of Medicine
Yale University School of Medicine
Department of Internal Medicine
Section of Pulmonary and Critical Care Medicine
New Haven, CT, USA

Margaret E. McAtee MN RN ACNP-BC CCRN
Cardiovascular Nurse Practitioner
Baylor All Saints Medical Center
Fort Worth, TX, USA

Scott E. Mimms MD
Advanced Laparoscopy and Bariatric Surgery Fellow
Indiana University
Indianapolis, IN, USA;
Indiana University Health Bariatics and Weight Loss,
Indiana University Health North,
Carmel, IN, USA

Alexander D. Miras MRCP BSc
Specialist Registrar in Endocrinology and Diabetes
Medical Research Council Clinical Research Fellow
Imperial Weight Centre
Imperial College London
London, UK

Mohammed Mogri MD
Pulmonary Critical Care Fellow
State University of New York at Buffalo
Buffalo, NY, USA

James M. O'Brien Jr MD MSc
Associate Professor
Division of Pulmonary, Allergy,
Critical Care & Sleep Medicine
Department of Internal Medicine
The Ohio State University Medical Center
Columbus, OH, USA

Pratik P. Pandharipande MD MSCI
Associate Professor of Anesthesiology
Vanderbilt Medical Center and VA TVHCS
Nashville, TN, USA

Anthony Passannante MD
Professor of Anesthesiology
Department of Anesthesiology
University of North Carolina Hospitals
Chapel Hill, NC, USA

Amani D. Politano MD
Department of Surgery
University of Virginia Health System
Charlottesville, VA, USA

Jahan Porhomayon MD
Assistant Professor
Department of Anesthesia,
State University of New York
Buffalo School of Medicine
and Biomedical Sciences and School
of Public Health and Health Professions
Buffalo, NY, USA

Srinivasa R. Prasad MD
Professor of Radiology
University of Texas Health Science Center
San Antonio, TX, USA

Hallie C. Prescott MD
Chief Resident
Department of Internal Medicine
The Ohio State University Medical Center
Columbus, OH, USA

Carlos S. Restrepo MD
Department of Radiology
University of Texas
Health Science Center
San Antonio, TX, USA

Laura H. Rosenberger MD
Department of Surgery
University of Virginia Health System
Charlottesville, VA, USA

Yasser Sakr MD PhD
Consultant
Department of Anaesthesiology
and Intensive Care
Friedrich Schiller University Hospital
Jena, Germany

Susana Sangiao-Alvarellos PhD
Investigation Department
University Hospital A Coruña
University of A Coruña
A Coruña, Spain

Robert G. Sawyer MD
Professor of Surgery
University of Virginia Health System
Charlottesville, VA, USA

Marcus J. Schultz MD PhD
Professor of Intensive Care Medicine
Academic Medical Center
University of Amsterdam
Amsterdam, The Netherlands

Dorry L. Segev MD PhD
Associate Professor of Surgery and
Epidemiology
Director of Clinical Research
Transplant Surgery
Department of Surgery
Johns Hopkins School of Medicine
Baltimore MD, USA;
Department of Epidemiology
Johns Hopkins Bloomberg School
of Public Health
Baltimore, MD, USA

Mark D. Siegel MD
Associate Professor
Pulmonary & Critical Care Section
Department of Internal Medicine
Yale School of Medicine
New Haven, CT, USA

Michael Tielborg MD MSc
Assistant Professor
Department of Anesthesiology
University of North Carolina
Chapel Hill, NC, USA

Terence K. Trow MD
Director, Yale Pulmonary Vascular
Disease Program
Associate Professor of Medicine
Yale University School of Medicine
Department of Internal Medicine
Section of Pulmonary and
Critical Care Medicine
New Haven, CT, USA

Kristin Turza Campbell MD
Department of Surgery
University of Virginia Health System
Charlottesville, VA, USA

Eline R. van Slobbe-Bijlsma MD
Anesthesiologist-Intensivist
Department of Intensive Care Adults
Academic Medical Center
Amsterdam, The Netherlands

Joseph Varon MD FACP FCCP FCCM
Chief of Critical Care Services
University General Hospital
Houston, TX, USA;
Clinical Professor of Medicine and
Professor of Acute and
Continuing Care
The University of Texas
Health Science Center at Houston
Houston, TX, USA;
Clinical Professor of Medicine
The University of Texas Medical Branch
at Galveston
Houston, TX, USA

Lisa Weavind MD
Associate Professor of Anesthesiology
Vanderbilt University School of Medicine
Nashville, TN, USA

Mohamed Zeiden MD PhD
Department of Anaesthesiology and Intensive Care
Theodor Bilharz Institute
Cairo, Egypt

Preface

Obesity has risen at an epidemic rate over the past 20 years. The number of overweight people is higher than ever, and the pervasiveness of obesity across age groups irrespective of racial and ethnic differences has raised the awareness of scientists, health professionals, and health organizations worldwide. The most recent National Health and Nutrition Examination Survey (NHANES) data document a dramatic rise in the prevalence of obesity, with a prevalence estimate of approximately 68% for overweight and obese adults combined. Obesity increases the risk for many chronic diseases including diabetes mellitus, cardiovascular diseases, and respiratory and sleep disorders. As such, the proportion of morbidly obese patients requiring critical care services is rising exponentially. A thorough knowledge of the underlying physiology and complications of morbid obesity is therefore essential for the proper management of these patients in order to achieve a satisfactory outcome.

Critically ill obese patients require a multidisciplinary approach with input from multiple allied health specialties including internal medicine, cardiology, pulmonary, infectious disease, surgery, nutrition, pharmacy, and rehabilitation therapy among others. Caring for a morbidly obese patient also poses a significant challenge for the nursing staff both physically and psychologically. This book is an attempt to develop a working framework between different disciplines on the challenges posed by critically ill obese patients in an attempt to provide comprehensive but clinically relevant knowledge to health care practitioners from different backgrounds. The combination of state of the art expertise and insightful editorial execution provides practitioners and trainees of critical care specialties with a comprehensive resource for everyday use.

The contents of the book address most aspects of care of the critically ill obese patient as well as serving as a resource to facilitate the management of services, use of clinical information, and negotiation of ethical issues that occur during the stay in the intensive care unit. The initial chapters review the physiological derangements of obesity. Subsequent chapters focus on the clinical management of organ dysfunction and hemodynamic alterations in critically ill obese patients and the role of pharmacy and nutrition in providing therapeutic support during the acute phase of illness. A section on bariatric surgery and its complications is included to reflect the growing trend in these innovative procedures. The last few chapters address the controversies in prognosticating the outcome of these patients, organ donation, and the ethical issues that face the critical care specialists in these settings.

The book has been organized in a consistent format to ease identification of relevant material. Extensive use of tables, figures, and practice tips is located throughout each chapter to identify areas of care that are particularly pertinent for readers. It is not the intent that readers progress sequentially through the book, but rather explore chapters or sections that are relevant for daily practice.

I trust that this book will be a valuable resource in guiding the care of the critically ill obese patient.

Ali El Solh, MD, MPH

Part I

Physiology and Consequences of Obesity

1

Cardiovascular Physiology in Obesity

Eric J. Chan and Martin A. Alpert

University of Missouri-Columbia School of Medicine, University of Missouri, Health Sciences Center, Columbia, MO, USA

> **KEY POINTS**
> - Obesity, particularly class III obesity, produces central hemodynamic changes that cause alterations in cardiac morphology and ventricular function which may lead to heart failure.
> - In the absence of systemic hypertension, hemodynamic changes include increased total and circulating blood volume, high cardiac output, low systemic vascular resistance, left ventricular dilatation, eccentric left ventricular hypertrophy and elevated left ventricular end-diastolic pressure.
> - Left ventricular function in long-standing obesity is often characterized by impaired diastolic filling and infrequently associated with systolic dysfunction.

INTRODUCTION

Obesity is a growing epidemic in the United States and worldwide [1–4]. In the United States, 33 of the 50 states have a prevalence of obesity $\geq 25\%$ [2]. Ten years ago the prevalence of obesity was $< 25\%$ in all 50 states [2,3]. Worldwide the prevalence of obesity ranges from 12 to 80%, with the highest rates occurring in the more industrialized nations [1]. Obesity is traditionally categorized in terms of body mass index (BMI). Current definitions of overweight and obesity in adults are as follows: overweight: BMI of 25.0–29.9 kg/m²; class I obesity: BMI of 30.0–34.9 kg/m²; class II obesity: BMI of 35.0–39.9 kg/m²; and class III obesity: BMI ≥ 40 kg/m². Class III obesity is sometimes referred to as severe, extreme or morbid obesity [1–4]. The term "super obesity" is used to describe patients whose BMI is ≥ 50 kg/m² [4].

A relationship between obesity and the heart has been recognized since ancient times, as noted by Senac (aphorism no. 11) and Hippocrates in his oft quoted aphorism no. 44: "Sudden death is more common in those that are naturally fat than in the lean" [5]. In 1806 Corvisart described adipose surrounding the heart in obese subjects and suggested that in obese people the heart was "oppressed by enveloping fat" [5]. In 1847 William Harvey reported a post-mortem examination of a corpulent man and wrote that "the heart was large, thick and fibrous, with a considerable quantity of adhering fat, both in its circumference and over its septum" [5]. Harvey reported that shortly before his death this patient developed facial lividity, difficult breathing and orthopnea, perhaps the first description of obesity cardiomyopathy. During this period of time it was presumed that excessive epicardial fat was responsible for cardiac dysfunction in patients with severe obesity. The term "adipositas cordis" was used to describe this phenomenon. In 1933 Smith and Willius published autopsy findings of 136 obese subjects whose excess weight ranged from 14 to 175% [6]. In nearly all of the obese subjects heart weight exceeded that predicted for normal body weight [6]. Subsequent studies established that myocardial fat content in obese persons is no different than that of lean individuals [5,7,8]. In addition, several case reports and small series characterized what would subsequently become known as the sleep apnea/obesity hypoventilation syndrome or "Pickwickian" syndrome [9–11]. Renewed interest in the cardiovascular physiology and pathophysiology of obesity occurred with publication of hemodynamic studies of extremely obese adults by Alexander and colleagues in 1959 [12]. The purpose of this chapter is to review cardiovascular physiology and pathophysiology in obesity, based primarily on research performed and published during the last half-century. This chapter will focus on central and peripheral hemodynamics, emphasizing their effects on cardiac morphology and ventricular function and the development of heart failure. The pathophysiological effects of systemic hypertension and the sleep apnea/obesity hypoventilation syndrome on the heart will also be discussed, as will the effects of weight reduction. The relationship between obesity and coronary artery disease is complex and is beyond the scope of this review. Neither this issue nor the matter of ventricular arrhythmias and sudden death in obesity will be addressed in this chapter.

CARDIOVASCULAR HEMODYNAMIC ALTERATIONS ASSOCIATED WITH OBESITY

Obesity, particularly morbid obesity, produces a variety of hemodynamic changes that may predispose to alterations in cardiac morphology and ventricular function [12–22]. Figure 1.1 summarizes the major cardiovascular hemodynamic alterations associated with obesity and their pathophysiological sequelae. This figure may be used for reference in this section and in subsequent sections on cardiac morphology and ventricular function.

Central cardiovascular hemodynamics

Obesity produces an increase in total and circulating blood volume [4,12–14]. This phenomenon was originally attributed entirely to excessive adipose accumulation, but recent evidence indicates that increased fat-free mass plays an important role [4,15,16]. In normotensive obese individuals, systemic vascular resistance is lower than in normotensive lean persons [4,12–14,17,18]. The increase in circulating blood volume together with reduced systemic vascular resistance results in an increase in cardiac output. Indeed, Alexander et al. demonstrated that cardiac output increased in proportion to the excess in body weight in obese subjects [12–14]. Heart rate did not differ from that predicted with ideal body weight in this study and stroke volume increased in proportion to the excess in body weight [12–14]. Thus, the increase in cardiac output associated with obesity is entirely attributable to an increase in left ventricular (LV) stroke volume [12–14]. Oxygen consumption and arteriovenous oxygen difference are reportedly increased in moderately to

severely obese patients despite the high cardiac output state [4,12–14]. In a study of 10 moderately to severely obese subjects, DeDivitiis and colleagues confirmed these findings and noted the presence of increased LV work and stroke work [17]. DeDivitiis and coworkers also reported a decrease in LV Dp/dt in this study, possibly suggesting the presence of an intrinsic defect of myocardial contractility [17]. They reported right ventricular (RV) end-diastolic pressure and mean pulmonary artery pressure values in excess of those predicted for ideal body weight [17]. In actuality, right heart pressures associated with obesity reported in the literature are somewhat variable, depending in part on the contribution of left heart failure, sleep apnea/obesity hypoventilation and other pulmonary disorders [12–19]. Pulmonary capillary wedge pressure and LV end-diastolic pressure values reported in the literature are similarly variable, ranging from high-normal to markedly elevated [12–14,17–19]. However, studies assessing central hemodynamics during exercise have uniformly noted a marked increase in LV filling pressure even with modest exertion, often reaching levels sufficient to produce pulmonary edema [4,13,18]. Whether extreme physiological stresses such as those encountered in the critical care setting produce similar results is unproven, but likely. Thus, it appears that moderate to severe obesity raises cardiac output at the expense of LV filling pressure. The aforementioned pathophysiological observations are applicable primarily to normotensive obese patients. Systemic hypertension tends to intensify these hemodynamic responses and will be discussed in a later section.

Distribution of obesity may be an important issue as individuals with central obesity have been shown to have higher systemic vascular resistance and lower cardiac output than those with a centripetal fat distribution [4,19]. It is also important to emphasize that central hemodynamic studies have been performed predominantly on class II and III obese subjects. The applicability of data derived from these studies to overweight and class I obese patients is uncertain.

Peripheral hemodynamics

Adipose tissue is surrounded by an extensive capillary network [4]. Adipocytes are located close to vessels with high permeability and low hydrostatic pressure. This, coupled with a short distance for transport, facilitates movement of molecules to and from adipocytes [4]. The resting blood flow in adipose tissue is 2–3 ml/min/100 g of fat and can increase up to 10-fold [4]. Adipose tissue

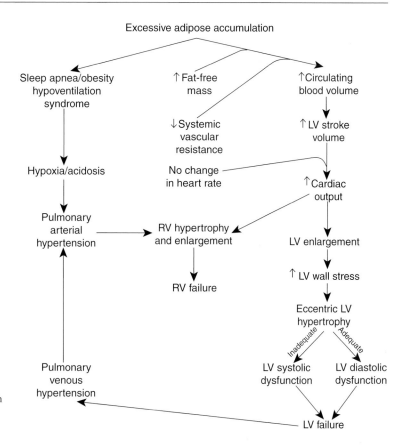

Figure 1.1 Major cardiovascular hemodynamic alterations associated with uncomplicated obesity and their pathophysiological sequelae.

makes up a substantial proportion of total body weight. The interstitial portion of adipose tissue contains a large quantity of fluid [4]. This fluid, however, is not readily accessible to the central circulation because blood flow per unit of adipose tissue is reduced by the vasodilatory effect of B1 receptors [4]. Although cardiac output increases with total fat mass the perfusion per unit of adipose tissue actually decreases with increasing percentage body fat [4]. Because the enlarged bed of adipose tissue in the obese is less vascularized than other tissue, the observed increase in stroke volume and cardiac output cannot be explained by fat mass alone [4]. As previously noted, recent studies have confirmed that fat-free mass plays an important and possibly predominant role in the previously-noted central hemodynamic alterations [4,15,16].

An important concept in peripheral hemodynamics in obesity is the role of the adipocyte as an endocrine and paracrine organ. Adipokines released by adipocytes play an important role in modulating peripheral hemodynamics. Leptin helps modulate energy expenditure and

sympathetic tone through the hypothalamus. In the obese, a pattern of selective leptin resistance has been identified [20]. It is characterized by continued leptin resistance to satiety, but not to its effect on sympathetic tone [20]. Leptin resistance is thought to be mediated by down regulation of the leptin receptor by leptin itself, producing increased circulating leptin levels, increased sympathetic tone, and peripheral vasoconstriction [20]. Three decades ago Messerli et al. demonstrated that plasma renin activity was higher in normotensive obese subjects than in normotensive lean subjects, suggesting activation of the renin-angiotensin-aldosterone system in obesity [21]. More recently, Massiera and colleagues reported increased expression of adipose angiotensinogen in rats with increased fat mass sufficient to be detected in the circulation [22]. This study provides additional evidence of renin-angiotensin-aldosterone system activation in obesity. These endocrine and paracrine activities of adipose may produce vasoconstriction and an increase in systemic vascular resistance. In doing so they may predispose to obesity-related hypertension.

Little information exists concerning regional distribution of blood flow in other organ beds in obesity. Older studies in extremely obese adults suggest that cerebral blood flow is mildly reduced, splanchnic blood flow is mildly increased and renal blood flow is low-normal to normal [13].

EFFECT OF OBESITY ON CARDIAC MORPHOLOGY

Left ventricle

Post-mortem studies of extremely obese subjects have uniformly shown increased LV wall thickness and microscopic LV hypertrophy [23–25]. However, these studies did not exclude patients with hypertension and other comorbidities. Early echocardiographic studies in morbidly obese subjects reported LV enlargement in 8–40%, increased LV wall thickness in 6–56%, and increased LV mass in 64–87% [23]. The wide ranges reported may be attributable to differences in comorbidities and in the severity and duration of obesity [23]. Numerous studies have compared various measures of LV morphology in obese and lean subjects [23–28]. The severity of obesity ranged from mild to severe. In most of these studies the measure of LV morphology (diastolic chamber size, ventricular septal thickness, posterior wall thickness, mass, mass index, mass/height index) was significantly higher/greater in obese than in lean subjects. A study by Kasper and colleagues of 409 lean patients and 43 patients whose BMI was $> 35\,kg/m^2$ with heart failure showed a higher prevalence of dilated cardiomyopathy in obese than in lean patients [29]. A specific cause was noted in 64% of obese and only 23% of lean patients [29]. Myocyte hypertrophy was identified on 67% of myocardial biopsies of obese patients [29]. In the Framingham study, BMI strongly correlated with LV wall thickness, LV internal dimension in diastole, and LV mass even after adjusting for age and blood pressure, particularly in patients whose BMI was $> 30\,kg/m^2$ [30]. In a study of 50 normotensive morbidly obese patients, Alpert et al. reported that LV mass/height index correlated positively and significantly with the LV internal dimension in diastole, systolic blood pressure and LV end-systolic wall stress, and duration of morbid obesity (emphasizing the important role that loading conditions and duration play in the development of LV hypertrophy) [31,32].

Figure 1.1 shows the evolution of LV morphological changes in obesity. The hypercirculatory state characterized by increased circulating blood volume and cardiac output leads to LV dilatation. This in turn predisposes to increased LV wall stress in accordance with the law of LaPlace. Morphologically this may be manifested as increased LV radius:thickness or volume:mass ratio. In the normotensive obese patient persistent elevation of wall stress may produce eccentric LV hypertrophy, which is effectively a mechanism to normalize wall stress. Whether the patient develops LV remodeling and hypertrophy depends on the severity of obesity, the presence or absence of hypertension, and the duration of obesity. Recent studies have suggested that concentric LV remodeling and hypertrophy may occur to a variable extent in normotensive obese persons. The mechanism for this is uncertain [28].

Left atrium

Post-mortem studies of morbidly obese patients have reported left atrial enlargement in virtually all cases, particularly when hypertension was present [23–25]. Echocardiographic studies have reported an incidence of left atrial enlargement that ranges from 10 to 50%, depending on the severity and duration of obesity [23]. Sasson and colleagues reported an incidence of left atrial enlargement in 37% of class I obese patients and 6% of 35 lean patients [33]. Wang et al. demonstrated a significant association between BMI and the development of atrial fibrillation [34]. With each unit increase in BMI, the risk of atrial fibrillation increased 5% [34]. Adjustment for left atrial diameter attenuated this correlation, suggesting that left atrial size rather than BMI was more directly involved in the genesis of the arrhythmia [34].

Right ventricle

Early post-mortem studies of morbidly obese subjects commonly reported excessive quantities of epicardial fat (33–100%), predominantly covering the right ventricle [5,23]. Not infrequently cords of fat penetrated RV myocardium (a form of metaplasia) [4,5,23]. RV enlargement and hypertrophy have been described to a variable extent, depending in part on the presence of left heart failure and pulmonary hypertension from the sleep apnea/obesity hypoventilation syndrome [5,23,25]. Increased circulating blood volume and elevated cardiac output associated with class II and III obesity may also contribute to RV enlargement [5,13,23,25]. Rare cases of restrictive physiology have also been described [36,37]. Little information exists concerning RV morphology in asymptomatic obese subjects. Alpert and coworkers reported RV enlargement by echocardiography in 32% of asymptomatic normotensive morbidly obese patients [39].

LEFT VENTRICULAR DIASTOLIC FUNCTION

Left ventricular end-diastolic pressure

As noted in the section on central hemodynamics LV end-diastolic pressure (LV filling pressure) in patients with class III obesity is frequently elevated, often markedly so, particularly during exercise. Whether the physiological stresses encountered in the intensive care setting produce similar elevations of LV end-diastolic pressure in such patients is uncertain. LV filling pressures in class I and II obese patients have not been extensively reported in the literature.

Left ventricular diastolic filling

While LV end-diastolic pressure is the most specific clinical measure of LV diastolic function, a variety of non-invasive cardiac indices have been developed to assess early and late LV diastolic filling [38,40]. These include radionuclide indices (peak filing rate, time to peak filling, isovolumic relaxation time), transmitral echocardiographic/Doppler indices (E:A ratio, deceleration time, and deceleration half-time), and tissue Doppler indices (E:Ea, Ea:Aa). These non-invasive indices have facilitated evaluation of LV diastolic function in patients with all classes of obesity. Studies comparing LV diastolic filling based on noninvasive indices in patients with class I, II, and III obesity with lean patients consistently showed greater impairment of LV diastolic filling in patients at all stages of obesity than in lean patients [41–45]. Studies by Alpert and coworkers in normotensive morbidly obese subjects showed that there was a significant positive correlation between transmitral E wave deceleration time (or half time) and LV mass height index, LV internal dimension in diastole, systolic blood pressure, and LV end-systolic wall stress [46,47]. Conversely, transmitral E:A ratio correlated negatively and significantly with these variables [46,47]. This confirms that in normotensive obese patients LV hypertrophy and the loading conditions that predispose to hypertrophy underlie impairment of LV diastolic filling (see Figure 1.1). Studies by Alpert et al. indicates that duration of obesity also plays an important role in the development of LV diastolic dysfunction [32]. All of the aforementioned invasive

and noninvasive indices of diastolic function are load dependent. Tissue Doppler is ostensibly free from the effects of loading conditions. Recent studies assessing diastolic function indices with tissue Doppler have shown lower myocardial velocities and E:Ea ratios (a surrogate for LV filling pressure) in lean than in obese patients [38,40].

LEFT VENTRICULAR SYSTOLIC FUNCTION

As noted in Figure 1.1, increased circulating blood volume coupled with increased cardiac output in the setting of obesity leads to LV dilation, which in the absence of systemic hypertension predisposes to LV hypertrophy. LV hypertrophy contributes to LV diastolic dysfunction, as noted in the last section. LV hypertrophy contributes to normalization of LV wall stress. In patients with class I and class II obesity and in many patients with class III obesity hypertrophy is adequate, wall stress normalizes, and LV systolic function remains preserved [48]. In a minority of class III obese patients LV wall stress remains high due to inadequate hypertrophy and LV systolic dysfunction ensues [48].

Multiple studies have compared LV systolic function (by measuring LV ejection fraction or LV fractional shortening) in class I–III obese patient with lean controls [48]. Most have shown normal LV systolic function in both groups and no significant difference between groups. However, a study by Iacobellis and coworkers reported an average 5% greater LV ejection fraction in obese than in lean patients [49]. In a study of 50 normotensive morbidly obese patients reported by Alpert and coworkers, LV fractional shortening correlated negatively and significantly with LV mass/height index, LV internal dimension in diastole, systolic blood pressure, and LV end-systolic wall stress, indicating that LV mass and loading conditions that contribute to LV hypertrophy may adversely affect LV systolic function [50]. Duration of morbid obesity was also identified as an important determinant of LV systolic function in morbid obesity [32]. Alpert and colleagues noted that exercise produced an increase in LV ejection fraction in patients with normal LV mass, but no change in those with elevated LV mass [51]. Tissue Doppler studies of systolic function in obese subjects have produced conflicting results [38,52]. Liptoxicity involving myocardium has been described in obese animals, but has not been documented to occur in humans [28].

OBESITY, HYPERTENSION, AND THE HEART

System hypertension has been estimated to occur in up to 60% of obese persons and is severe in up to 10% [53]. The physiological mechanisms responsible for obesity hypertension are incompletely understood. Epidemiological and genetic factors are thought to play a role in some cases [53,54]. An interplay involving activation of the renin-angiotensin-aldosterone system, increased adrenergic activity, hyperinsulinemia/insulin resistance, alterations in intracellular calcium and sodium-potassium distribution, increased smooth muscle tone and vascular resistance, increased sodium sensitivity and absorption, elevated cardiac output, and expanded intravascular and cardiopulmonary volume are thought to contribute to the development of hypertension in the setting of obesity [53,54]. A detailed discussion of the pathophysiology of obesity hypertension is beyond the scope of this review.

The effect of systemic hypertension on LV morphology depends on the relative contributions of obesity and hypertension [53,55,56]. In healthy normotensive lean persons, LV chamber size, wall thickness, and mass are normal. In lean hypertensive persons, LV wall thickness increases, chamber size decreases or remains unchanged, and LV mass increases due to concentric LV hypertrophy [53,55,56]. In most normotensive obese persons, as discussed previously, eccentric LV hypertrophy develops, characterized by chamber dilation and initial thinning of wall thickness followed by secondary hypertrophy [53,55,56]. LV mass, however, is increased. In hypertensive obese patients, LV chamber dilation occurs to a lesser degree than in normotensive obese persons [53,55,56]. Wall thickness is often increased in such patients. This is in essence a "hybrid" form of LV hypertrophy, previously referred to as "eccentric–concentric" hypertrophy [55,56] and now classified as a form of concentric hypertrophy. LV mass may be substantially elevated in such patients [55,56]. In reality, the patterns of hypertrophy noted depend on the predominant hemodynamic stress. For example, a patient with class I obesity and long-standing severe hypertension may present with concentric LV hypertrophy, whereas a patient with class III obesity and mild hypertension may present with eccentric or eccentric–concentric LV hypertrophy. Patients with long-standing obesity hypertension with eccentric–concentric hypertrophy typically have higher systemic vascular resistance and higher LV filling pressure values than normotensive obese patients with eccentric LV hypertrophy alone [53,57].

HEART FAILURE AND OBESITY

The cardiovascular hemodynamic morphological changes and alterations in ventricular function described previously may begin to develop in class I and II obesity. Indeed, obesity clearly serves as a risk factor for heart failure in such individuals [58]. However, in the absence of comorbidities such as coronary artery disease, valvular heart disease or hypertensive heart disease, heart failure resulting exclusively from obesity occurs almost exclusively in patients with class III obesity and super-obesity [4,13,59–61]. The pathophysiological basis for heart failure in such patients is shown in Figure 1.1. In normotensive morbidly obese patients, LV hypertrophy produces LV diastolic and in some cases LV systolic dysfunction [4,59–61]. This predisposes to pulmonary venous hypertension, leading to increased pulmonary capillary pressure and pulmonary edema [4,59–61]. Pulmonary arterial hypertension then ensues, leading to RV hypertrophy and dilation, and eventually right heart failure [4,59–61]. Hypoxemia related to sleep apnea/obesity hypoventilation may contribute to pulmonary hypertension and right heart decompensation [4,59–61]. In morbidly obese patients right heart failure rarely occurs in the absence of left heart failure. Although the term "obesity cardiomyopathy" is often applied to the pathophysiological process described in this review, it more properly should be defined as heart failure due entirely or predominantly to severe obesity [61]. Not unexpectedly, studies comparing cardiac structure and function in morbidly obese patients with and without heart failure have shown that LV mass is significantly higher, LV diastolic filling is more significantly impaired and LV systolic function is more frequently abnormal in those with than in those without heart failure [59].

EFFECT OF WEIGHT REDUCTION

Weight reduction is the single most effective measure for reversing the cardiovascular pathophysiological changes associated with obesity. Weight loss-related changes have been reported in all classes of obesity, but mainly in class III obese patients [62–72].

The effects of weight reduction on central resting hemodynamics have been evaluated in class II and class III obese patients [62–65]. These studies have consistently shown that substantial weight loss decreases oxygen consumption, arteriovenous oxygen difference, total and circulating blood volume, cardiac output, LV stroke work, and LV work. LV stroke volume consistently decreased in these studies, but not always significantly [62–65]. The response of systemic vascular resistance has been more variable [62–65]. Heart rate and mean pulmonary artery pressure did not change significantly with weight loss in most studies [62–65]. Mean pulmonary capillary wedge pressure/LV end-diastolic pressure decreased with weight loss in some studies, but not in others [62–65]. Systemic blood pressure responses in normotensive patients have been variable. In hypertensive obese patients, the hemodynamic response to weight reduction is similar to that of normotensive patients, except that blood pressure more consistently decreases and stoke volume and systemic vascular resistance do not consistently change significantly [62,66]. After weight loss, LV stroke volume and cardiac output increase to a significantly greater extent with exercise than before weight loss [66].

Most studies exploring the effects of weight loss on LV morphology have reported significant decreases in LV mass, LV mass index, LV mass/height index, LV wall thickness, and LV diastolic chamber size, regardless of the severity of obesity prior to weight loss or the modality used to achieve weight loss [62,67–70]. The mechanisms by which these occur are not entirely clear, but favorable alterations in adverse loading conditions appear to play an important role.

Little information exists concerning the effect of weight loss on left atrial and right heart morphology.

In studies of morbidly obese patients with LV hypertrophy and impaired diastolic filling using transmitral Doppler flow indices, LV diastolic filling improved following substantial weight loss [62,67,69,72]. This improvement was associated with regression of LV hypertrophy and favorable alterations in LV loading conditions. Patients without LV hypertrophy experienced no change in LV diastolic filling with weight loss.

Because LV systolic function is usually normal in most obese individuals, most studies assessing the effect of weight reduction on this variable have shown no significant change [62,67,69,72]. In a study of normotensive morbidly obese subjects, however, those with depressed LV systolic function prior to weight loss experienced a significant improvement in LV systolic function with substantial weight reduction [50]. This was attributed in part to afterload reduction resulting from weight loss [50].

CONCLUSION

In conclusion, obesity, particularly class III obesity, is associated with cardiovascular hemodynamic changes that predispose to alterations in cardiac morphology and ventricular function which may lead to heart failure (obesity cardiomyopathy). Systemic hypertension and the sleep apnea/obesity hypoventilation syndrome may further contribute to the development of cardiac decompensation in such patients. An understanding of cardiovascular pathophysiology in obesity may assist the intensivist in managing critically ill patients who are at particularly high risk by virtue of the alterations in cardiac structure and function related to excessive adipose accumulation.

BEST PRACTICE TIPS

1 In most normotensive class III obese patients, cardiac output and LV filling pressure are elevated and systemic vascular resistance is reduced. Intensivists should take these hemodynamic alterations into consideration in fluid management and in selecting drugs for blood-pressure support.

2 The combination of systemic hypertension and class III obesity commonly produces concentric or eccentric–concentric LV hypertrophy with elevated LV filling pressure and normal or increased systemic vascular resistance. Such patients may be at risk for LV failure and pulmonary edema. Lowering blood pressure in such patients may attenuate this risk.

3 In class III and super-obese patients, it may be difficult to confirm the diagnosis of heart failure based on the medical history, physical examination, chest X-ray or natriuretic peptide values. In some critically ill patients it may be necessary to perform bedside pulmonary artery catheterization to establish this diagnosis.

4 In class III and super-obese patients, right heart failure rarely if ever occurs in the absence of left heart failure, even in patients with the sleep apnea/obesity hypoventilation syndrome. Thus, therapy in such individuals should be designed to treat biventricular failure as well as pulmonary complications.

5 LV systolic function is normal or increased in most obese persons, even when heart failure is present. Thus, inotropic therapy is of limited value in the treatment of heart failure in most obese persons and should be reserved for those with reduced LV systolic dysfunction or atrial fibrillation (digitalis).

REFERENCES

1 World Health Organization. Obesity: Preventing and managing the global epidemic. WHO Technical report series No. 894. Geneva, World Health Organization. 2000.

2 Obesity and Overweight for Professionals: Data and Statistics: US Obesity Trends DNPAO CDC. Available at: http://www.cdc.gov/obesity/data/trends.html1 [Accessed December 4, 2010].

3 Flegal KM, Carroll MD, Kuczmarski RJ, Johnson CL. Overweight and obesity in the United States: prevalence and trends, 1960–1994. Int J Obes Relat Metab Disord. 1998 Jan;22(1):39–47.

4 Poirier P, Giles TD, Bray GA, Hong Y, Stern JS, Pi-Sunyer X, Eckel RH. Obesity and cardiovascular disease: pathophysiology, evaluation, and effect of weight loss. Circulation. 2006; 113:898–918.

5 Alexander JK, Alpert MA. Historical notes. In Alpert MA, Alexander JK, editors. The Heart and Lung in Obesity. Armonk, NY, Futura Publishing Co. 1998. pp. 1–10.

6 Smith HL, Willius FA. Adiposity of the heart: a clinical and pathologic study of one hundred and thirty-six obese patients. Arch Intern Med. 1933;52:911–31.

7 Saphir O, Corrigan M. Fatty infiltration of myocardium. Arch Intern Med. 1993;52:410–28.

8 Carpenter HM. Myocardial fat infiltration. Am Heart J. 1962;63:491–6.

9 Ester EH Jr, Sieker HO, McIntosh HD, Kelser GA. Reversible cardiopulmonary syndrome with extreme obesity. Circulation. 1957 Aug;16(2):179–87.

10 Lillington GA, Anderson MA, Brandenberg RO. The cardiorespiratory syndrome of obesity. Dis Chest. 1957 Jul;32(1):1–20.

11 Bickelmann AG, Burwell CS, Robin ED, Whaley RD, et al. Extreme obesity associated with hypoventilation – a Pickwickian syndrome. Am J Med. 1956 Nov;21(5):811–18.

12 Alexander JK. Obesity and cardiac performance. Am J Cardiol. 1959 Dec;14:860–5.

13 Alexander JK, Alpert MA. Hemodynamic alterations associated with obesity in man. In Alpert MA, Alexander JK, editors. The Heart and Lung in Obesity. Armonk, NY, Futura Publishing Co. 1998. pp. 45–56.

14 Alexander JK, Dennis EW, Smith WG, Amad KH, Duncan WC, Austin RC. Blood volume, cardiac output and distribution of systemic blood flow in extreme obesity. Cardiovascular Res Center Bull. 1962–3 Winter;1:39–44.

15 Collis T, Devereux RB, Roman MJ, de Simone G, Yeh J, Howard BV, Fabsitz RR, Welty TK. Relations of stroke volume and cardiac output to body composition: the Strong Heart Study. Circulation. 2001 Feb;103(6):820–5.

16 Bella JN, Devereux RB, Roman MJ, O'Grady MJ, Welty TK, Lee ET, Fabsitz RR, Howard BV. Relations of left ventricular mass to fat-free and adipose body mass: the Strong Heart Study: the Strong Heart Study Investigators. Circulation. 1998 Nov;98(23):2538–44.

17 De Divitiis O, Fazio S, Petitto M, Maddalena G, Contaldo F, Mancini M. Obesity and cardiac function. Circulation. 1981 Sep;64(3):477–82.

18 Kaltman AJ, Goldring RM. Role of circulatory congestion in the cardiorespiratory failure of obesity. Am J Med. 1976 May;60(5):645–53.

19 Jern S, Bergbrant A, Bjorntorp P, Hansson L. Relation of central hemodynamics to obesity and body fat distribution. Hypertension. 1992 Jun;19(6 Part 1):520–7.

20 Mark AL, Correia ML, Rahmouni K, Haynes WG. Selective leptin resistance: a new concept in leptin physiology with cardiovascular implications. J Hypertens. 2002 Jul;20 (7):1245–50.

21 Messerli FH, Christie B, DeCarvalho JG, Aristimuno GG, Suarez DH, Dreslinski GR, Frohlich ED. Obesity and essential hypertension: hemodynamics, intravascular volume, sodium excretion, and plasma renin activity. Arch Intern Med. 1981 Jan;141(1):81–5.

22 Massiera F, Block-Faure M, Ceiler D, Murokami K,Fukamizu, Gase JM, Quigrard-Boulange A, Negrel R, Ailhoud G, Seydoux J, Meneton P, Teboul M. Adipose angiotensinogen is involved in adipose tissue growth and blood pressure regulation. FASEB J. 2001 Dec;15(14):2727–9.

23 Alpert MA, Alexander JK. Cardiac morphology and obesity in man. In Alpert MA, Alexander JK, editors. The Heart and Lung in Obesity. Armonk, NY, Futura Publishing Co. 1998. pp. 25–44.

24 Amad KH, Brennan JC, Alexander JK. The cardiac pathology of chronic exogenous obesity. Circulation. 1965 Nov;32(5):740–5.

25 Warnes CA, Roberts WC. The heart in massive (more than 300 pounds or 136 kilograms) obesity: analysis of 12 patients studied at necropsy. Am J Cardiol. 1984 Nov;54 (8):1087–91.

26 Crisostomo LL, Araújo LM, Câmara E, Carvahlo C, Silva FA, Viera M, Mendes CM, Rabelo A. Left ventricular mass and function in young obese women. Int J Obes Relat Metab Disord. 2001 Feb;25(2):233–8.

27 Iacobellis G, Ribaudo MC, Zappaterreno A, Iannucci CV, Vecci E, DiMario U. Adapted changes in left ventricular structure and function in severe uncomplicated obesity. Obes Res. 2004 Oct;12(10):1616–21.

28 Abel ED, Litwin SE, Sweeney G. Cardiac remodeling in Obesity. Physiol Rev. 2008 Apr;88(4):389–419.

29 Kasper EK, Hruban RH, Baughman KL. Cardiomyopathy of obesity: a clinicopathologic evaluation of 43 obese patients with heart failure. Am J Cardiol. 1992 Oct;70(9): 921–4.

30 Lauer MS, Anderson KM, Kannel WB, Levy D. The impact of obesity on left ventricular mass and geometry: the Framingham Heart Study. JAMA. 1991 Jul;266(2):231–6.

31 Alpert MA, Lambert CR, Terry BE, Kelly DL, Panayiotou H, Mukerji V, Massey CV, Cohen MV. Effect of weight loss on left ventricular mass in non-hypertensive morbidly obese patients. Am J Cardiol. 1994 May;73(12):918–21.

32 Alpert MA, Lambert CR, Panayiotou H, Terry BE, Cohen MV, Massey CV, Hashimi MW, Mukerji V. Relation of duration of morbid obesity to left ventricular mass, systolic function and diastolic filling, and effect of weight loss. Am J Cardiol. 1995 Dec;76(16):1194–7.

33 Sasson Z, Rasooly Y, Gupta R, Rasooly I. Left atrial enlargement in healthy obese: prevalence and relation to left ventricular mass and diastolic function. Can J Cardiol. 1996 Mar;12(3):257–63.

34 Wang TJ, Parise H, Levy D, D'Agostino RB Sr, Wolf PA, Vasan RS, Benjamin EJ. Obesity and the risk of new-onset atrial fibrillation. JAMA. 2004 Nov;292(20):2471–7.

35 Her C, Cerabona T, Bairamian M, McGoldrick KE. Right ventricular systolic function is not depressed in morbid obesity. Obes Surg. 2006 Oct;16(10):1287–93.

36 Wong CY, O'Moore-Sullivan T, Leano R, Strudwick M, Marwick TH. Association of subclinical right ventricular dysfunction with obesity. J Am Coll Cardiol. 2006 Feb;47 (3):611–16.

37 Dervan JP, Ilercil A, Kane PB, Anagnostopoulos C. Fatty infiltration: another restrictive cardiomyopathic pattern. Cathet Cardiovasc Diagn. 1991 Mar;22(3):184–9.

38 Willens HJ, Chakko S, Lowery MH, Bryers P, Labrador E, Gallagher A, Castrillon JC, Myerburg RJ. Tissue Doppler imaging of the right and left ventricle in severe obesity (body mass index >35 kg/m). Am J Cardiol. 2004 Oct;94(8):1087–90.

39 Alpert MA, Singh A, Terry BE, Kelly DL, el Deane MS, Mukerji V, Villareal D, Artis AK. Effect of exercise and cavity size on right ventricular function in morbid obesity. Am J Cardiol. 1989 Jun;64(20):1361–5.

40 Ommen SR, Nishimura RA, Appleton CP, Miller FA, Oh JK, Redfield MM, Tajik AJ. Clinical utility of Doppler echocardiography and tissue Doppler imaging in the estimation of left ventricular filling pressures: a comparative simultaneous Dopper-catheterization study. Circulation. 2000 Oct;102(15):1788–94.

41 Chakko S, Alpert MA, Alexander JK. Obesity and ventricular function in man: diastolic function. In Alpert MA, Alexander JK, editors. The Heart and Lung in Obesity. Armonk, NY, Futura Publishing Co. 1998. pp. 57–76.

42 Zarich SW, Kowalchuk GHJ, McGuire MP, Benotti PN, Mascioli EA, Nesto RW. Left ventricular abnormalities in asymptomatic morbid obesity. Am J Cardiol. 1991 Aug;68(4):377–81.

43 Scaglione R, Dichiara MA, Indovina R, Lipara R, Ganguzza A, Capuano G, Merlimo G, Licata G. Left ventricular diastolic and systolic function in normotensive obese subjects: influence of degree and duration of obesity. Eur Heart J. 1992 Jun;13(6):138–42.

44 Ku CS, Lin SL, Wang DJ, Chang SK, Lee WJ. Left ventricular filling in young normotensive obese adults. Am J Cardiol. 1994 Mar;73(8):613–15.

45 Stoddard MF, Tsedo K, Thomas B, Dillon S, Kupersmith J. The influence of obesity on left ventricular filling and systolic function. Am Heart J. 1992 Sep;124(3):694–9.

46 Alpert MA, Lambert CR, Terry BE, Cohen MV, Mulekar M, Massey CV, Hashimi MW, Panayiotou H, Mukerji V. Effect of weight loss on left ventricular diastolic filling in morbid obesity. Am J Cardiol. 1995 Dec;76(16):1198–201.

47 Alpert MA, Lambert CR, Terry BE, Cohen MV, Mukerji V, Massey CV, Hashimi MW, Panayiotou H. Influence of left ventricular mass on left ventricular diastolic filling in normotensive morbidly obese patients. Am Heart J. 1995 Nov;130(5):1068–73.

48 Alpert MA, Alexander JK, Chakko S. Obesity and ventricular function in man: systolic function. In Alpert MA, Alexander JK, editors. The Heart and Lung in Obesity. Armonk, NY, Futura Publishing Co. 1998. pp. 77–94.

49 Iacobellis G. True uncomplicated obesity is not related to increased left ventricular mass and systolic dysfunction. J Am Coll Cardiol. 2004 Dec;44(11):2257–8.

50 Alpert MA, Terry BE, Lambert CR, Kelly DL, Panayiotou H, Mukerji V, Massey CV, Cohen MV. Factors influencing left ventricular systolic function in non-hypertensive morbidly obese patients and effect of weight loss induced by gastroplasty. Am J Cardiol. 1993 Mar;71(8):733–7.

51 Alpert MA, Singh A, Terry BE, Kelly DL, Villarreal D, Mukerji V. Effect of exercise on left ventricular systolic function and reserve in morbid obesity. Am J Cardiol. 1989 Jun;63(20): 1478–82.

52 Wong CY, O'Moore-Sullivan T, Leano R, Byrne N, Bellis E, Marwick TH. Alterations of left ventricular myocardial characteristics associated with obesity. Circulation. 2004 Nov;110(19):3081–7.

53 Reisin E, Cook E. Obesity hypertension and the heart. In Alpert MA, Alexander JK, editors. The Heart and Lung in Obesity. Armonk, NY, Futura Publishing Co. 1998. pp. 95–107.

54 Reisin E, Messerli FH. Obesity-related hypertension: mechanisms, cardiovascular risks, and heredity. Curr Opin Nephrol-Hyperten. 1995 Jan;4(1):67–71.

55 Messerli FH, Sundgaard-Riise K, Reisin ED, Dreslinski GR, Ventura HO, Oigman W, Frohlick ED, Dunn FG. Dimorphic cardiac adaptation to obesity and arterial hypertension. Ann Intern Med. 1983 Dec;99(6):757–61.

56 Messerli FH, Sundgaard-Reise K, Reisin E, Dreslinski G, Dunn FG, Frohlich E. Disparate cardiovascular effects of obesity and arterial hypertension. Am J Med. 1983 May;74 (5):808–12.

57 Garavaglia GE, Messerli FH, Nunez BJ, Schmieder RE, Grossman E. Myocardial contractility and left ventricular function in obese patients with essential hypertension. Am J Cardiol. 1988;62:594–7.

58 Kenchaiah S, Evans JC, Levy D, Wilson PW, Benjamin EJ, Kannel WS, Vason RS. Obesity and the risk of heart failure. N Engl J Med. 2002 Aug;347(5):305–13.

59 Alpert MA, Terry BE, Mulekar M, Cohen MV, Massey CV, Fan TM, Panayiotou H, Mukerji V. Cardiac morphology and left ventricular function in morbidly obese patients with and

without congestive heart failure and effects of weight loss. Am J Cardiol. 1997 Sep;80(6):736–46.

60 Wong C, Marwick TH. Obesity cardiomyopathy pathogenesis and pathophysiology. Nat Clin Pract Cardiovasc Med. 2007 Aug;4(8):436–43.

61 Alpert MA. Obesity cardiomyopathy: pathophysiology and evolution of the clinical syndrome. Am J Med Sci. 2001 Apr;321(4):225–36.

62 Alpert MA, Alexander JK. Treatment of obesity cardiomyopathy. In Alpert MA, Alexander JK, editors. The Heart and Lung in Obesity. Armonk, NY, Futura Publishing Co. 1998. pp. 199–212.

63 Alexander JK, Peterson KL. Cardiovascular effects of weight reduction. Circulation. 1972 Feb;45(2):310–18.

64 Alaud-din A, Meterissian S, Lisbona R, Maclean LD, Forse RA. Assessment of cardiac function in patients who were morbidly obese. Surgery. 1990 Oct;108(4):809–20.

65 Backman L, Freyschuss U, Hallberg D, Melcher A. Reversibility of cardiovascular changes in extreme obesity: effects of weight reduction through jejunoileostomy. Acta Med Scand. 1979 May;205(5):367–73.

66 Reisin E, Frohlich ED, Messerli FH, Dreslinkski GR, Dunn FG, Jones MM, Batson HM Jr. Cardiovascular changes after weight loss in obesity hypertension. Ann Intern Med. 1983 Mar;98(3):315–19.

67 Alpert MA, Terry BE, Kelly DK. Effect of weight loss on cardiac chamber size, wall thickness and left ventricular function in morbid obesity. Am J Cardiol. 1985 Mar;55 (6):783–86.

68 Himeno E, Nishino K, Nakashima Y, Kuroiwa A, Ikeda M. Weight reduction regresses left ventricular mass regardless of blood pressure level in obese subjects. Am Heart J. 1996 Feb;131(2):313–19.

69 Karason K. Wallentin I, Larsson B, Sjostron L. Effects of obesity and weight loss on cardiac function and valvular performance. Obes Res. 1998 Nov;6(6):422–9.

70 MacMahon SW, Wilcken DEL, MacDonald GJ. The effect of weight reduction on left ventricular mass: a randomized, controlled trial in young, overweight, hypertensive patients. N Engl J Med. 1986 Feb;314(6):334–9.

71 Das Gupta P, Ramhanmdany E, Bridgen G, Lahiri A, Baird IM, Raftery EB. Improvement of left ventricular function after rapid weight loss in obesity. Eur Heart J. 1992 Aug;13(8):1060–6.

72 Willens HJ, Chakko SC, Byers P, Chirinos JA, Labrador E, Castrillon JC, Lowery MH. Effects of weight loss after gastric bypass on right and left ventricular function assessed by tissue Doppler imaging. Am J Cardiol. 2005 Jun;95 (12):1521–4.

2 Effects of Obesity on Respiratory Physiology

Philippe Abou Jaoude, Jahan Porhomayon, and Ali A. El Solh

State University of New York at Buffalo, Buffalo, NY, USA

KEY POINTS

- There is an exponential decrease of functional residual capacity and expiratory reserve volume with increasing body mass index, even for mild obesity and overweight.
- The effect of obesity on lung volumes is more prominent in subjects with predominant upper body fat distribution compared with those with lower body fat distribution.
- The apparent reduction in airway caliber in the obese is attributable to the reduction in lung volumes rather than to airway obstruction.

INTRODUCTION

For several decades, the global prevalence of obesity has been rising dramatically [1,2]. The greatest increase has been noted in the USA; the prevalence of obesity in the USA is three times greater than in France, and one and a half times greater than in the UK [3]. Between 1980 and 2004, the prevalence of obesity in the USA more than doubled in adults and more than tripled in children [3]. The greatest relative increase has been in the proportion of individuals with a body mass index (BMI) greater than 50 kg/m². This chapter describes the mechanisms whereby obesity brings about functional abnormalities on resting and exercise-related respiratory physiology.

LUNG MECHANICS

Obesity decreases total respiratory compliance by as much as two-thirds of the normal value measured in nonobese individuals [4]. The decrease in compliance was thought to result primarily from a reduced chest-wall compliance associated with the deposition of fat in and around the ribs, the diaphragm, and the abdomen. Subsequent investigations in healthy obese subjects revealed higher total respiratory system and chest-wall elastances during voluntary muscle relaxation than during paralysis [5], suggesting that incomplete relaxation may have contributed to the lower chest-wall compliance reported in earlier studies. Actually, the chest-wall compliance is usually normal in obese subjects and the decrease in total respiratory compliance is that of the lung. The reduction in lung compliance in obese individuals is exponentially related to BMI [6]. This decrement is the result of increased pulmonary blood volume, closure of dependent airways [7], and increased alveolar surface tension due to the reduction in functional residual capacity (FRC) [8–10].

LUNG VOLUMES AND SPIROMETRY

The most common and consistent characteristic of obesity in lung function is a reduction in the FRC (Figure 2.1). This derangement reflects the mass load of adipose tissue around the rib cage and abdomen [11]. In contrast, residual volume (RV) is usually well preserved, and the RV:TLC ratio remains normal or slightly increased [12]. As a result, expiratory reserve volume (ERV) decreases exponentially with increasing BMI, even in mild obesity or overweight due to displacement of the diaphragm into the thorax and increased chest-wall mass. ERV reduction is greatest in the supine position. The reduction is often so marked that FRC approaches RV. At that point, regional thoracic gas trapping may take place, causing an elevated RV/TLC ratio [13].

Total lung capacity (TLC) and vital capacity (VC) decrease linearly with a rising BMI, but the changes are small, and TLC is usually maintained above the lower limit of normal. A marked abnormality of lung volumes in mild to moderate obesity should raise

Critical Care Management of the Obese Patient, First Edition. Edited by Ali A. El Solh.
© 2012 John Wiley & Sons, Ltd. Published 2012 by John Wiley & Sons, Ltd.

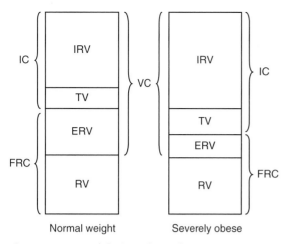

Normal weight   Severely obese

Figure 2.1 Impact of obesity on lung volumes.

suspicion of an underlying intrinsic lung disease or neuromuscular pathology, except in those with morbid obesity or those with excessive central adiposity (waist: hip ratio ≥ 0.95) [14].

Spirometry is normal in mild obesity. As BMI increases, there is a reduction in expiratory flow and a decrease in forced expiratory volume in 1 second (FEV1) and forced vital capacity (FVC) [15]. The ratio of FEV1 to FVC is preserved and even increased, which is attributed to peripheral airway closure and gas trapping, which reduces the VC. However, the reduction in FEV1 and FVC is strongly correlated with abdominal obesity. FVC, FEV1, and TLC were found to be significantly lower in subjects with upper body fat distribution or central obesity [16]. Abdominal obesity is responsible for a reduced FEV1:FVC ratio, suggesting an effect of obesity on large airway caliber as well. In addition to these spirometric derangements, tidal volume is reduced in severe obesity, and breathing follows a rapid, shallow pattern [17]. This functional change is typically due to the elastic load, which can be replicated in normal-weight subjects with elastic strapping of the chest [18]. As FRC becomes less than the closing volume, airway closure occurs during tidal breathing. Together with alveolar collapse, this leads to decreased ventilation of the lung bases, ventilation–perfusion mismatch, and hypoxemia. For these reasons, both the arterial pressure of oxygen (PaO_2) and the alveolar–arterial gradient are related to FRC.

The improvement of lung function with weight loss supports the causative effects of obesity on respiratory physiology. Following bariatric surgery, restrictive pulmonary mechanics improve significantly, with corresponding increases in FEV1, FVC, and $FEV_{25-75\%}$. Additionally, the obstructive lung pattern (FEV1:FVC ratio less than 0.8) tends to normalize [19]. In one program, weight loss was accompanied by an improvement of 73 ml in FEV1 and 92 ml in FVC for every 10% relative loss of pretreatment weight [20].

The effect of obesity on lung volumes and chest compliance can be worsened by anesthesia and muscular paralysis, which is manifested by decreased lung volumes, and higher lung and respiratory system elastances. This deterioration in lung function is more pronounced with abdominal surgeries [21] but is also seen in other types of non-abdominal procedures. Although the postoperative spirometry of obese patients shows a decrease in FEV1, FVC, and peak expiratory flow, the reduction in VC is the most prominent abnormality in both abdominal and nonabdominal surgery, and is greater with increasing BMI.

Various methods have been tried to compensate for the effects of obesity on lung function, ranging from positional changes, to adopting altered intraoperative ventilation strategies, to the use of prophylactic bilevel positive airway pressure (BiPAP) postoperatively [22]. The reverse Trendelenburg (RT) position is one measure that seems to improve the respiratory compliance and gas exchange in morbidly obese patients during bariatric surgery. However, it is not yet clear if the beneficial effect of this position can be replicated for all abdominal and non-abdominal surgeries in obese patients. Similarly, in intubated patients with large abdomen, a 45° RT position is associated with larger tidal volume and lower respiratory rate compared with a 90° position [23]. These results suggest that the RT may be the optimal position for use in obese patients, particularly in intubated intensive care unit (ICU) patients or those undergoing or recovering from anesthesia and surgery [21–23].

In addition to body positioning, different ventilation strategies are used to improve respiratory function in obese patients. Increasing positive end-expiratory pressure (PEEP) to 10 cm H_2O in anesthetized or paralyzed patients significantly reduces elastances of the respiratory system, lung and chest wall, and improves oxygenation [24]. In one study that used computed tomography to assess atelectasis in morbidly obese anesthetized patients undergoing gastroplasty, recruitment maneuver with 55 cm H_2O inspiratory pressure for 10 seconds, followed by 10 cm of PEEP, reduced atelectasis and improved oxygenation, while recruiting maneuver alone without PEEP yielded only a transient reduction of atelectasis that was not sustained 20 minutes later [25].

In addition, 10 cm of PEEP alone did not affect atelectasis. Repeating the recruitment maneuver every 10 minutes, in addition to PEEP of $10\,cm\,H_2O$, had better results in terms of improving respiratory compliance and oxygenation. Whether such ventilation strategies can be applied to medical obese patients in the ICU is to be determined [24–26].

The use of BiPAP as a prophylactic measure to improve pulmonary function after surgery has been studied in obese patients following gastroplasty. The prophylactic use of BiPAP System 12/4 (but not 8/4) during the first 24 hours postoperatively reduces pulmonary dysfunction after gastroplasty, and accelerates reestablishment of preoperative pulmonary function, which is reflected in improved FVC and FEV1, as well as SpO_2. The BiPAP acts by enhancing the alveolar recruitment during inspiration, while preventing the expiratory alveolar collapse and thus reducing the postoperative restrictive syndrome [27].

RESPIRATORY MUSCLES/WORK OF BREATHING

Studies on the respiratory muscles of obese individuals are scarce. Overall, obese subjects demonstrate inefficiency of respiratory muscles, most notably the diaphragm. The maximum inspiratory and expiratory pressures at all lung volumes are lower in obese patients compared to controls, without reaching statistical significance, except in patients with obesity hypoventilation syndrome (OHS). The maximal voluntary ventilation, a measurement of respiratory muscle endurance, is reduced by 20% in healthy obese individuals and by 45% in patients with OHS [28]. It is suggested that the additional load causes a length–tension disadvantage for the diaphragm due to fiber overstretching placing the diaphragmatic fibers at suboptimal length. Furthermore, analysis of the diaphragmatic electromyogram reveals a persistence of electrical activity into early expiration, the length of which also depends on the degree of obesity. These findings indicate that the diaphragm's volume-generating function in the obese is reduced, and furthermore the persistence of its activity in expiration serves to attenuate the rate of expiratory flow [28–30]. On a cellular level, obesity with high intake-associated lipid accumulation in muscle interferes with cellular mitochondrial function through the generation of reactive oxygen species (ROS) [31]. These compounds lead to lipid membrane peroxidative injury and disruption of mitochondrial-dependent enzymes, resulting in decreased oxidative metabolism. A reduced ability to oxidize fatty acids has

also been reported in skeletal muscle of obese individuals both before and after weight loss, which would support an intrinsic abnormality of fatty acid oxidation [32].

After weight loss, there is a significant increase and return to normal reference values, with regard to both the strength and the endurance of respiratory muscles, with the latter showing greater improvement. This improvement in respiratory muscle endurance is related to increased chest-wall compliance and pulmonary volumes, as a consequence of weight reduction [33].

AIRWAY RESISTANCE

Obese subjects have an increased total respiratory resistance due to a predominantly increased airway resistance rather than chest-wall resistance. However, when airway resistance is adjusted for the lung volume at which the measurements are made, specific airway resistance is in the normal range, indicating that the apparent reduction in airway caliber in the obese is attributable to the reduction in lung volumes rather than to airway obstruction [34]. Recent investigations have suggested that the increase in resistance may not be entirely due to reduction of FRC since differences between obese and nonobese may persist after lung volume adjustment [35,36]. The mechanism by which obesity could cause increased airway resistance is not well understood. The possible hypotheses include increased atopy related to an enhanced inflammatory state secondary to obesity [37]. Some in vitro studies, as well as human studies, suggest that lower lung volumes secondary to obesity lead to a reduction in peripheral airway diameter, which over time causes smooth muscle dysfunction, and causes both airways obstruction and hyperresponsiveness. In addition, leptin has been suggested to be involved in the airway dysfunction associated with obesity through its proinflammatory properties and/or via a direct effect on airways smooth muscles [38]. However, the data addressing this question have been inconclusive so far and further studies are needed to understand the mechanism of increased airway resistance and responsiveness in obesity [37,39–45].

The effect of obesity on airway hyperresponsiveness (AHR) has been inconsistently demonstrated. Investigators simulated obesity-related lung volume reductions in nonasthmatic subjects by externally mass-loading the chest wall and abdomen and documented an augmentation of airway responsiveness to methacholine relative to that of control [46]. The relationship between

BMI and AHR has also been reported in the European Community Respiratory Health Survey [47]. However, the association between asthma and obesity in adults and children has so far failed to show a consistent increase in AHR [37]. In addition, weight-loss programs did not result in substantial change in AHR despite documented improvements in lung function. Therefore, there is a plausible mechanism to explain how obesity is implicated in AHR but is not consistently reproducible in clinical studies.

CONTROL OF BREATHING

Although some studies investigating ventilatory drive in simple obesity have demonstrated that the ventilatory responses to inhalation of carbon dioxide ($DVE/DPCO_2$) are normal, others have indicated a reduced response, particularly in patients with OHS [48,49]. These abnormalities were initially attributed to the mechanical limitations and decreased chest compliance preventing adequate ventilation. However, the anticipated response to CO_2 did not improve in OHS patients following weight loss. Further, VD/VT (ratio of dead space to tidal volume) did not correlate with subjects' resting PCO_2 [50]. One theory proclaims that the diminished responsiveness may represent an adaptive process sparing O_2 for non-ventilatory demands. Yet there is an inherent problem with using ventilatory responses as a marker of respiratory drive because minute ventilation response to a stimulus may also be influenced by respiratory muscle function and respiratory system mechanics. The mouth occlusion pressure (P0.1) believed to reflect neurogenic drive is twice the normal value in mild obesity and increases normally with CO_2 inhalation. In contrast, the P0.1 response to CO_2 in patients with OHS is half that in subjects with simple obesity [49]. The fact that OHS subjects can normalize their arterial pressure of carbon dioxide (PaCO_2) by hyperventilation provides supportive evidence that ventilatory control is abnormal in OHS [51]. Hence, the cumulative data indicate that subjects with simple obesity have an enhanced respiratory drive while the respiratory drive of subjects with OHS is either depressed or *inappropriately suppressed*.

OXYGEN COST OF BREATHING

In nonobese individuals, the percentage of cardiac output and total body oxygen consumption (VO_2) dedicated to respiratory muscle work during quiet

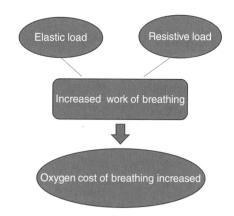

Figure 2.2 Interplay of respiratory mechanics on oxygen consumption in obese patients.

breathing is very small (less than 3%). In contrast, the oxygen cost of breathing is 4–10-fold higher than normal among subjects with eucapneic obesity (Figure 2.2). In one study of obese patients undergoing bariatric surgery, a 16% reduction in mean VO_2 in obese patients was observed compared to less than 1% reduction in the nonobese during the transition from spontaneous breathing to positive pressure ventilation. This suggests that morbidly obese patients dedicate a disproportionately high percentage of total VO_2 for respiratory work. Of interest, the obese patients demonstrate a significantly lower VO_2 when standardized by BMI, which has been attributed to the lower blood flow and metabolic rate of adipose tissue compared with lean body tissue. Nevertheless, the lower VO_2 standardized to body size does not ameliorate the detrimental impact of morbid obesity on oxygen consumption. This respiratory inefficiency results in a limited ventilatory reserve, which predisposes these patients to respiratory failure in the setting of acute pulmonary or systemic illnesses [52,53].

VENTILATION/PERFUSION

Ventilation in nonobese patients is greatest in dependent lung zones and decreases toward the upper zones; however, this distribution may be reversed in obesity. When lung ventilation and perfusion were examined in obese subjects with ERV at 21% of predicted, the normal tidal breath predominantly distributed to the upper zones, while perfusion was predominant in the lower zones. In contrast, subjects who had an average ERV of

49% of predicted value had normal ventilation distribution [54]. Thus, impairment of the ventilation/perfusion (V/Q) relationship depends on the location of the excess body weight. Individuals with central obesity seem the most affected. Similar results were reproduced in the lateral decubitus position [55]. This V/Q mismatch results from airway closure in the lungs' dependent areas of obese patients.

DIFFUSING CAPACITY AND GAS EXCHANGE

The diffusing capacity (DLCO) of obese subjects is usually preserved, although studies have reported increased and decreased values [56]. An increased DLCO in obese patients is probably related to increased pulmonary blood volume and flow, while a decreased DLCO may result from structural changes in the interstitium from lipid deposition or decreased alveolar surface area. In either scenario, weight loss appears to have little effect on DLCO as values remained unchanged following surgical or medical treatment [57,58].

Morbid obesity is associated with low PaO_2 and increased alveolar–arterial oxygen partial pressure difference [58]. These changes are usually more prominent in men than in women secondary to gender differences in waist : hip ratio. $PaCO_2$ is usually normal in obese patients who do not have OHS. While the gas exchanges improve with peak exercise, obese subjects have a poor compensatory hyperventilation, resulting in low exercise tolerance and premature termination of exercise [59]. The mechanism by which obesity impairs blood gas exchange and oxygenation is related to lower lung volumes and basilar atelectasis secondary to airway closure and alveolar collapse. Increased airway resistance has little to do with impaired gas exchange at rest (normal $PaCO_2$); it may however play a role in the poor exercise tolerance through increased expiratory airflow limitation and dynamic hyperinflation.

Therapeutic measures that are used to improve lung volumes and decrease atelectasis are also associated with improvement of oxygenation and blood gas exchange. In fact, both PaO_2 and alveolar–arterial oxygen difference were ameliorated when a PEEP of $10\,cm\,H_2O$ was applied to paralysed and anesthetized postoperative obese patients after abdominal surgery, compared to PEEP of zero. Similarly, the alveolar–arterial oxygen difference was significantly reduced when morbidly obese patients undergoing bariatric surgery were placed

in RT position. In addition, the application of BiPAP 12/4 improved oxygen saturation when used prophylacticly in obese patients for 24 hours after undergoing gastroplasty [56,60].

ALTERED EXERCISE RESPIRATORY PHYSIOLOGY

At rest, the baseline VO_2 is approximately 25% greater than the VO_2 for nonobese individuals. Because adipose tissue has a lower metabolic rate than other tissues, peak VO_2 uptake adjusted for true body weight is reduced, but peak VO_2 is usually normal or increased when adjusted for ideal body weight [61]. Interestingly, the slope of the VO_2 work-rate relationship is unchanged but is shifted upward by approximately $6\,ml/min/kg$ of extra body weight on a cycle ergometer. This means that an appropriate peak VO_2 standard reference for an obese subject can be predicted by increasing the standard peak VO_2 from the reference body weight by $6\,ml/min$ for each kilogram greater than the reference weight. Other responses may vary depending on the exercise protocol and severity of obesity. Parameters including peak O_2 pulse (VO_2/heart rate (HR)) and anaerobic threshold are usually normal in mild to moderate obesity [62]. The resting HR is usually elevated, reflecting an increase in cardiac output at rest. With exercise, there is a normal HR–VO_2 relationship, reflected by a normal HR–VO_2 slope and attainment of the predicted HR with no HR reserve.

It is unusual for obese individuals to demonstrate ventilatory limitation despite the abnormalities imposed on the respiratory system at rest. Because the ventilation perfusion relationship normalizes during exercise, dead space ventilation usually responds normally with a decrease toward the normal range with exercise [63].

PULMONARY VASCULATURE

Pulmonary artery systolic pressure (PASP) correlates echocardiographically with BMI independently of age, gender or comorbid diseases. Using echocardiography, PASP $\geq 30\,mm\,Hg$ and $\geq 35\,mm\,Hg$ occurred in up to 66% and 36% of obese subjects, respectively. For each unit increase in BMI, the PASP increases by 0.1–$0.4\,mm\,Hg$. The exact mechanism of increased PASP in obesity is not clear, but is likely related to increased blood volume. Obstructive sleep apnea and pulmonary capillary spasm secondary to nocturnal hypoxia are other possible contributing factors. However, in the absence of right heart catheterization, echocardiographic findings should be interpreted with caution [64].

CONCLUSION

Obesity affects respiratory physiology in many ways, with significant clinical implications. There are few measures that have been shown to improve respiratory function in obese patients undergoing medical or surgical treatment. These include RT position, higher PEEP with recruitment maneuvers, pressure control mode in ventilated patients and prophylactic use of BiPAP after surgery/sedation.

BEST PRACTICE TIPS

1 Pulmonary mechanics improve significantly after weight loss with increase in FEV1, FVC, and FEV$_{25-75\%}$.
2 The RT position is a recognized measure that improves respiratory compliance and gas exchange in morbidly obese patients during surgery and mechanical ventilation.
3 The effects of obesity on lung volumes can be worsened by anesthesia and paralysis.
4 Increasing PEEP to 10 cm H$_2$O significantly reduced elastances of the respiratory system, lung and chest wall in obese patients.
5 Application of BiPAP 12/4 improves oxygen saturation in obese patients for 24 hours after gastroplasty.

REFERENCES

1 Mokdad AH, Ford ES, Bowman BA, et al. Prevalence of obesity, diabetes, and obesity related health risk factors. JAMA. 2003;289:76–9.

2 Ogden C, Yanovski S, Carroll M, et al. The epidemiology of obesity. Gastroenterology. 2007;132:2087–102.

3 Sturm R. Increases in morbid obesity in the USA 2000–2005. Public Health. 2007;121:492–6.

4 Naimark A, Cherniack RM. Compliance of the respiratory system and its components in health and obesity. J Appl Phsyiol. 1960;15:377–82.

5 Van Lith P, Johnson FN, Sharp JT. Respiratory elastance in relaxed and paralyzed states in normal and abnormal men. J Appl Physiol. 1967;23:472–86.

6 Pelosi P, Croci M, Ravagnan I, et al. The effects of body mass on lung volumes, respiratory mechanics, and gas exchange during general anesthesia. Anesth Analg. 1998;87(3):654–60.

7 Ray C, Sue D, Bray G, Hansen J, et al. Effects of obesity on research function. Am Rev Respir Dis. 1983;128:501–6.

8 Pelosi P, Croci M, Ravagnan I, et al. Total respiratory system, lung, and chest wall mechanics in sedated-paralyzed postoperative morbidly obese patients. Chest. 1996; 109:144–51.

9 Hedenstierna G, Santesson J. Breathing mechanics, dead space and gas exchange in the extremely obese, breathing spontaneously and during anaesthesia with intermittent positive pressure ventilation. Acta Anaesthesiol Scand. 1976;20:248–54.

10 Suratt PM, Wilhoit SC, Hsiao HS, Atkinson RL, Rochester DF. Compliance of chest wall in obese subjects. J Appl Physiol. 1984;57:403–7.

11 Sharp JT, Henry JP, Swaeny SK, Meadows WR, Pietras RJ. Effects of mass loading the respiratory system in man. J Appl Physiol. 1964;19:959–66.

12 Watson RA, Pride NB. Postural changes in lung volumes and respiratory resistance in subjects with obesity. J Appl Physiol. 2005;98:512–17.

13 Jones RL, Nzekwu M. The effects of body mass index on lung volumes. Chest. 2006;130:827–33.

14 Lazarus R, Sparrow D, Weiss S. Effects of obesity and fat distribution on ventilator function: the normative aging study. Chest. 1997;111:891–8.

15 Rubinstein I, Zamel N, DuBarry L, et al. Airflow limitation in morbidly obese, nonsmoking men. Ann Intern Med. 1990; 112:828–32.

16 Leone N, Courbon D, Thomas F, et al. Lung function impairment and metabolic syndrome: the critical role of abdominal obesity. Am J Respir Crit Care Med. 2009;179:509–16.

17 Sampson MG, Grassino AE. Load compensation in obese patients during quiet tidal breathing. J Appl Physiol. 1983; 55:1269–76.

18 Caro CG, Butler J, DuBois AB. Some effects of restriction of chest cage expansion on pulmonary function man: an experimental study. J Clin Invest. 1960;39:573–83.

19 Nguyen N, Hinojosa M, Smith B, et al. Improvement of restrictive and obstructive pulmonary mechanics following laparoscopic bariatric surgery. Surg Endosc. 2009; 23:808–12.

20 Aaron SD, Fergusson D, Dent R, et al. Effect of weight reduction on respiratory function and airway reactivity in obese women. Chest. 2004;125:2046–52.

21 von Ungern-Sternberg BS, Regli A, Schneider M, et al. Effect of obesity and site of surgery on perioperative lung volumes. Brit J Anaesth. 2004;92:202–7.

22 Perilli V, Sollazzi L, Bozza P, et al. The effects of the reverse Trendelenburg position on respiratory mechanics and blood gases in morbidly obese patients during bariatric surgery. Anesth Analg. 2000;91:1520–5.

23 Burns SM, Egloff M, Ryan B, et al. Effect of body position on spontaneous respiratory rate and tidal volume in patients with obesity, abdominal distension and ascites. Am J Crit Care. 1994;3(2):102–6.

24 Pelosi P, Ravagnan I, Giurati G, et al. Positive end-expiratory pressure improves respiratory function in obese but not in

normal subjects during anesthesia and paralysis. Anesthesiology. 1999;91(5):1221–31.

25 Reinius H, Jonsson L, Gustafson S, et al. Prevention of atelectasis in morbidly obese patients during general anesthesia and paralysis. Anesthesiology. 2009;111:979–87.

26 Almarakbi WA, Fawzi H, Alhashemi J. Effects of four intraoperative ventilatory strategies on respiratory compliance and gas exchange during laparoscopic gastric banding in obese patients. Br J Anaesth. 2009;102(6):862–8.

27 Joris JL, Sottiaux TM, Chiche JD, et al. Effect of bi-level positive airway pressure (BiPAP) nasal ventilation on the postoperative pulmonary restrictive syndrome in obese patients undergoing gastroplasty. Chest. 1997;111(3):665–70.

28 Magnami C, Cataneo A. Respiratory muscle strength in obese individuals and influence of upper body fat distribution. Sao Paulo Med J. 2007;125(4).

29 Kelly TM, Jensen RL, Elliott CG, Crapo RO. Maximum respiratory pressures in morbidly obese subjects. Respiration. 1988;54(2):73–7.

30 Koenig SM. Pulmonary complications of obesity. Am J Med Sci. 2001;321(4):249–79.

31 Peterson K, Dufour S, Befroy D, et al. Impaired mitochondrial activity in the insulin-resistant offspring of patients with type 2 diabetes. N Engl J Med. 2004;350:664–71.

32 Kelley D, Goodpaster B, Wing R, et al. Skeletal muscle fatty acid metabolism in association with insulin resistance, obesity and weight loss. Am J Physiol. 1999;277:E1130–41.

33 Weiner P, Waizman J, Weiner M, Rabnet M, Magadle R, Zamir D. Influence of excessive weight loss after gastroplasty for morbid obesity on respiratory muscle performance. Thorax. 1998;53(1):39–42.

34 Zerah F, HArf A, Perlemuter L, et al. Effects of obesity on respiratory resistance. Chest. 1993;103:1470–6.

35 King C, Brown N, Diba C, Thorpe C, et al. The effects of body weight on airway caliber. Eur Respir J. 2005;25:896–901.

36 Watson R, Pride N. Postural changes in lung volumes and respiratory resistance in subjects with obesity. J Appl Physiol. 2005;98:512–17.

37 Schachter L, Salome C, Peat J, et al. Obesity is a risk for asthma and wheeze but not airway hyperresponsiveness. Thorax. 2001;56:4–8.

38 Gunst SJ, Tang DD, Opazo Saez A. Cytoskeletal remodeling of the airway smooth muscle cell: a mechanism for adaptation to mechanical forces in the lung. Respir Physiol Neurobiol. 2003;137:151–68.

39 Bibi H, Shoseyov D, Figenbaum D, et al. The relationship between asthma and obesity in children: is this real or a case of overdiagnosis? J Asthma. 2004;41:403–10.

40 Hakala K, Mustajoki P, Aittomaki J, et al. Effects of weight loss on peak flow variability, airways obstruction, and lung volumes in obese patients with asthma. Chest. 2000;118:1315–21.

41 Maniscalco M, Zedda A, Faraone S, et al. Weight loss and asthma control in severely obese asthmatic females. Respir Med. 2008;102:102–8.

42 Huang SL, Shiao G, Chou P. Association between body mass index and allergy in teenage girls in Taiwan. Clin Exp Allergy. 1999;29:323–9.

43 Shore SA, Schwartzman IN, Mellema MS, et al. Effect of leptin on allergic airway responses in mice. J Allergy Clin Immunol. 2005;115:103–9.

44 Shore SA. Obesity and asthma: possible mechanisms. J Allergy Clin Immunol. 2008;121:1087–93.

45 Nair P, Radford K, Fanat A, et al. The effects of leptin on airway smooth muscle responses. Am J Respir Cell Mol Biol. 2008;39:475–81.

46 Wang L, Cerny F, Kufel T, et al. Simulated obesity-related changes in lung volume increases airway responsiveness in lean, nonasthmatic subjects. Chest. 2006;130:834–40.

47 Chin S, Jarvis D, Burney P. Relation of bronchial responsiveness to body mass index in the ECRHS (European Community Respiratory Health Survey). Thorax. 2002;57:1028–33.

48 Burki NK, Baker RW. Ventilatory regulation in eucapnic morbid obesity. Am Rev Respir Dis. 1984;129:538–43.

49 Lopata M, Onal E. Mass loading, sleep apnea, and the pathogenesis of obesity hypoventilation. Am Rev Respir Dis. 1982;126:640–5.

50 Kaufman BJ, Ferguson MH, Cherniack RM. Hypoventilation in obesity. J Clin Invest. 1959;38:500–11.

51 Leech J, Onal E, Aronson R, et al. Voluntary hyperventilation in obesity hypoventilation. Chest. 1991;100:1334–8.

52 Rochester D. Obesity and pulmonary function. In Alpert M, Alexander J, editors. The Heart and Lung in Obesity. Armonk, NY, Futura Publishing Co. 1998. pp. 108–32.

53 Refsum HE, Holter P, Lovig T, et al. Pulmonary function and energy expenditure after marked weight loss in obese women: observations before and one year after gastric banding. Int J Obesity. 1990;14:175–83.

54 Holley HS, Milic-Emili J, Becklake MR, Bates DV. Regional distribution of pulmonary ventilation and perfusion in obesity. J Clin Invest. 1967;46:475–81.

55 Hurewitz AN, Susskind H, Harold WH. Obesity alters regional ventilation in lateral decubitus position. J Appl Physiol. 1985;59:774–83.

56 Thomas P, Cowen E, Hulands G, et al. Respiratory function in the morbidly obese before and after weight loss. Thorax. 1989;44:382–6.

57 Li A, Chan D, Wong E, et al. The effects of obesity on pulmonary function. Arch Dis Child. 2003;88:361–3.

58 Womack C, Harris D, Katzel L, et al. Weight loss, not aerobic exercise, improves pulmonary function in older obese men. J Gerontol A Biol Sci Med Sci. 2000;55:M453–7.

59 Zavorsky G, Kim Do J, Sylvestre J, et al. Alveolar membrane diffusing capacity improves in the morbidly obese after bariatric surgery. Obes Surg. 2008;18:256–63.

60 Zavorsky G, Hoffman S. Pulmonary gas exchange in the morbidly obese. Obes Rev. 2008;9:326–39.

61 Buskirk E, Taylor H. Maximal oxygen intake and its relation to body composition, with special reference to chronic physical activity and obesity. J Appl Phys. 1957;11:72–8.

62 American Thoracic Society/American College of Chest Physicians Joint Committee. ATS/ACCP statement on cardiopulmonary exercise testing. Am J Respir Crit Care Med. 2003;167:211–77.

63 Johnson BD, Weisman IM, Zeballos RJ, Beck KC. Emerging concepts in the evaluation of ventilatory limitation during exercise: the exercise tidal flow-volume loop. Chest. 1999;116:488–503.

64 Weyman A, Davidoff R, Gardin J, et al. Echocardiographic evaluation of pulmonary artery pressure with clinical correlates in predominantly obese adults. J Am Soc Echocardiogr. 2002;15:454–62.

3 Gastrointestinal Physiology in Obesity

Alexander D. Miras and Carel W. le Roux

Imperial Weight Centre, Imperial College London, London, UK

> **KEY POINTS**
> - Obesity affects every single gastrointestinal tract organ and increases the risk of gastrointestinal disease.
> - Obese acutely unwell patients may present with more severe forms of gastrointestinal conditions.
> - Currently the most effective long-term treatment for obesity is bariatric surgery.

INTRODUCTION

The gastrointestinal tract is the largest endocrine organ and together with the brain and adipose tissue plays a vital role in the regulation of body weight. The gut communicates with the brain regions that control energy balance through neural connections and gut hormones. This complex but remarkably efficient metabolic machinery regulates food intake, absorption and excretion. In times of health, robust feedback pathways regulate the gut's function within tight physiological control. The disease state of obesity not only arises from disruption of a delicate hormonal, neural and mechanical balance but also exacerbates gastrointestinal pathophysiology in a vicious-circle manner. This chapter will attempt to explore these pathological processes in more detail in order to provide a better understanding of their clinical consequences.

OBESITY AND GASTROINTESTINAL TRACT KINETICS

A number of studies have examined the association between obesity and gastroesophageal reflux disease (GERD). Even though some of the results are conflicting, the majority of the literature suggests a positive correlation between body mass index (BMI) and GERD. The Progression of Gastroesophageal Reflux Disease (ProGERD) study, which is one of the largest in the field, reported an association between BMI and symptoms of GERD, but also the presence of erosive esophagitis [1]. Interestingly, the differences were observed in women but not in men. There are insufficient data in terms of oesophageal gastric exposure; however, it has been shown that the majority of obese patients have abnormal 24 hour ambulatory measurements and an increase in postprandial episodes of reflux [2,3]. More alarmingly, patients with a BMI of over $25 \, kg/m^2$ have a higher risk of developing erosive esophagitis leading to adenocarcinoma [4]. Weight loss achieved through lifestyle modification can lead to symptomatic improvements but improvements in endoscopic findings have not been demonstrated [5]. Gastric bypass surgery reduces acid production and results in reduced symptoms [6].

The two most important mechanisms leading to GERD are dysfunction of the lower esophageal sphincter (LES) and decrease of the LES pressure secondary to lower esophageal sphincter relaxation (TLESR). Obesity is associated with higher TLESR and the frequency of TLESR episodes is directly related to higher BMI [7].

The raised intraabdominal pressure in obesity leads to the proximal migration of a hiatus hernia and increases in the pressure gradient along the gastroesophageal sphincter [8]. Measurements of gastric capacity using intragastric water-filled balloons have demonstrated an increase in patients with obesity [9]. These two changes in physiology can exacerbate GERD.

The rate of gastric emptying relates to the development of GERD or even contributes to the development of

Critical Care Management of the Obese Patient, First Edition. Edited by Ali A. El Solh.
© 2012 John Wiley & Sons, Ltd. Published 2012 by John Wiley & Sons, Ltd.

obesity. To study gastric emptying, radioisotope scintigraphy has been used. The results of studies in obesity and weight loss are controversial. However, obese patients consume more high-calorie foods, which delay gastric emptying [10], which may lead to reflux disease.

Changes in the local acid environment can also exacerbate the above mechanical disturbances. In obesity, acid sensitivity is increased [11], there is higher maximal gastric acid production following intravenous pentagastrin, and gastric contents are richer in bile and gastrin [12]. In obese individuals following intravenous secretin administration, basal acid production is not suppressed [12].

The contractility of the small bowel is more prominent in the fasting state in patients with obesity, potentially leading to more efficient absorption of nutrients [13]. The orocaecal transit times are controversial, but the most recent data suggest that there is no difference in the intestinal transit of either low- or high-fat food between obese and normal-weight subjects [14].

OBESITY AND THE BILIARY TRACT

Obesity has long been considered a major risk factor for the development of gallstones. Increased BMI, waist : hip ratio and skinfold thickness are strongly correlated with gallstone formation [15,16]. The Nurses' Health Study showed that the incidence of symptomatic gallstones increased when BMI exceeded $30 \, kg/m^2$ [17]. The prevalence of gallbladder disease in the obese population is approximately 87–97% [18]. Obese patients also have more asymptomatic gallbladder disease compared to normal-weight controls [19].

Three steps are necessary for cholesterol gallstone formation: first the cholesterol supersaturation of bile; second derivatives of gallbladder mucin (nucleating and antinucleating factors) accelerating cholesterol crystal nucleation and growth in supersaturated bile; and third gallbladder hypomotility, promoting stasis [20]. Cholesterol production is linearly related to body fat and indeed obese patients have been shown to have a higher hepatic production of cholesterol [21]. High cholesterol concentrations compared to bile acids and phospholipids in bile (i.e. a high cholesterol saturation index) lead to stone precipitation in the gallbladder. The only available investigation of nucleating factors in obesity has led to the conclusion that obesity is not associated with a nucleation defect [22]. Many but not all studies on gallbladder motility have shown a decreased motility and emptying together with a higher fasting volume in obesity [23,24].

During weight loss, and especially rapid and excessive weight loss through dieting, the risk of gallstone development increases. It is thought, but not consistently shown, that the biliary lipid content might become favorable for stone synthesis during a hypocaloric diet [25]. The nucleation time decreases with weight loss [26], whereas low-calorie and low-fat diets decrease gallbladder motility, as demonstrated by increased fasting and resting gallbladder volumes [23].

OBESITY AND THE LIVER

Together with insulin resistance and dyslipidemia, obesity is associated with a range of chronic liver conditions, the commonest of which is hepatic steatosis [27]. Through the use of abdominal imaging it has been estimated that a third of the population of the USA suffers from fatty liver disease, and its prevalence correlates with increasing BMI [28]. Nonalcoholic steatohepatitis (NASH) is a more sinister form of liver disease in which hepatocytes are damaged or die, causing localized inflammation and eventually fibrosis. The presence of NASH on liver biopsy increases the risk of progression to cirrhosis, something which is rare in cases of simple steatosis.

Patients often present late in the course of their disease as signs of early hepatic liver damage can be subtle. Early physical signs include abdominal obesity, which can make hepatomegaly difficult to detect, acanthosis nigricans or even androgenic alopecia, and hirsutism in women with coexisting polycystic ovarian syndrome. Signs of decompensated disease include jaundice, ascites and encephalopathy, all conferring a worse prognosis. It is much more common for steatosis to be detected on routine biochemical investigations by an elevated AST : ALT ratio. Physicians have to exclude the presence of other causes of hepatic pathology (i.e. vital, autoimmune) before proceeding to the diagnosis of nonalcoholic fatty liver disease (NAFLD). In terms of imaging, ultrasonography is considered the least sensitive of all modalities but is cheap and easily accessible. More sensitive techniques include computer tomography (CT) and magnetic resonance imaging (MRI), with proton nuclear imaging MR spectroscopy considered the most sensitive of all. However, liver biopsy is still the gold standard for confirmation of the diagnosis, and also provides useful information on the degree of fibrosis and therefore the prognosis [29]. Serum markers of fibrosis may eventually obviate the need for liver biopsy, which still carries morbidity and mortality.

The commonest causes of mortality in patients with NAFLD include cardiovascular disease, cancer and liver disease itself [30]. Even though only 5% of patients with steatosis progress to cirrhosis, NAFLD is the commonest cause of liver failure in the USA as a result of the obesity epidemic [31].

Histologically, the diagnosis of NAFLD requires the presence of a intrahepatic triglyceride (IHTG) content of more than 5% of liver volume, or more than 5% of hepatocytes containing intracellular triglycerides [32,33]. The presence of hepatic triglycerides depends on four pathological mechanisms: 1) hepatic fatty acid (FA) uptake, 2) de novo FA synthesis, 3) FA oxidation and 4) FA export [34].

1 The rate of FA uptake by the liver depends on the rate of delivery of free fatty acid (FFA). Interestingly, the major source of portal vein FFA is the subcutaneous fat and not the visceral fat. Postprandially, the release of FFA is directly dependent on fat mass and therefore greater in the obese [35]. Additionally, the gene expression of both hepatic lipase and FAT/CD36 – a regulator of FFA uptake – is increased in obesity and leads to higher hepatic FFA uptake and steatosis [36].

2 The liver is capable of synthesizing FA de novo, but the contribution of this to the FA incorporated into the very-low-density lipoprotein (VLDL) particles is less than 5% in healthy individuals. However, this process becomes much more significant in NAFLD and accounts for up to 23% of the IHTG [37]. In the presence of insulin resistance this phenomenon is exacerbated and consumption of a high-carbohydrate meal leads to a postprandial shift of glucose from muscle glycogen storage toward de novo liver FA synthesis [38].

3 The liver requires a considerable amount of energy even for basal functioning. FA and amino acid oxidation provide the vast majority of this energy in the basal state. Inhibition of FA oxidation in rodents can lead to an increased IHTG content [39]; however, it is unknown whether this process is present in humans. Indirect measurement of hepatic mitochondrial FA oxidation through serum ketone levels has shown that it is either normal or increased in patients with NAFLD [40].

4 FAs are esterified into triglycerides and secreted as VLDL particles from the liver, in an attempt to lower IHTG content. Interestingly, the VLDL-triglyceride secretion is increased in patients with NAFLD [41]. However, this reaches a plateau even in the presence of increasing IHTG content and thus leads to further hepatic steatosis [42].

One way of treating NAFLD is through lifestyle modification and weight loss. Even within 48 hours of caloric restriction, IHGT content and hepatic insulin resistance decrease [43]. Sustained weight loss of 5–10% leads to improvements in liver enzyme biochemistry and even reduction of hepatic steatosis and inflammation on histology [44]. There is no evidence from controlled clinical trials to support the use of a specific dietary manipulation in order to improve NAFLD, even though observation studies advocate the use of low-carbohydrate diets [45].

Weight loss through behavioral means is successful only in the short term, as the vast majority of patients cannot maintain this reduced weight. The only long-term effective weight-loss therapy is obesity surgery [46]. Observational cohort studies have reported improvements or complete resolution of steatosis, inflammation and fibrosis after surgically induced weight loss [47]. These are accompanied by positive metabolic effects including decreased hepatic glucose production, VLDL-TG secretion and gene expression of inflammation/fibrosis factors [48]. As is the case with other pathologies ameliorated by obesity surgery, there is a lack of randomized controlled trials comparing the effects of surgically induced weight loss on NAFLD with conservative or medical management.

OBESITY AND THE PANCREAS

The hypothesis of chronic inflammation encompasses the association of a chronic inflammatory state and the development of cancer [49]. Obesity is linked with the development of pancreatitis and pancreatic cancer, which may be exacerbated by the chronic inflammatory hypothesis.

Both prospective studies and metaanalysis support that acute pancreatitis is more severe in the obese population [50]. Patients with a $BMI > 30\,kg/m^2$ have higher Acute Physiology and Chronic Health Evaluation (APACHE) scores and higher levels of interleukin 6 (IL-6) compared to lean patients.

Obese mice have been found to have a more severe form of caerulin-induced pancreatitis, with serum adiponectin levels inversely related to disease severity [51]. In humans, adiponectin is thought to be a more useful marker for distinguishing pancreatic cancer from chronic pancreatitis, with a specificity of 97% compared to 90% with CA 19–9 [52].

A history of pancreatitis confers a sevenfold risk of developing pancreatic cancer [53]. However, the same investigators did not find a correlation between BMI and the presence of genetic polymorphisms of the proinflammatory genes TNF-alpha-308 and RANTES-403.

Investigators have focused on the study of IL-6 as it is elevated in both obesity and cancer. IL-6 induced colonic tumor cell proliferation in an in vitro study of preneoplastic epithelial colonocytes treated with leptin [54]. The study of IL-6 in patients with pancreatic cancer showed levels correlating with disease degree and more specifically weight loss [55]. It is unclear if IL-6 has a role in the rate of pancreatic cancer progression and the metastatic process.

OBESITY AND THE COLON

The National Health and Nutrition Examination Survey (NHANES) was a large epidemiological study that followed up individuals in the USA for 15 years and reported that baseline BMI is associated with colon cancer in both men and women [56]. The distribution of adiposity affected the risk of developing neoplasia, with subscapular skin thickness conferring a higher risk compared to triceps skinfold thickness. The Framingham cohort study also showed that both sexes with a high waist circumference had a 70% increased risk of colon cancer, while those with an extra large circumference had an impressive 90% increased risk of developing the condition [57]. Obesity has also been linked with the development of colorectal adenomas. In the Insulin Resistance Atherosclerosis Study (IRAS) a cohort of 600 subjects underwent colonoscopy, and BMI at the time was found to be associated with a 2.16 risk of a colonic adenoma; the risk increased in patients with recent weight gain [58].

Obesity in patients with insulin resistance leads to hyperinsulinemia, low levels of insulin growth factor binding protein (IGFBP) and elevated insulin-like growth factor 1 (IGF-1). The latter inhibits colonic apoptosis and promotes epithelial cell proliferation. In a similar manner, elevated levels of the adipocyte hormone leptin stimulate the ObRb receptor on colonic cells, causing expression of transcription factors, proinflammatory cytokines and cell proliferation [59]. Interestingly, another mechanism potentially contributing to the development of colorectal cancer is a reduced intake of calcium and vitamin D. These are also lower in excess adiposity and it has been suggested that vitamin D is sequestrated in adipose tissue, leading to lower serum levels and reduced antiinflammatory and anticarcinogenic effects [60].

A small retrospective study of patients who developed complications of diverticulosis showed that the mean BMI was associated with a higher rate of abscess and perforation and recurrent attacks [61]. The more recent Health Professionals Follow-up Study of 47 228 male participants also reported that obese men had a higher risk of diverticulosis complications associated with physical inactivity [62].

OBESITY AND THE GUT FLORA

Interest in the study of gut organisms as potential contributors to obesity stemmed from the observation that members of the same family, with similar genetic makeup and dietary habits, have different amounts of total body fat. The intestine contains 10^{14} bacteria, mainly anaerobes, with three dominant species: Bacteroidetes, which are gram negative, and Firmicutes and Actinobacteria, which are gram positive. Following birth, the composition and characteristics of gut bacteria evolve rapidly up to the age of 4 and remain remarkably constant until the 7th decade. The use of antibiotics is one of the few interventions that intermittently affects the stable community of these microorganisms. In between subjects, however, there is large variability in the composition of gut bacteria, making the study of their contribution to the development of obesity more complex.

Initial experiments in mice showed that those that were raised conventionally had more total body fat and gonadal fat compared to bacteria-free mice, even though the former group had a lower energy intake [63]. The mechanism proposed as an explanation for these results is that gut bacteria increase the energy intake from the host organism's diet. Physiologically, gut colonization causes suppression of lipoprotein lipase inhibitor, through suppression of the expression of the fasting-induced adipose factor, leading to higher absorption of fatty acids and storage in adipose tissue [63]. On the other hand, bacteria-free mice have higher levels of phosphorylated AMP-activated protein kinase in skeletal muscle and liver cells, which in turn stimulate fatty acid oxidation [64]. In terms of identifying the culprit bacteria, there is a reduction in the numbers of the Bacteroidetes and a simultaneous increase in Firmicutes in obese mice [65]. Through the increased fermentation of dietary carbohydrates and production of monosaccharides and short-chain fatty acids (SCFAs), the caecal microbiota contribute to weight gain in these ob/ob mice [66].

The relative presence of different classes of gut bacteria in obese humans remains a matter of debate. Some investigators have shown that Bacteroidetes decrease and Firmicutes increase in obese subjects, and more interestingly that weight loss through caloric and fat restriction causes the opposite trend [67]. The low Bacteroidetes/

high Firmicutes explanation has not however been supported by data from other studies, which show instead that the amount of SCFA produced as a result of bacterial fermentation is more important in promoting weight gain [68].

The gut microbiota is implicated in the inflammatory state, which is active in both obesity and type 2 diabetes mellitus. Most of the available data again come from animal models. A high-fat diet as well as a decrease in the numbers of bifidobacteria increases the plasma levels of lipopolysaccharide, which triggers secretion of proinflammatory cytokines [69]. Butyrate is an energy source for colonocytes but also acts as an antinflammatory agent. Obese humans are deficient in plasma butyrate and diets with high amounts of carbohydrates that cannot be ingested are thought to stimulate gut bacteria to produce butyrate [70].

The fascinating interplay between diet, bacteria and gut hormones can also affect total body fat mass and predispose to obesity. The gut hormones glucagon-like peptide 1 (GLP-1) and peptide YY (PYY) are secreted mainly from the distal intestinal L cells and increase satiety, reduce hunger and finally improve glucose homeostasis postprandially. The addition of the prebiotic fibre oligofructose in diet has been shown to increase GLP-1 production in rats [71] and to increase satiety and prevent weight gain and fat mass accumulation in humans [72]. It is also postulated that the higher levels of gut hormones after gastric bypass surgery may be partly due to an altered composition of the gut microbiota, which postoperatively includes a larger number of Enterobacteriaceae and fewer Firmicutes and methanogens [73].

It remains to be seen whether manipulation of the gut flora can be used therapeutically to decrease the energy yield from our high-fat, high-calorie diets and eventually promote weight loss in patients suffering from obesity.

CONCLUSION

The gut is not only involved in the pathogenesis of obesity but is affected by its presence. The latter is implicated in numerous gastrointestinal complications and diseases ranging from GERD to colonic cancer and liver cirrhosis. The available literature suggests that obesity has a causative role in the development of these sinister clinical conditions with poor outcomes; however, the mechanisms underlying the pathophysiology are still not fully understood. The elucidation of the mechanisms may not only lead to effective treatment for diseases of the gut, but potentially to new therapies for obesity itself.

> **BEST PRACTICE TIPS**
>
> 1 Have a low threshold for investigating obese patients for gastrointestinal organ cancers.
> 2 Be aware that weight loss can paradoxically increase the likelihood of gallstone formation.
> 3 Obese patients with pancreatitis may present with a more severe form of the condition.
> 4 Computer tomography and magnetic resonance imaging are more sensitive modalities for the diagnosis of NAFLD compared to simple ultrasonography.
> 5 Treat obesity as a disease not as a failure of patient self control.

REFERENCES

1 Nocon M, et al. Association of body mass index with heartburn, regurgitation and esophagitis: results of the Progression of Gastroesophageal Reflux Disease study. J Gastroenterol Hepatol. 2007;22(11):1728–31.

2 Talley NJ, Howell S, Poulton R. Obesity and chronic gastrointestinal tract symptoms in young adults: a birth cohort study. Am J Gastroenterol. 2004;99(9):1807–14.

3 El-Serag HB, et al. Obesity increases oesophageal acid exposure. Gut. 2007;56(6):749–55.

4 Hampel H, Abraham NS, El Serag HB. Meta-analysis: obesity and the risk for gastroesophageal reflux disease and its complications. Ann Intern Med. 2005;143(3):199–211.

5 Kjellin A, et al. Gastroesophageal reflux in obese patients is not reduced by weight reduction. Scand J Gastroenterol. 1996;31(11):1047–51.

6 Smith SC, Edwards CB, Goodman GN. Symptomatic and clinical improvement in morbidly obese patients with gastroesophageal reflux disease following Roux-en-Y gastric bypass. Obes Surg. 1997;7(6):479–84.

7 Wu JC, et al. Obesity is associated with increased transient lower esophageal sphincter relaxation. Gastroenterology. 2007;132(3):883–9.

8 Sugerman HJ, et al. Increased intra-abdominal pressure and cardiac filling pressures in obesity-associated pseudotumor cerebri. Neurology. 1997;49(2):507–11.

9 Geliebter A. Gastric distension and gastric capacity in relation to food intake in humans. Physiol Behav. 1988;44(4–5):665–8.

10 Calbet JA, MacLean DA. Role of caloric content on gastric emptying in humans. J Physiol. 1997;498(Pt 2):553–9.

11 Mercer CD, et al. Lower esophageal sphincter pressure and gastroesophageal pressure gradients in excessively obese patients. J Med. 1987;18(3–4):135–46.

12 Anand G, Katz PO. Gastroesophageal reflux disease and obesity. Gastroenterol Clin North Am. 2010;39(1):39–46.

13 Pieramico O, et al. Interdigestive gastroduodenal motility and cycling of putative regulatory hormones in severe obesity. Scand J Gastroenterol. 1992;27(7):538–44.

14 Wisen O, Johansson C. Gastrointestinal function in obesity: motility, secretion, and absorption following a liquid test meal. Metabolism. 1992;41(4):390–5.

15 Ruhl CE, Everhart JE. Relationship of serum leptin concentration and other measures of adiposity with gallbladder disease. Hepatology. 2001;34(5):877–83.

16 Barbara L, et al. A population study on the prevalence of gallstone disease: the Sirmione Study. Hepatology. 1987;7(5):913–17.

17 Stampfer MJ, et al. Risk of symptomatic gallstones in women with severe obesity. Am J Clin Nutr. 1992;55(3):652–8.

18 Calhoun R, Willbanks O. Coexistence of gallbladder disease and morbid obesity. Am J Surg. 1987;154(6):655–8.

19 Dittrick GW, et al. Gallbladder pathology in morbid obesity. Obes Surg. 2005;15(2):238–42.

20 Everhart JE. Contributions of obesity and weight loss to gallstone disease. Ann Intern Med. 1993;119(10):1029–35.

21 Bray GA. Medical consequences of obesity. J Clin Endocrinol Metab. 2004;89(6):2583–9.

22 Whiting MJ, Watts J. Supersaturated bile from obese patients without gallstones supports cholesterol crystal growth but not nucleation. Gastroenterology. 1984;86(2):243–8.

23 Marzio L, et al. Gallbladder kinetics in obese patients: effect of a regular meal and low-calorie meal. Dig Dis Sci. 1988;33(1):4–9.

24 Vezina WC, et al. Increased volume and decreased emptying of the gallbladder in large (morbidly obese, tall normal, and muscular normal) people. Gastroenterology. 1990;98(4):1000–7.

25 Liddle RA, Goldstein RB, Saxton J. Gallstone formation during weight-reduction dieting. Arch Intern Med. 1989;149(8):1750–3.

26 Marks JW, et al. The sequence of biliary events preceding the formation of gallstones in humans. Gastroenterology. 1992;103(2):566–70.

27 Angulo P. Obesity and nonalcoholic fatty liver disease. Nutr Rev. 2007;65(6 Pt 2):S57–63.

28 Browning JD, et al. Prevalence of hepatic steatosis in an urban population in the United States: impact of ethnicity. Hepatology. 2004;40(6):1387–95.

29 Wieckowska A, Feldstein AE. Diagnosis of nonalcoholic fatty liver disease: invasive versus noninvasive. Semin Liver Dis. 2008;28(4):386–95.

30 Adams LA, et al. The natural history of nonalcoholic fatty liver disease: a population-based cohort study. Gastroenterology. 2005;129(1):113–21.

31 Adams LA, Lindor KD. Nonalcoholic fatty liver disease. Ann Epidemiol. 2007;17(11):863–9.

32 Hoyumpa AM Jr, et al. Fatty liver: biochemical and clinical considerations. Am J Dig Dis. 1975;20(12):1142–70.

33 Kleiner DE, et al. Design and validation of a histological scoring system for nonalcoholic fatty liver disease. Hepatology. 2005;41(6):1313–21.

34 Fabbrini E, Sullivan S, Klein S. Obesity and nonalcoholic fatty liver disease: biochemical, metabolic, and clinical implications. Hepatology. 2010;51(2):679–89.

35 Nielsen S, et al. Splanchnic lipolysis in human obesity. J Clin Invest. 2004;113(11):1582–8.

36 Greco D, et al. Gene expression in human NAFLD. Am J Physiol Gastrointest Liver Physiol. 2008;294(5):G1281–7.

37 Diraison F, Moulin P, Beylot M. Contribution of hepatic de novo lipogenesis and reesterification of plasma non esterified fatty acids to plasma triglyceride synthesis during non-alcoholic fatty liver disease. Diabetes Metab. 2003;29(5):478–85.

38 Petersen KF, et al. The role of skeletal muscle insulin resistance in the pathogenesis of the metabolic syndrome. Proc Natl Acad Sci U S A. 2007;104(31):12587–94.

39 Zhang D, et al. Mitochondrial dysfunction due to long-chain Acyl-CoA dehydrogenase deficiency causes hepatic steatosis and hepatic insulin resistance. Proc Natl Acad Sci U S A. 2007;104(43):17075–80.

40 Bugianesi E, et al. Insulin resistance in non-diabetic patients with non-alcoholic fatty liver disease: sites and mechanisms. Diabetologia. 2005;48(4):634–42.

41 Adiels M, et al. Overproduction of large VLDL particles is driven by increased liver fat content in man. Diabetologia. 2006;49(4):755–65.

42 Fabbrini E, et al. Alterations in adipose tissue and hepatic lipid kinetics in obese men and women with nonalcoholic fatty liver disease. Gastroenterology. 2008;134(2):424–31.

43 Kirk E, et al. Dietary fat and carbohydrates differentially alter insulin sensitivity during caloric restriction. Gastroenterology. 2009;136(5):1552–60.

44 Mittendorfer B, Patterson BW, Klein S. Effect of weight loss on VLDL-triglyceride and apoB-100 kinetics in women with abdominal obesity. Am J Physiol Endocrinol Metab. 2003;284(3):E549–56.

45 Clark JM. Weight loss as a treatment for nonalcoholic fatty liver disease. J Clin Gastroenterol. 2006;40(Suppl 1): S39–43.

46 Buchwald H, et al. Bariatric surgery: a systematic review and meta-analysis. JAMA. 2004;292(14):1724–37.

47 Dixon JB, et al. Nonalcoholic fatty liver disease: improvement in liver histological analysis with weight loss. Hepatology. 2004;39(6):1647–54.

48 Klein S, et al. Gastric bypass surgery improves metabolic and hepatic abnormalities associated with nonalcoholic fatty liver disease. Gastroenterology. 2006;130(6):1564–72.

49 Cottam DR, et al. The chronic inflammatory hypothesis for the morbidity associated with morbid obesity: implications and effects of weight loss. Obes Surg. 2004;14(5):589–600.

50 Papachristou GI, et al. Obesity increases the severity of acute pancreatitis: performance of APACHE-O score and correlation with the inflammatory response. Pancreatology. 2006;6(4):279–85.

51 Pitt HA. Hepato-pancreato-biliary fat: the good, the bad and the ugly. HPB (Oxford). 2007;9(2):92–7.

52 Chang MC, et al. Adiponectin as a potential differential marker to distinguish pancreatic cancer and chronic pancreatitis. Pancreas. 2007;35(1):16–21.

53 Duell EJ, et al. Inflammation, genetic polymorphisms in proinflammatory genes TNF-A, RANTES, and CCR5, and risk of pancreatic adenocarcinoma. Cancer Epidemiol Biomarkers Prev. 2006;15(4):726–31.

54 Fenton JI, et al. Interleukin-6 production induced by leptin treatment promotes cell proliferation in an Apc (Min/+) colon epithelial cell line. Carcinogenesis. 2006;27(7):1507–15.

55 Okada S, et al. Elevated serum interleukin-6 levels in patients with pancreatic cancer. Jpn J Clin Oncol. 1998;28(1):12–15.

56 Ford ES. Body mass index and colon cancer in a national sample of adult US men and women. Am J Epidemiol. 1999;150(4):390–8.

57 Moore LL, et al. BMI and waist circumference as predictors of lifetime colon cancer risk in Framingham Study adults. Int J Obes Relat Metab Disord. 2004;28(4):559–67.

58 Sedjo RL, et al. Change in body size and the risk of colorectal adenomas. Cancer Epidemiol Biomarkers Prev. 2007;16(3):526–31.

59 Fenton JI, et al. Microarray analysis reveals that leptin induces autocrine/paracrine cascades to promote survival and proliferation of colon epithelial cells in an Apc genotype-dependent fashion. Mol Carcinog. 2008;47(1):9–21.

60 Harris SS, Dawson-Hughes B. Reduced sun exposure does not explain the inverse association of 25-hydroxyvitamin D with percent body fat in older adults. J Clin Endocrinol Metab. 2007;92(8):3155–7.

61 Dobbins C, et al. The relationship of obesity to the complications of diverticular disease. Colorectal Dis. 2006;8(1):37–40.

62 Strate LL, et al. Obesity increases the risks of diverticulitis and diverticular bleeding. Gastroenterology. 2009;136(1):115–122 e1.

63 Backhed F, et al. The gut microbiota as an environmental factor that regulates fat storage. Proc Natl Acad Sci U S A. 2004;101(44):15718–23.

64 Backhed F, et al. Mechanisms underlying the resistance to diet-induced obesity in germ-free mice. Proc Natl Acad Sci U S A. 2007;104(3):979–84.

65 Turnbaugh PJ, et al. An obesity-associated gut microbiome with increased capacity for energy harvest. Nature. 2006;444(7122):1027–31.

66 Turnbaugh PJ, et al. Diet-induced obesity is linked to marked but reversible alterations in the mouse distal gut microbiome. Cell Host Microbe. 2008;3(4):213–23.

67 Ley RE, et al. Microbial ecology: human gut microbes associated with obesity. Nature. 2006;444(7122):1022–3.

68 Schwiertz A, et al. Microbiota and SCFA in lean and overweight healthy subjects. Obesity (Silver Spring). 2010;18(1):190–5.

69 Cani PD, Delzenne NM. Gut microflora as a target for energy and metabolic homeostasis. Curr Opin Clin Nutr Metab Care. 2007;10(6):729–34.

70 Louis P, et al. Understanding the effects of diet on bacterial metabolism in the large intestine. J Appl Microbiol. 2007;102(5):1197–208.

71 Kok NN, et al. Insulin, glucagon-like peptide 1, glucose-dependent insulinotropic polypeptide and insulin-like growth factor I as putative mediators of the hypolipidemic effect of oligofructose in rats. J Nutr. 1998;128(7):1099–103.

72 Cani PD, et al. Oligofructose promotes satiety in healthy human: a pilot study. Eur J Clin Nutr. 2006. 60(5):567–72.

73 Zhang H, et al. Human gut microbiota in obesity and after gastric bypass. Proc Natl Acad Sci U S A. 2009;106(7):2365–70.

4 Metabolic and Endocrine Physiology in Obesity

Paula Alvarez-Castro,[1] Susana Sangiao-Alvarellos,[2] and Fernando Cordido[2]

[1]Xeral Lugo Hospital, Lugo, Spain
[2]University Hospital A Coruña, A Coruña, Spain

> **KEY POINTS**
> - Obesity is associated with important disturbances in metabolic and endocrine function.
> - In obesity there is an impaired growth hormone secretion, either stimulated or spontaneous.
> - Ghrelin is the only known circulating orexigenic factor and has been found decreased in obese humans.

INTRODUCTION

The etiology of obesity is an imbalance between the energy ingested in food and the energy expended. The excess energy is stored in fat cells. Enlarged adipose tissue produces the clinical problems associated with obesity, diseases such as diabetes mellitus, gallbladder disease, osteoarthritis, heart disease, and some forms of cancer. The spectrum of medical, social, and psychological disabilities includes a range of medical and behavioral problems. A variety of endocrine and metabolic changes are associated with overweight and obesity (Table 4.1). Most of these changes are secondary because they can be induced by overfeeding and reversed by weight loss. It is not completely clear if some of the hormonal changes may contribute to the pathophysiology or perpetuate the obese state. In this chapter we discuss the metabolic and endocrine disturbances present in obesity.

ENDOCRINE PANCREAS

The most characteristic endocrine and metabolic alteration in obesity is altered insulin secretion. Insulin concentrations are increased in persons with obesity.

Basal and total 24-hour rates of insulin secretion are three to four times higher in obese subjects than in lean controls. Both obesity and type 2 diabetes are associated with insulin resistance [1].

The release of nonesterified fatty acids (NEFAs) by the adipose tissue may be the single most critical factor in modulating insulin sensitivity. Increased NEFA levels are observed in obesity and type 2 diabetes, and are associated with the insulin resistance observed in both [1]. NEFAs are important for normal β-cell function, and potentiate insulin release in response to glucose and nonglucose secretagogues.

The distribution of body fat is itself a critical determinant of insulin sensitivity. Lean individuals with a more peripheral distribution of fat are more insulin sensitive than lean individuals who have their fat distributed predominantly centrally. Intraabdominal and subcutaneous fat are also different. Intraabdominal fat is more lipolytic than subcutaneous fat and is less sensitive to the antilypolitic effect of insulin [2].

ADIPOSE TISSUE

The identification and characterization of leptin in 1994 firmly established adipose tissue as an endocrine organ. Adipose tissue is now known to express and secrete a variety of bioactive peptides, known as adipokines, which act at both the local (autocrine/paracrine) and systemic (endocrine) levels. The best characterized of the proteins secreted by the adipose tissue is leptin [3,4]. Leptin is a 16 kDa polypeptide containing 167 amino acids with structural homology to cytokines. Adipocytes secrete leptin in direct proportion to adipose tissue mass as well

Critical Care Management of the Obese Patient, First Edition. Edited by Ali A. El Solh.
© 2012 John Wiley & Sons, Ltd. Published 2012 by John Wiley & Sons, Ltd.

Table 4.1 Principal endocrine and metabolic changes in obesity.

Endocrine Gland	Hormonal Alteration
Endocrine pancreas	Hyperinsulinemia
Adipose tissue	Hyperleptinemia. Decreased Adiponectin
Pituitary	Decreased basal and stimulated GH Decreased response to stimuli of Prolactin
Gonads	Woman: Decreased SHBG. Increased estrogens and androgens Man: Decreased SHBG. Decreased testosterone
Adrenals	Free urinary cortisol increased and normal plasmatic cortisol
Gastrointestinal hormones	Decreased ghrelin
Thyroid	Increased TSH and free T3

as nutritional status, and this secretion is greater from subcutaneous relative to visceral adipose tissue.

The effects of leptin on energy homeostasis are well documented. Many of these effects, particularly on energy intake and expenditure, are mediated via hypothalamic pathways, while others are mediated via direct action on peripheral tissues including muscle and pancreatic ß-cells. Although initially viewed as an antiobesity hormone, leptin's primary role is to serve as a metabolic signal of energy sufficiency rather than excess. Leptin levels rapidly decline with caloric restriction and weight loss. This decline is associated with adaptive physiological responses to starvation, including increased appetite and decreased energy expenditure. These same responses are observed in leptin-deficient mice and humans, despite massive obesity. Furthermore, these responses are readily normalized by low-dose leptin replacement. In contrast, common forms of obesity are characterized by elevated circulating leptin. The mechanism for leptin resistance is unknown but may result from defects in leptin signaling or transport across the blood–brain barrier [3].

Adiponectin is secreted exclusively from adipose tissue and is an abundant plasma protein. Structurally, adiponectin is related to the complement 1q family and contains a carboxyl-terminal globular domain and an amino-terminal collagenous domain. It also shares extensive sequence homology with collagen VIII and X. With the exception of severe cases of undernutrition and in the newborn, there is a strong negative correlation between plasma adiponectin concentration in humans and fat mass, with obesity reducing adiponectin levels and weight reduction increasing adiponectin. Adiponectin has been shown to improve whole-body insulin sensitivity in models of genetic and diet-induced obesity [3,5].

Other proteins that are secreted by adipose tissue with important metabolic effects include resistin, TNFα, IL-6, proteins of the renin angiotensin system, adipsin and acylation-stimulating protein (ASP), macrophages, and monocyte chemoattractant protein (MCP)-1.

PITUITARY

The most clearly established alteration of the hypothalamus–pituitary system in obesity involves growth hormone (GH). GH secretion is mainly dependent on the interaction between GHRH and somatostatin. Ghrelin, the endogenous ligand of the GH-secretagogues (GHSs) receptor, probably also has a role in this interaction [6]. In addition, several neurotransmitters, peripheral hormones, and metabolic signals influence GH secretion [7]. In obesity there is a markedly decreased GH secretion. For both children and adults, the greater the body mass index (BMI), the lower the GH response to provocative stimuli [8], including the response to GHRH. This relative GH deficiency may contribute to develop or maintain the obese state.

The altered somatotroph function of obesity is not permanent: it can be reversed by a return to normal weight or by short-term calorie restriction [9]. The most striking example of reversibility appeared when obese subjects were treated with GHRH plus GHRP-6, both at saturating doses, which resulted in a massive GH response [8]. The primary cause of the impaired GH secretion of obesity could be an altered hypothalamus, abnormal pituitary function, or a perturbation of the peripheral signals acting at either the pituitary or hypothalamic level. Elevated insulin levels seem capable of reducing GH release and the hyperinsulinemia which is a frequent finding in obesity could be related to the impaired GH secretion [10,11]. The somatotroph sensitivity to the inhibitory effect of rhIGF-I is preserved in obesity, making it less likely that the GH hyposecretion of obesity is due to a greater somatotroph inhibition by circulating IGF-I levels. Some data suggest that the decreased GH secretion of obesity is not due to the increased leptin levels of overweight [12]. Free fatty acid (FFA) reduction with acipimox, a lipid-lowering drug with minimal side effects, notably increased pyridostigmine-, GHRH-, and GHRH plus GHRP-6-mediated GH secretion, restores

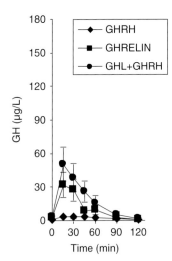

Figure 4.1 Mean ± SEM serum GH (μg/l) levels after the administration of GHRH, ghrelin or ghrelin plus GHRH (GHL + GHRH) in obese patients.

the level of this secretion to 50–70% of normal [13]. These and other results indicate that elevated FFA levels play an important role in causing GH insufficiency in obesity. On the other hand, arginine and pyridostigmine, a drug thought to reduce somatostatinergic tone, increase GHRH-stimulated GH secretion in obese subjects. Together with the nearly preserved GH response to hypoglycemia in obesity, the effects of arginine and pyridostigmine suggest that an enhanced somatostatinergic tone could partially explain the altered somatotroph function in obese patients. Although in obesity the defect responsible for GH hyposecretion is probably multifactorial [14], we have also shown that in obese patients ghrelin, the new hormone implicated in the regulation of GH secretion, is the most potent GH stimulus so far known and that after the combined administration of ghrelin and GHRH there is a massive GH secretion in obese subjects (Figure 4.1). The GH response to ghrelin or GHRH plus ghrelin is modestly diminished in obese patients when compared with normal; in contrast the response to GHRH is markedly decreased in obese patients when compared with normal [15]. The persistence of a decreased response in obese subjects after ghrelin alone or combined with GHRH suggests the existence of another defect implicated in the altered GH secretion of obesity. The massive GH discharge that followed the administration of GHRH plus ghrelin was not observed after any stimulus in obesity,

clearly indicating that the impaired GH secretion is a functional and potentially reversible state and suggesting that decreased ghrelin secretion could be responsible at least in part for the GH hyposecretion.

GHSs may well be considered analogues of ghrelin [16]. However, the knowledge accumulated with these compounds cannot be automatically transferred to ghrelin. The response of obese patients to the natural GHS ghrelin was greater than the response to the synthetic GHS GHRP-6, both alone and combined with GHRH. When considered on a molar basis, the data suggest that ghrelin is more potent in releasing GH than synthetic nonnatural GHSs. As previously hypothesized, based on the effect of synthetic GHSs [8], the additive interaction between ghrelin and GHRH indicates that these peptides act, at least partially, via different mechanisms. In summary, in obesity there is a decreased GH secretion; the altered somatotroph function of obesity is functional as it can be reversed in different situations. The pathophysiological mechanism responsible for the hyposecretion of obesity is probably multifactorial. There are many data which strongly suggest that a chronic state of somatostain hypersecretion results in an inhibition of GH release, that increased FFA probably contributes to the altered GH secretion, and that there is probably a defect in ghrelin secretion (Figure 4.2).

The biochemical diagnosis of adult GH deficiency is established by provocative testing of GH secretion. The insulin hypoglycemia (tolerance) test (ITT) is the diagnostic test of choice for adult GHD (GHDA). A reference for the ITT is yet to be standardized. It may be impossible to evaluate the possible influences of sex, age, body composition, and cortisol levels in ITT-stimulated GH levels, as patients find the ITT unpleasant. Obesity is probably the most important confounding factor for the diagnosis of GHDA. The GH response of obese normal patients and of obese adults with hypopituitarism was similar after GHRH alone. In contrast, the GH response after GHRH plus acipimox (GHRH + Ac) was markedly decreased in obese adults with hypopituitarism compared with obese normal patients [13]. After GHRH + GHRP-6 the maximal response in hypopituitary subjects was lower than the minimal response in normal subjects and lower than the minimal response in obese subjects. In contrast, after ITT, GHRH or GHRH + Ac, the maximal response in hypopituitarism was lower than the minimal response in normal subjects, but higher than the minimal response in obese subjects. Moreover, the differential between normal subjects or obese patients and hypopituitary patients for

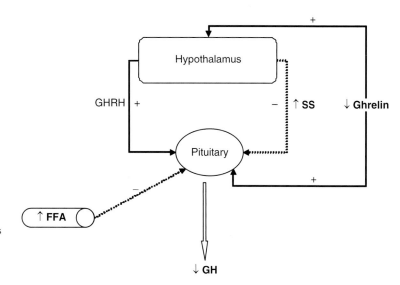

Figure 4.2 Pathophysiological alterations in the hyposomatotropism of obesity. Somatostatin (SS), free fatty acids (FFA), growth hormone (GH).

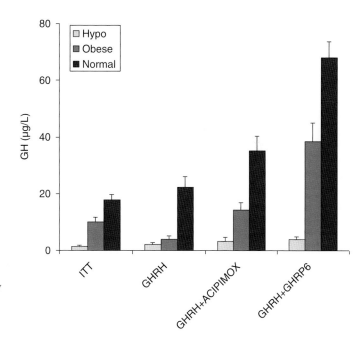

Figure 4.3 Mean ± SEM peak serum GH (µg/l) levels in normal subjects, obese, and hypopituitary patients after the administration of ITT, GHRH, GHRH + Ac or GHRH + GHRP-6. Insulin tolerance test (ITT).

GHRH + GHRP-6 was higher than for ITT, GHRH or GHRH + Ac. The fact that both acipimox and GHRP-6 partially reverse the functional hyposomamotropism of obesity after GHRH, but not the organic hyposomatotropism of hypopituitarism, makes the combined GHRH + GHRP-6 the most reliable test to distinguish between both entities [17] (Figure 4.3).

GONADS

Ovary

In women, obesity is associated with important alterations in steroid plasmatic levels. Blood production rates of testosterone, dihydrotestosterone, and androstenedione are elevated in morbidly obese women. The distribution of body fat is an important factor. Women with upper-body obesity have higher androgen production rates and higher free testosterone and free estradiol levels, whereas women with lower-body obesity make increased amounts of estrone from peripheral aromatization. Other studies found that in obese premenopausal women, an abundance of visceral fat was significantly associated with diminished levels of sex hormone-binding globulin (SHBG) and free 17 β-estradiol:free testosterone ratios and with elevated levels of free testosterone after adjustment for age and total fat mass. In women, loss of visceral fat was significantly related to rises in the SHBG level and the free 17 β-estradiol:free testosterone ratio, independent of total fat loss [18].

The dramatic fall in serum estrogen levels together with relative hyperandrogenism may contribute to weight gain and changes in adipose tissue distribution after menopause.

Testis

Obesity in men is associated with a reduction in serum total testosterone and SHBG levels [19,20]. The major pathogenic factors suggested as being responsible for testosterone reduction in obesity are the decrease in the binding capacity of SHBG, the reduction of LH pulse amplitude, and hyperestrogenemia.

Evaluation of sex hormone profile in obese subjects showed that plasma free testosterone levels were subnormal either in moderate or massively obese men, despite reduced SHBG concentrations [21]. The decline of androgens in obese men is inversely correlated with indexes of body weight, representing a continuum across varying degrees of obesity. In addition, there is an inverse relationship between plasma total testosterone level, free testosterone, SHBG, and visceral fat [22].

ADRENAL GLAND

Due to the occurrence of obesity and central distribution of fat with hypercortisolemia (Cushing's syndrome), many studies have sought to determine whether cortisol plays a role in the manifestation of obesity in the general population and in the distribution of central fat in men and women [23–25].

In obese women with abdominal body fat distribution, daily urinary free cortisol excretion rates (per g creatinine) were significantly higher than in women with peripheral body fat distribution or than in normal-weight healthy women [26]. Basal levels of ACTH rose significantly after CRH plus arginine vasopressin administration and this increase was significantly higher

in men with obesity than in normal-weight healthy men [24]. These results suggest that obese men and women with abdominal body fat distribution may have hyperactivity of the hypothalamic–pituitary–adrenal axis.

Although it is generally assumed that plasma cortisol levels appear normal in obesity, there are exaggerated dynamic cortisol responses [24]. In particular, abdominal obesity is associated with increased urinary free cortisol excretion and increased total cortisol production rates [27]. Other recent studies have also found similarly increased cortisol production in obese polycystic ovary syndrome women and obese control women [25].

GASTROINTESTINAL HORMONES

Ghrelin is a 28-amino-acid peptide, predominantly produced by the stomach, showing a unique structure with an n-octanoyl ester at its third serine residue, which is essential for its potent stimulatory activity on somatotroph secretion. It displays strong GH-releasing activity mediated by the hypothalamus–pituitary GHS receptors [8,15]. Besides stimulating GH secretion, ghrelin has other endocrine and nonendocrine actions including stimulation of lactotroph and corticotroph secretion, inhibition of the gonadal axis, stimulation of appetite and a positive energy balance, control of gastric motility and acid secretion, influence on both endocrine and exocrine pancreatic function, cardiovascular actions, influence on behavior and sleep, and modulation of cell proliferation and of the immune system [6].

Ghrelin seems to play a role in the neuroendocrine and metabolic response to food intake. Indeed, its circulating levels are increased in anorexia and cachexia but reduced in obesity [28,29], and plasma ghrelin levels are negatively correlated with BMI, body fat mass, and plasma leptin, insulin, and glucose levels. Different studies suggest the importance of ghrelin in feeding and weight homeostasis [28,30–34]. Circulating plasma ghrelin levels increase before a meal and decrease following the consumption of nutrients (Figure 4.4). Gastric distension achieved by infusion of water into the stomach does not lead to ghrelin reduction, but ingestion of nonnutritive fiber does decrease ghrelin levels [35,36].

Separately, plasma ghrelin levels are decreased in obese humans when compared with lean [28,37]. More interestingly, it has been demonstrated that obese subjects do not exhibit the decline in plasma ghrelin levels seen after a meal in lean subjects [38]. Insulin resistance has been postulated to play a role in determining this lower plasma ghrelin in the obese. The increase in the plasma ghrelin level with diet-induced

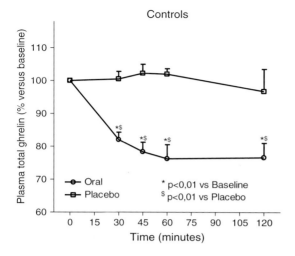

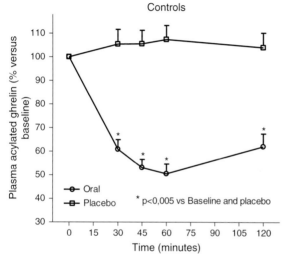

Figure 4.4 Plasma circulating total and acylated ghelin after the ingestion of a mixed meal versus placebo in normal subjects.

weight loss is consistent with the hypothesis that ghrelin has a role in the long-term regulation of body weight in humans [39]. After gastric bypass, ghrelin levels are markedly suppressed, possibly contributing to the weight-reducing effect of the procedure.

PYY is a 36-amino-acid peptide that is synthesized and released into the circulation from specialized enteroendocrine cells, called L-cells, predominantly located in the distal gastrointestinal (GI) tract. Circulating PYY levels increase in response to nutrient ingestion, with caloric load, food consistency, and nutrient composition all affecting circulating PYY concentrations [40]. PP is a 36-amino-acid peptide produced predominantly by a population of cells, F-cells, located in the periphery of pancreatic islets of Langerhans and to lesser extent the colon. Circulating PP concentrations increase following nutrient ingestion in a biphasic manner in proportion to the caloric load and concentrations remain elevated up to 6 hours after a meal [41]. Oxyntomodulin (OXM) is a 37-amino-acid peptide hormone released from L-cells in response to food ingestion and in proportion to the caloric load. Amylin is a neuroendocrine peptide hormone composed of 37 amino acids. It is cosecreted with insulin from pancreatic islet β-cells in response to nutrient ingestion, incretin hormones, and neural input. Amylin exerts glucoregulatory actions that complement the effects of insulin, suppressing postprandial glucagon secretion and delaying gastric emptying [42]. Glucagon-like peptide-1 (GLP-1) is produced from the L-cells of the small intestine and is secreted in response to nutrients. It is known as incretin hormone and is released into circulation approximately 30 minutes after nutrient ingestion. Its main effect is displayed in stimulating glucose-dependent insulin release from the pancreatic islets, and restoring first- and second-phase insulin response to glucose [43]. Other actions are the inhibition of post-meal glucagon release, slowing of gastric emptying, and reduction of food intake. Therapy with GLP-1 and its analogs is associated with weight loss, owing in part to the effects on gastric emptying and its side effects of nausea and vomiting.

THYROID GLAND

Hypothyroidism is usually associated with a modest weight gain and decreased thermogenesis and metabolic rate, whereas hyperthyroidism is related with weight loss despite increased appetite and elevated metabolic rate. Although thyroid function is usually normal in obese subjects, it is known that thyrotropin (TSH) and BMI are positively correlated. In fact, many studies in children, adolescents, and adults have demonstrated that TSH levels are slightly increased in obese subjects as compared to normal-weight humans [44].

While it has been found that obesity increases the susceptibility to autoimmune thyroid disease, it has been suggested that leptin may have a role as a peripheral determinant [45]. More research is necessary to determine whether mild thyroid hormone deficiency and the consequent mild TSH increase, to the upper limit of the reference range, are involved in the development of obesity [46]. Although thyroid hormones have been inappropriately and frequently used in attempts to induce weight loss in obese euthyroid subjects, this practice is not encouraged except in obese hypothyroid subjects [46].

METABOLIC SYNDROME

The metabolic syndrome (MS) is a cluster of metabolic abnormalities including obesity (particularly central adiposity), hyperglycemia, dyslipidemia, and hypertension. These interrelated alterations confer risk for cardiovascular disease and diabetes [47]. Various diagnostic criteria have been proposed by different organizations over the past decade. Most recently, these have come from the International Diabetes Federation (IDF) and the American Heart Association/National Heart, Lung, and Blood Institute (AHA/NHLBI). The main difference concerns the measure for central obesity, which is an obligatory component in the IDF definition, lower than in the AHA/NHLBI criteria, and ethnic-specific. There has been a meeting between several major organizations in an attempt to unify criteria [47]. It was agreed that there should not be an obligatory component, but that waist measurement would continue to be a useful preliminary screening tool. Three abnormal findings out of five would qualify a person for the metabolic syndrome (Table 4.2). A single set of cut points would be used for all components except waist circumference, for which further work is required. In the interim, national or regional cut points for waist circumference can be used. Two levels of abdominal obesity in men or women of European origin are identified. An increased risk occurs at waist circumferences of ≥94 cm in men and ≥80 cm in women, but risk is substantially higher at ≥102 cm in men and 88 cm in women. Higher thresholds are generally used to define abdominal obesity in the USA and Canada. It is recommended that the IDF cut points be used for non-Europeans [47]. It has been shown that, regardless of which definition was used, both men and women with the MS were characterized by increased subclinical atherosclerosis, as measured with six different noninvasive measurements, compared with participants without any component of the definitions of the MS present [48].

Although the prevalence of the MS depends on the definition used and population studied, it has clearly been increasing globally [49]. In a recent study based on the MS defined by the National Cholesterol Education Program Adult Treatment Panel III with data from the Third National Health and Nutrition Examination Survey, there was an estimated MS prevalence of 32.6 and 28.8% for male and female subjects aged 40 years or older respectively [49]. In the previous study MS was associated with all-cause, cardiovascular, cardiac, and even noncardiovascular mortality in women aged 40 years or older, but surprisingly no significant association was observed in men [49].

Table 4.2 Criteria for clinical diagnosis of the metabolic syndrome. Three abnormal findings out of five would qualify a person for the metabolic syndrome.

Measure	Categorical Cut Points
Elevated waist circumference	Population-specific definitions
Elevated triglycerides (or drug treatment)	≥150 mg/dl (1.7 mmol/l)
Reduced HDL-C (or drug treatment)	<40 mg/dL (1.0 mmol/l) in males or <50 mg/dl (1.3 mmol/l) in females
Elevated blood pressure (or drug treatment)	Systolic ≥130 and/or diastolic ≥85 mm Hg
Elevated fasting glucose (or drug treatment)	≥100 mg/dl

It is unclear whether there is a unifying pathophysiological mechanism resulting in the MS. Insulin resistance explains most of the MS. No other mechanisms have emerged that come close to justifying the individual components of their clustering. There is evidence that all the components of the MS begin with excess central adiposity [50]. Insulin resistance in the adipose tissue, the liver, and muscle is an important contributor to the MS [51]. Proinflammatory molecules, endoplasmic reticulum stress, genetic predisposition, and vitamin D deficiency are other possible contributors [50,51].

The MS is not exclusive to adults. In fact, the prevalence of the MS in younger populations is increasing in parallel with childhood obesity. This will likely be associated with increased risk for cardiovascular disease and type 2 diabetes in adulthood. Most studies show that the MS is associated with an approximate doubling of cardiovascular disease risk and that the risk for incident type 2 diabetes is more than five times higher in individuals with the MS compared with those without the syndrome [51]. In addition, the MS is associated with a number of other comorbidities such as nonalcoholic fatty liver disease, sleep disorders, reproductive tract disorders, and microvascular disease [51]. In a longitudinal and multicenter study, carried out in a large sample size of elderly subjects from the general population, the fasting blood glucose component potentiated the excess mortality risk associated with lipid abnormality. This finding strongly supports a causal impact of the multicomponent MS on mortality risk in the elderly and suggests that assessing MS in clinical practice and ensuring the optimal management of the hyperglycemia or dyslipidemia in older subjects by the medical practitioner may help to delay age-related morbidity and mortality [52]. MS prevalence is modulated by other diseases. For example, MS prevalence in GH-deficiency patients was higher than in the general population in the USA (and was higher in the USA than Europe). Prevalence was unaffected by GH replacement, but baseline MS status and obesity were strong predictors of MS after GH treatment [53].

CONCLUSION

Obesity is associated with important disturbances in metabolic and endocrine function. Hyperinsulinemia and insulin resistance are the most well known alterations in obesity. In obesity there is a decreased GH secretion; the pathophysiological mechanism responsible for the GH hyposecretion of obesity is probably multifactorial. In women, abdominal obesity is associated with hyperandrogenism and low SHBG levels. Obese men have low testosterone and gonadotropin concentrations. Ghrelin has been found in reduced levels in obese humans. The metabolic syndrome (MS) is a cluster of metabolic abnormalities including obesity (particularly central adiposity), hyperglycemia, dyslipidemia, and hypertension. These interrelated alterations confer risk for cardiovascular disease and diabetes.

ACKNOWLEDGEMENT

Supported in part by: FIS del Instituto de Salud Carlos III PI051024, PI070413, PI10/00088; Red de Grupos RGTO (G03/028, PI050983); Xunta de Galicia PS07/12, PGIDT05PXIC91605PN, INCITE08ENA916110ES; and Redes 2006/27 and 2009/20, Spain.

BEST PRACTICE TIPS

1 A variety of metabolic and endocrine changes are associated with overweight and obesity. Most of these changes can be induced by overfeeding and reversed by weight loss.

2 Hyperinsulinism is common in obesity and insulin resistance is characteristic when major weight gain occurs.

3 Although initially viewed as an antiobesity hormone, leptin's primary role is to serve as a metabolic signal of energy sufficiency rather than excess. The increased leptin levels of obesity rapidly decline with caloric restriction and weight loss.

4 The pathophysiological mechanism responsible for the GH hyposecretion of obesity is probably multifactorial. Obesity is probably the most important confounding factor for the diagnosis of GH deficiency of the adult.

5 In obesity, ghrelin levels are reduced.

REFERENCES

1 Kahn SE, Hull RL, Utzschneider KM. Mechanisms linking obesity to insulin resistance and type 2 diabetes. Nature. 2006;444:840–6.

2 Montague CT, O'Rahilly S. The perils of portliness: causes and consequences of visceral adiposity. Diabetes. 2000;49:883–8.

3 Kershaw EE, Flier JS. Adipose tissue as an endocrine organ. J Clin Endocrinol Metab. 2004;89:2548–56.

4 Peino R, Fernandez Alvarez J, Penalva A, et al. Acute changes in free-fatty acids (FFA) do not alter serum leptin levels. J Endocrinol Invest. 1998;21:526–30.

5 Galic S, Oakhill JS, Steinberg GR. Adipose tissue as an endocrine organ. Mol Cell Endocrinol. 2010;316:129–39.

6 van der Lely AJ, Tschop M, Heiman ML, Ghigo E. Biological, physiological, pathophysiological, and pharmacological aspects of ghrelin. Endocr Rev. 2004;25:426–57.

7 Alvarez P, Isidro L, Peino R, et al. Effect of acute reduction of free fatty acids by acipimox on growth hormone-releasing hormone-induced GH secretion in type 1 diabetic patients. Clin Endocrinol (Oxf). 2003;59:431–6.

8 Cordido F, Penalva A, Dieguez C, Casanueva FF. Massive growth hormone (GH) discharge in obese subjects after the combined administration of GH-releasing hormone and GHRP-6: evidence for a marked somatotroph secretory capability in obesity. J Clin Endocrinol Metab. 1993;76:819–23.

9 De Marinis L, Bianchi A, Mancini A, et al. Growth hormone secretion and leptin in morbid obesity before and after biliopancreatic diversion: relationships with insulin and body composition. J Clin Endocrinol Metab. 2004;89:174–80.

10 Clasey JL, Weltman A, Patrie J, et al. Abdominal visceral fat and fasting insulin are important predictors of 24-hour GH release independent of age, gender, and other physiological factors. J Clin Endocrinol Metab. 2001;86:3845–52.

11 Cordido F, Garcia-Buela J, Sangiao-Alvarellos S, Martinez T, Vidal O. The decreased growth hormone response to growth hormone releasing hormone in obesity is associated to cardiometabolic risk factors. Mediators Inflamm. 2010;2010:434–562.

12 Ozata M, Dieguez C, Casanueva FF. The inhibition of growth hormone secretion presented in obesity is not mediated by the high leptin levels: a study in human leptin deficiency patients. J Clin Endocrinol Metab. 2003;88:312–16.

13 Cordido F, Fernandez T, Martinez T, et al. Effect of acute pharmacological reduction of plasma free fatty acids on growth hormone (GH) releasing hormone-induced GH secretion in obese adults with and without hypopituitarism. J Clin Endocrinol Metab. 1998;83:4350–4.

14 Alvarez P, Isidro L, Leal-Cerro A, Casanueva FF, Dieguez C, Cordido F. Effect of withdrawal of somatostatin plus GH-releasing hormone as a stimulus of GH secretion in obesity. Clin Endocrinol (Oxf). 2002;56:487–92.

15 Alvarez-Castro P, Isidro ML, Garcia-Buela J, et al. Marked GH secretion after ghrelin alone or combined with GH-releasing hormone (GHRH) in obese patients. Clin Endocrinol (Oxf). 2004;61:250–5.

16 Kojima M, Hosoda H, Matsuo H, Kangawa K. Ghrelin: discovery of the natural endogenous ligand for the growth hormone secretagogue receptor. Trends Endocrinol Metab. 2001;12:118–22.

17 Cordido F, Alvarez-Castro P, Isidro ML, Casanueva FF, Dieguez C. Comparison between insulin tolerance test, growth hormone (GH)-releasing hormone (GHRH), GHRH plus acipimox and GHRH plus GH-releasing peptide-6 for the diagnosis of adult GH deficiency in normal subjects, obese and hypopituitary patients. Eur J Endocrinol. 2003;149:117–22.

18 Leenen R, van der Kooy K, Seidell JC, Deurenberg P, Koppeschaar HP. Visceral fat accumulation in relation to sex hormones in obese men and women undergoing weight loss therapy. J Clin Endocrinol Metab. 1994;78:1515–20.

19 Kaufman JM, Vermeulen A. The decline of androgen levels in elderly men and its clinical and therapeutic implications. Endocr Rev. 2005;26:833–76.

20 Mah PM, Wittert GA. Obesity and testicular function. Mol Cell Endocrinol. 2010;316:180–6.

21 Isidro ML, Alvarez P, Martinez T, Cordido F. [Neuroendocrine disturbances in obesity]. Rev Med Univ Navarra. 2004; 48:24–9.

22 Haffner SM. Sex hormones, obesity, fat distribution, type 2 diabetes and insulin resistance: epidemiological and clinical correlation. Int J Obes Relat Metab Disord. 2000;24 (Suppl 2):S56–8.

23 Andrew R, Phillips DI, Walker BR. Obesity and gender influence cortisol secretion and metabolism in man. J Clin Endocrinol Metab. 1998;83:1806–9.

24 Pasquali R, Gagliardi L, Vicennati V, et al. ACTH and cortisol response to combined corticotropin releasing hormone-arginine vasopressin stimulation in obese males and its relationship to body weight, fat distribution and parameters of the metabolic syndrome. Int J Obes Relat Metab Disord. 1999;23:419–24.

25 Roelfsema F, Kok P, Pereira AM, Pijl H. Cortisol production rate is similarly elevated in obese women with or without the polycystic ovary syndrome. J Clin Endocrinol Metab. 2010;95:3318–24.

26 Pasquali R, Cantobelli S, Casimirri F, et al. The hypothalamic-pituitary-adrenal axis in obese women with different patterns of body fat distribution. J Clin Endocrinol Metab. 1993;77:341–6.

27 Stewart PM, Boulton A, Kumar S, Clark PM, Shackleton CH. Cortisol metabolism in human obesity: impaired cortisone → cortisol conversion in subjects with central adiposity. J Clin Endocrinol Metab. 1999;84:1022–7.

28 Tschop M, Weyer C, Tataranni PA, Devanarayan V, Ravussin E, Heiman ML. Circulating ghrelin levels are decreased in human obesity. Diabetes. 2001;50:707–9.

29 Otto B, Cuntz U, Fruehauf E, et al. Weight gain decreases elevated plasma ghrelin concentrations of patients with anorexia nervosa. Eur J Endocrinol. 2001;145:669–73.

30 Tschop M, Smiley DL, Heiman ML. Ghrelin induces adiposity in rodents. Nature. 2000;407:908–13.

31 Wren AM, Seal LJ, Cohen MA, et al. Ghrelin enhances appetite and increases food intake in humans. J Clin Endocrinol Metab. 2001;86:5992–5995.

32 Cummings DE, Frayo RS, Marmonier C, Aubert R, Chapelot D. Plasma ghrelin levels and hunger scores in humans initiating meals voluntarily without time- and food-related cues. Am J Physiol Endocrinol Metab. 2004;287:E297–304.

33 Diz-Lois MT, Garcia-Buela J, Suarez F, Sangiao-Alvarellos S, Vidal O, Cordido F. Altered fasting and postprandial plasma ghrelin levels in patients with liver failure are normalized after liver transplantation. Eur J Endocrinol. 2010;163:609–16.

34 Sangiao-Alvarellos S, Helmling S, Vazquez MJ, Klussmann S, Cordido F. Ghrelin neutralization during fasting-refeeding cycle impairs the recuperation of body weight and alters hepatic energy metabolism. Mol Cell Endocrinol. 2011;335:177–88.

35 Williams DL, Cummings DE, Grill HJ, Kaplan JM. Meal-related ghrelin suppression requires postgastric feedback. Endocrinology. 2003;144:2765–7.

36 Nedvidkova J, Krykorkova I, Bartak V, et al. Loss of meal-induced decrease in plasma ghrelin levels in patients with anorexia nervosa. J Clin Endocrinol Metab. 2003;88:1678–82.

37 Perez-Fontan M, Cordido F, Rodriguez-Carmona A, Peteiro J, Garcia-Naveiro R, Garcia-Buela J. Plasma ghrelin levels in patients undergoing haemodialysis and peritoneal dialysis. Nephrol Dial Transplant. 2004;19:2095–100.

38 English PJ, Ghatei MA, Malik IA, Bloom SR, Wilding JP. Food fails to suppress ghrelin levels in obese humans. J Clin Endocrinol Metab. 2002;87:2984.

39 Hansen TK, Dall R, Hosoda H, et al. Weight loss increases circulating levels of ghrelin in human obesity. Clin Endocrinol (Oxf). 2002;56:203–6.

40 Batterham RL, Heffron H, Kapoor S, et al. Critical role for peptide YY in protein-mediated satiation and body-weight regulation. Cell Metab. 2006;4:223–33.

41 Karra E, Batterham RL. The role of gut hormones in the regulation of body weight and energy homeostasis. Mol Cell Endocrinol. 2010;316:120–8.

42 Lutz TA. Amylinergic control of food intake. Physiol Behav. 2006;89:465–71.

43 Holst JJ. Glucagon-like peptide-1: from extract to agent. The Claude Bernard Lecture, 2005. Diabetologia. 2006;49:253–60.

44 Reinehr T. Obesity and thyroid function. Mol Cell Endocrinol. 2010;316:165–71.

45 Marzullo P, Minocci A, Tagliaferri MA, et al. Investigations of thyroid hormones and antibodies in obesity: leptin levels are associated with thyroid autoimmunity independent of bio-anthropometric, hormonal, and weight-related determinants. J Clin Endocrinol Metab. 2010;95:3965–72.

46 Biondi B. Thyroid and obesity: an intriguing relationship. J Clin Endocrinol Metab. 2010;95:3614–17.

47 Alberti KG, Eckel RH, Grundy SM, et al. Harmonizing the metabolic syndrome: a joint interim statement of the International Diabetes Federation Task Force on Epidemiology and Prevention; National Heart, Lung, and Blood Institute; American Heart Association; World Heart Federation; International Atherosclerosis Society; and International Association for the Study of Obesity. Circulation. 2009;120:1640–5.

48 Holewijn S, den Heijer M, Swinkels DW, Stalenhoef AF, de Graaf J. The metabolic syndrome and its traits as risk factors for subclinical atherosclerosis. J Clin Endocrinol Metab. 2009;94:2893–9.

49 Lin JW, Caffrey JL, Chang MH, Lin YS. Sex, menopause, metabolic syndrome, and all-cause and cause-specific mortality: cohort analysis from the Third National Health and Nutrition Examination Survey. J Clin Endocrinol Metab. 2010;95:4258–67.

50 Eckel RH, Alberti KG, Grundy SM, Zimmet PZ. The metabolic syndrome. Lancet. 2010;375:181–3.

51 Cornier MA, Dabelea D, Hernandez TL, et al. The metabolic syndrome. Endocr Rev. 2008;29:777–822.

52 Akbaraly TN, Kivimaki M, Ancelin ML, et al. Metabolic syndrome, its components, and mortality in the elderly. J Clin Endocrinol Metab. 2010;95:E327–32.

53 Attanasio AF, Mo D, Erfurth EM, et al. Prevalence of metabolic syndrome in adult hypopituitary growth hormone (GH)-deficient patients before and after GH replacement. J Clin Endocrinol Metab. 2010;95:74–81.

5 Renal Physiology in the Critically Ill Obese Patient

Eric A.J. Hoste[1,2] and Jan J. De Waele[1]

[1]Department of Intensive Care Medicine, Ghent University Hospital, Ghent University, Ghent, Belgium
[2]Research Foundation, Flanders, Belgium

KEY POINTS
- Obese patients are at greater risk for chronic kidney disease.
- Obese patients are also at greater risk for acute kidney injury.
- Obese patients with acute kidney injury have worse outcomes.

INTRODUCTION

Obese intensive care unit (ICU) patients are at greater risk for a wide range of complications, and are often affected by chronic comorbidities. This has a wide range of potential implications for renal function in these patients. Definitions that have been used in clinical studies may not be applicable for obese patients. Some have been based on changes in the serum creatinine concentration, others on the presence of oliguria and on the need for renal replacement therapy (RRT). These variations in definitions have confounded efforts to characterize the epidemiology of acute kidney injury (AKI) in critically ill morbidly obese patients. Interpretation and comparison of epidemiological studies must therefore take into consideration the particular criteria used to define AKI. Further, there are numerous technical implications, such as catheter type and insertion, and volume of replacement fluid in continuous veno-venous hemofiltration (CVVH), that pose particular challenges in the management of AKI in this population.

DEFINITION OF ACUTE KIDNEY INJURY

Numerous definitions for AKI have been used in the ICU literature, resulting in conflicting data on epidemiology and outcomes [1–3]. Since 2004, the RIFLE classification has been universally accepted as the new consensus definition for AKI [4]. This classification defines three grades of severity of AKI. Since then two modifications of this definition have been proposed based on new data in the literature (Table 5.1) [5]. The last modification, proposed by the Kidney Disease Improving Global Outcomes (KDIGO) group, has been communicated at several conferences, but was under external review and not yet published as a KDIGO clinical practice guideline at the time this chapter was written.

The RIFLE classification for AKI is defined by either an increase of serum creatinine or an episode of oliguria. In both arms of the definition, some specific considerations for obese patients are worth noting. The increase in serum creatinine can be either proportional (a 50% or greater increase of serum creatinine) or absolute (a 0.3mg/dl or greater increase within a 48-hour period). This absolute increase in creatinine was introduced after reports associating this criterion with worse outcomes [6]. However, the evidence for this criterion was not validated in an obese cohort. For example, an absolute increase of 0.3mg/dl represents a greater decrease in kidney function in lean patients compared to obese patients. In addition, the definition of oliguria is based on urine output of <0.5ml/kg for a period of ≥6 hours. However,

---

Table 5.1 Classification of acute kidney injury.

	Creatinine criteria	Urine output criteria
Stage 1	150–200% above the baseline within 7 days, or ≥0.3 mg/dl within 48 hours	<0.5 ml/kg per hour for >6 hours
Stage 2	200–300% above baseline	<0.5 ml/kg per hour for >12 hours
Stage 3	≥300% above baseline, or serum creatinine ≥4.0 mg/dl (354 μmol/L) with an increase of ≥0.5 mg/dl (44 μmol/L), or when treated with renal replacement therapy	<0.3 ml/kg per hour for >24 hours, or anuria for 12 hours

Adapted from the RIFLE classification [4], including the modifications proposed by the Acute Kidney Injury Network [5] and Kidney Disease Improving Global Outcomes.

there are no data to indicate what body weight is to be used. The lack of a standard definition has been a limiting factor in understanding the implications of AKI in critically ill obese patients.

EPIDEMIOLOGY OF AKI IN OBESE PATIENTS

With a well-recognized relationship between severity of illness, underlying comorbidities, and risk for AKI, it is not surprising that the incidence of AKI increases dramatically in obese patients requiring ICU setting. The incidence of AKI in critically ill morbidly obese patients is unknown. The estimate ranges between 2.8 and 14.3% in the postoperative observational cohorts, depending on the definition of AKI used, the type of surgery, and the population under study. In a large database of 310 208 patients, a stepwise increase of AKI, with adjusted odds ratios (AOR) of 1.64 for obese patients (body mass index (BMI)=30–39), 1.98 for morbidly obese patients (BMI=40–49), and 3.08 in super obese (BMI>50) [7], was observed. Similar findings were reported in specific surgical cohorts. The incidence of AKI treated with RRT was increased by sixfold after open abdominal aortic aneurysm repair in patients with BMI>40 [8]. In cardiac surgery, morbidly obese patients who underwent bypass or valvular surgery had a two to threefold higher incidence of AKI [9,10]. Yet, despite the increase in AKI, perioperative and 30-day mortality were not significantly different from the nonobese patients.

Obese patients who had bariatric surgery were also at increased risk for developing AKI. Three studies reported on AKI after gastric bypass surgery (both open and laparoscopic) [11–13]. McCullough, using a "liberal" definition for AKI (increase of serum creatinine >25% or 0.5 mg/dl above baseline), found that AKI occurred in 6.4% of 109 morbidly obese patients. In a cohort of 1800 patients who underwent laparoscopic gastric bypass surgery, Sharma et al. found that 2.3% of morbidly obese patients developed AKI. Of these, 14% were treated with RRT [12]. Thakar et al. reported an incidence of 8.5% when AKI was defined as a 50% increase in serum creatinine or RRT [13]. Higher BMI, hyperlipidemia, preoperative use of angiotensin-converting enzyme inhibitors (ACEIs) or angiotensin receptor blockers (ARBs), preoperative chronic kidney disease (CKD), longer operation times, and intraoperative hypotension were independently associated with occurrence of AKI.

Data on AKI in obese ICU patients are scarce. A relatively small multicenter study in mechanically ventilated patients could not establish that obese patients were at increased risk for developing AKI [14]. Similar, in a large surgical ICU cohort of 1373 patients, obese patients were not at greater risk for AKI (creatinine >2 mg/dl) [15].

EVALUATION OF KIDNEY FUNCTION

Assessment of kidney function by measurement of serum creatinine concentration

Serum creatinine concentration is considered the primary tool for assessment of kidney function in the ICU on a daily basis. Despite its widespread use, single-point creatinine concentration has important limitations as a biomarker for glomerular filtration rate (GFR) in critically ill morbidly obese patients [16]: 1) due to increased muscle mass, obese patients have a higher serum creatinine concentration compared to nonobese patients with comparable GFR; 2) because creatinine is filtered by the glomeruli and excreted by tubular secretion, a decline in GFR up to 50% may go unnoticed due to increased tubular secretion; 3) serum creatinine concentration may be falsely low in obese ICU patients who are volume overloaded, as creatinine is diluted by excess fluid [17]; and 4) creatinine is distributed in total body water, which means that it will take 1–2 days before a change in GFR is reflected in serum creatinine concentration (lag time) [18,19].

The GFR is considered to be the best indicator of the filtering capacity of the kidneys and the best overall measure of renal function. The most commonly used equations for estimating GFR (the Modification of Diet in Renal Disease (MDRD) and the Cockcroft–Gault) [20] are based on serum creatinine concentration (SCr). These equations provide practical and inexpensive methods for estimating GFR through the surrogate measure of creatinine clearance. However, their accuracy and precision are affected by factors such as age, muscle mass, diet, and proximal tubule secretion of creatinine [17,21]. Most of these equations have not been validated for use with obese patients. The exception is the Salazar–Corcoran [22] equation, which was developed using an obese rat model and then validated using data from obese patients [23]. However, in a recent analysis, Demirovic and colleagues [24] demonstrated a biased estimation of GFR in all three formulas when tested against measured creatinine clearance with timed urine collection in super-obese patients. Not surprisingly, these formulas perform poorly in ICU patients, as they were generated in a nonobese, non-ICU population with moderate CKD [25,26].

The gold standard for measurement of GFR is insulin clearance. Radioactive markers such as ^{125}I-iothalamate, ^{99m}Tc-DTPA, and ^{51}Cr-EDTA have also been utilized [16,20]. However, the technical requirements for an accurate measurement by these methods are so cumbersome that they cannot be recommended in the routine care of ICU patients. Creatinine clearance obtained by 24-hour urine collection provides a reliable and often useful assessment of GFR in obese critically ill patients [23]. Creatinine clearance rate (C_{Cr}) can be calculated from the concentration of creatinine in plasma (Pcr) and urine (Ucr) and from a timed urine collection according to the formula $C_{Cr} = $ (urine volume (ml) $\times$ Ucr) / (time (min) $\times$ Pcr). However, there are some caveats that should be kept in mind. First, the calculated C_{Cr} is usually corrected for body surface area (BSA) and expressed as ml/min/1.73 m^2 [27]. Unfortunately, the Du Bois and Du Bois formula for BSA was not validated in obese patients. Further, correction for BSA was introduced to correct for differences in kidney size, nephron number, and body size. A smaller person has smaller

kidneys and less nephrons. Obese patients, however, have a body habitus that exceeds their "programmed" body size, and it is therefore unlikely that C_{Cr} will be adequately adjusted for the "full" BSA of an obese patient [28].

Second, the standard for collecting urine volume occurs during a 24-hour observation period (C_{Cr}-24 h). However, C_{Cr} can only be measured correctly in patients whose renal function is in steady state, a condition that is not always present in ICU patients during a whole 24-hour period. It has been suggested that if a patient's renal function is in flux, C_{Cr} can be assessed by correcting for change in Pcr and by decreasing urine collection time. The correction in Pcr is made by replacing the Pcr with the mean of Pcr at the start and end time of the 24-hour urine collection. In addition, the use of shorter collection periods of 2 hours provides comparable results to C_{Cr}-24 h [21,27].

Alternative biomarkers for kidney function

In the last decade several alternative biomarkers for kidney function have been evaluated.

Cystatin C
Cystatin C, a 13 kDa protein, is produced by all nucleated cells at a relatively constant rate, and filtered by the glomeruli. In contrast to creatinine, cystatin C has a lower volume of distribution and appears to correlate better with GFR, especially at higher levels [18]. Cystatin C has been used successfully in critical care settings as a marker of AKI. However, like creatinine, cystatin C concentrations are increased in patients with higher muscle mass and BMI [29–31], and a single-point measurement of cystatin C should be interpreted with caution. At present, the reference range for cystatin C has not been standardized across laboratories, making its use for research purposes only. The levels of cystatin C can be affected by thyroid dysfunction and steroids therapy, although the effects of these diseases on serum concentrations in obese patients have not yet been delineated [32].

Neutrophil gelatinase-associated lipocalin
Neutrophil gelatinase-associated lipocalin (NGAL) has attracted a lot of interest in recent years for its potential use in diagnosis of AKI [33,34]. Kidney NGAL expression is enhanced in AKI, resulting in increased production of this small protein and increased serum and urine concentrations. Initial findings for the diagnostic performance of AKI by NGAL are promising [34]. However, given the

limitations of the available studies, and also given the limited sensitivity and specificity of NGAL in some cohorts, the exact place of NGAL measurement in urine or plasma for prediction or diagnosis of AKI is still a matter of debate. NGAL is also produced by adipose tissue, and it is associated with obesity, hypertriglyceridemia, hyperglycemia, and insulin resistance [35]. Further, NGAL is correlated with hypertriglyceridemia and LPS-binding protein in type 2 diabetics, a condition often present in obese patients [36]. How these mechanisms for NGAL production affect the diagnosis of AKI by NGAL concentrations in obese ICU patients is at this moment uncertain.

CHRONIC KIDNEY DISEASE IN OBESE PATIENTS

Obese patients have a higher incidence of diabetes and hypertension, well known conditions of CKD. The association between excess body weight and risk of CKD appears to persist even after accounting for the presence of comorbidities. Several molecular mechanisms have been proposed for obesity-related renal dysfunction.

Adipose tissue is now recognized as an active endocrine organ that generates and releases a number of proinflammatory cytokines, as well as growth factor and complement proteins known as adipokines. Leptin in particular stimulates activity of the sympathetic nervous system, endocapillary cell proliferation, and mesangial collagen deposition. It has a natriuretic effect besides inducing reactive oxygen species. In ICU patients, leptin is negatively correlated with IL-6. This correlation has significant impact on ICU prognosis because elevated levels of IL-6 portend a poor outcome whereas relatively low leptin levels may impair sympathetic system and immune functions [37].

The elevated metabolic demands on the kidney may also mediate the increased CKD risk in obese individuals. Obese patients have a higher incidence of increased C_{Cr}, glomerular hyperfiltration ($C_{Cr} > 140\,\mathrm{ml/min/1.73\,m^2}$) and increased renal plasma flow [38–40]. Renal hyperfiltration develops through renal vasodilation in a compensatory response to overcome the increased tubular reabsorption of sodium. However, vasodilation of afferent arterioles increases the hydrostatic pressure in the glomerulus, which can lead to hypertrophy over time and renal disease, even in patients without diabetes. In addition, hyperlipidemia and adipocyte-derived hormones contribute to the development of glomerular sclerosis. These structural changes occurring in human kidney as a consequence of obesity have been demon-

strated in large retrospective studies, which incorporated 6818 renal biopsies between 1986 and 2000. The obesity-associated focal and segmental glomerusclerosis (FSGS) differs from idiopathic FSGS in many ways. Distinct clinicopathological features such as glomerulomegaly, less-severe foot-process effacement, and the absence of features of the nephrotic syndrome despite nephrotic range proteinuria are helpful in differentiating this entity from the idiopathic FSGS [41–43].

Interestingly, weight loss after bariatric surgery is associated with normalization of hyperfiltration, and improvement of GFR and proteinuria, which may serve as indirect evidence that obesity plays a central role in the pathogenesis of FSGS [40,44–46].

INTRAABDOMINAL HYPERTENSION AND ITS EFFECT ON KIDNEY FUNCTION IN OBESE PATIENTS

Intraabdominal hypertension (IAH) is defined as a sustained pathological elevation in intraabdominal pressure (IAP) of 12 mm Hg or higher on three measurements obtained 4–6 hours apart [47]. One extreme of IAH, the abdominal compartment syndrome (ACS), was described more than a century ago in the surgical literature, but the recent consensus on a unified definition has made this clinical entity a frequent event in critically ill patients. Whereas in nonobese healthy subjects the IAP is around 0–5 mm Hg [48], the reported IAP in patients undergoing bariatric surgery has been estimated between 4 and 14 mm Hg [49], with the highest value recorded in the super-obese patients. In obesity, the abdominal fat mass is responsible for the increase in IAP, which is reflected by an increase in sagittal abdominal diameter (SAD). Increasingly, SAD is considered a better marker of intraabdominal adiposity and cardiometabolic risk [50].

The clinical implication of IAH is its association with significant kidney injury [51]. Blood flow both to and from the kidney is impaired in patients with IAH as IAH decreases cardiac output (to a variable extent) [52], leading to reduced arterial blood flow to the renal system. More importantly, it is thought that AKI may be attributed to IAH-induced venous congestion resulting from decreased venous outflow [52].

The effect of IAH on renal function has exclusively been studied in severely ill or postoperative patients. There are no studies to our knowledge evaluating the epidemiology of IAP or ACS in morbidly obese patients requiring intensive care. However, in the critically ill obese patients, abdominal obesity (defined as a SAD higher than the 75th percentile) was associated with twice the risk of requiring RRT compared to patients with lower SAD [53]. The risk of death was also higher in the abdominally obese group, with an adjusted odds ratio of 2.12. Given the higher baseline IAP, obese patients may reach the IAP criterion for IAH or ACS much sooner than nonobese patients. Abdominal decompression is the mainstay of therapy, often necessitating another round of surgical intervention, paracentesis, and aggressive management of ileus.

OUTCOME IN OBESE AKI PATIENTS

In the general population, BMI and outcome have an inverse relationship, resulting in worse outcomes in obese subjects [54]. In contrast, higher BMI confers a survival advantage in ICU settings [13,55–60]. This remarkable and incompletely understood phenomenon is called the obesity paradox.

A departure from these observations is seen in the subgroup of obese ICU patients who have severe AKI and are treated with RRT. Druml et al. demonstrated a J-shaped relationship between BMI and mortality in 5232 AKI patients treated with RRT [61]. A similar finding of higher mortality (4.8 vs 0%, p=0.007) and greater length of hospital stay was also noted in those with less severe AKI [13].

CONCLUSION

Obesity has a clear and reversible pathophysiological effect on the kidneys. The available literature suggests that AKI is not an uncommon phenomenon in critically ill morbidly obese patients. Current information on the epidemiology, diagnosis, and management of AKI in this population remains scarce. Further research exploring the role of novel biomarkers, optimal management, and outcome analysis is urgently needed.

BEST PRACTICE TIPS

1 Kidney function in obese patients should be assessed by measured urinary creatinine clearance.
2 Equations for the assessment of kidney function, such as the Cockcroft–Gault or MDRD, should not be used in obese ICU patients.
3 Single-point serum creatinine measurements may under- or overestimate kidney function.
4 AKI should be defined according to the modified RIFLE classification.
5 Obese patients are at greater risk for AKI and have worse outcomes

---

REFERENCES

1 Kellum JA, Levin N, Bouman C, Lameire N. Developing a consensus classification system for acute renal failure. Curr Opin Crit Care. 2002;8:509–14.
2 Hoste EA, Cruz DN, Davenport A, et al. The epidemiology of cardiac surgery-associated acute kidney injury. Int J Artif Organs. 2008;31:158–65.
3 Hoste EAJ, Schurgers M. Epidemiology of AKI: how big is the problem? Crit Care Med. 2008;36:S1–4.
4 Bellomo R, Ronco C, Kellum JA, Mehta RL, Palevsky P. Acute renal failure: definition, outcome measures, animal models, fluid therapy and information technology needs: the Second International Consensus Conference of the Acute Dialysis Quality Initiative (ADQI) Group. Crit Care. 2004;8:R204–12.
5 Mehta RL, Kellum JA, Shah SV, et al. Acute Kidney Injury Network: report of an initiative to improve outcomes in acute kidney injury. Crit Care. 2007;11:R31.
6 Chertow GM, Burdick E, Honour M, Bonventre JV, Bates DW. Acute kidney injury, mortality, length of stay, and costs in hospitalized patients. J Am Soc Nephrol. 2005;16:3365–70.
7 Glance LG, Wissler R, Mukamel DB, et al. Perioperative outcomes among patients with the modified metabolic syndrome who are undergoing noncardiac surgery. Anesthesiology. 2010;113:859–72.
8 Johnson ONr, Sidawy AN, Scanlon JM, et al. Impact of obesity on outcomes after open surgical and endovascular abdominal aortic aneurysm repair. J Am Coll Surg. 2010;210:166–77.
9 Wigfield CH, Lindsey JD, Munoz A, Chopra PS, Edwards NM, Love RB. Is extreme obesity a risk factor for cardiac surgery? An analysis of patients with a BMI > or = 40. Eur J Cardiothorac Surg. 2006;29:434–40.
10 Yap CH, Mohajeri M, Yii M. Obesity and early complications after cardiac surgery. Med J Aust. 2007;186:350–4.
11 McCullough PA, Gallagher MJ, Dejong AT, et al. Cardiorespiratory fitness and short-term complications after bariatric surgery. Chest. 2006;130:517–25.
12 Sharma SK, McCauley J, Cottam D, et al. Acute changes in renal function after laparoscopic gastric surgery for morbid obesity. Surg Obes Relat Dis. 2006;2:389–92.
13 Thakar CV, Kharat V, Blanck S, Leonard AC. Acute kidney injury after gastric bypass surgery. Clin J Am Soc Nephrol. 2007;2:426–30.
14 Frat JP, Gissot V, Ragot S, et al. Impact of obesity in mechanically ventilated patients: a prospective study. Intensive Care Med. 2008;34:1991–8.
15 Nasraway SAJ, Albert M, Donnelly AM, Ruthazer R, Shikora SA, Saltzman E. Morbid obesity is an independent determinant of death among surgical critically ill patients. Crit Care Med. 2006;34:964–70; quiz 971.
16 Lameire N, Hoste E. Reflections on the definition, classification, and diagnostic evaluation of acute renal failure. Curr Opin Crit Care. 2004;10:468–75.

17 Hoste EA, Damen J, Vanholder RC, et al. Assessment of renal function in recently admitted critically ill patients with normal serum creatinine. Nephrol Dial Transplant. 2005;20:747–53.

18 Herget-Rosenthal S, Marggraf G, Husing J, et al. Early detection of acute renal failure by serum cystatin C. Kidney Int. 2004;66:1115–22.

19 Moran SM, Myers BD. Course of acute renal failure studied by a model of creatinine kinetics. Kidney Int. 1985;27:928–37.

20 K/DOQI clinical practice guidelines for chronic kidney disease: evaluation, classification, and stratification. Part 5: Evaluation of laboratory measurements for clinical assessment of kidney disease. Am J Kidney Dis. 2002;39:S76–110.

21 Herrera-Gutierrez ME, Seller-Perez G, Banderas-Bravo E, Munoz-Bono J, Lebron-Gallardo M, Fernandez-Ortega JF. Replacement of 24-h creatinine clearance by 2-h creatinine clearance in intensive care unit patients: a single-center study. Intensive Care Med. 2007;33:1900–6.

22 Salazar DE, Corcoran GB. Predicting creatinine clearance and renal drug clearance in obese patients from estimated fat-free body mass. Am J Med. 1988; 84:1053–60.

23 Snider DR, Kruse JA, Bander JJ, et al. Accuracy of estimated creatinine clearance in obese patients with stable renal function in the intensive care unit. Pharmacotherapy. 1995; 15:747–53.

24 Demirovic J, Pai A, Pai M. Estimation of creatinine clearance in morbidly obese patients. Am J Health Syst Pharm. 2009; 66:642–8.

25 Cockcroft DW, Gault MH. Prediction of creatinine clearance from serum creatinine. Nephron. 1976;16:31–41.

26 Levey AS, Bosch JP, Lewis JB, Greene T, Rogers N, Roth D. A more accurate method to estimate glomerular filtration rate from serum creatinine: a new prediction equation. Modification of Diet in Renal Disease Study Group. Ann Intern Med. 1999;130:461–70.

27 K/DOQI clinical practice guidelines for chronic kidney disease: evaluation, classification, and stratification. Part 4. Defintion and classification of stages of chronic kidney disease. Am J Kidney Dis. 2002;39:S46–75.

28 Levey AS, Kramer H. Obesity, glomerular hyperfiltration, and the surface area correction. Am J Kidney Dis. 2010;56:255–8.

29 Kottgen A, Selvin E, Stevens LA, Levey AS, Van Lente F, Coresh J. Serum cystatin C in the United States: the Third National Health and Nutrition Examination Survey (NHANES III). Am J Kidney Dis. 2008;51:385–94.

30 Muntner P, Winston J, Uribarri J, Mann D, Fox CS. Overweight, obesity, and elevated serum cystatin C levels in adults in the United States. Am J Med. 2008;121:341–8.

31 Young JA, Hwang SJ, Sarnak MJ, et al. Association of visceral and subcutaneous adiposity with kidney function. Clin J Am Soc Nephrol. 2008;3:1786–91.

32 Westhuyzen J. Cystatin C: a promising marker and predictor of renal function. Ann Clin Lab Sci. 2006;36:387–94.

33 Mishra J, Dent C, Tarabishi R, et al. Neutrophil gelatinase-associated lipocalin (NGAL) as a biomarker for acute renal injury after cardiac surgery. Lancet. 2005;365:1231–8.

34 Haase M, Bellomo R, Devarajan P, Schlattmann P, Haase-Fielitz A. Accuracy of neutrophil gelatinase-associated lipocalin (NGAL) in diagnosis and prognosis in acute kidney injury: a systematic review and meta-analysis. Am J Kidney Dis. 2009;54:1012–24.

35 Wang Y, Lam KS, Kraegen EW, et al. Lipocalin-2 is an inflammatory marker closely associated with obesity, insulin resistance, and hyperglycemia in humans. Clin Chem. 2007;53:34–41.

36 Moreno-Navarrete JM, Manco M, Ibanez J, et al. Metabolic endotoxemia and saturated fat contribute to circulating NGAL concentrations in subjects with insulin resistance. Int J Obes (Lond). 2010;34:240–9.

37 Patricia Fernández-Riejos, Souad Najib, Jose Santos-Alvarez, ConsueloMartín-Romero, Antonio Pérez-Pérez, Carmen González-Yanes, and Víctor Sánchez-Margalet. Role of leptin in the activation of immune cells. Mediators of Inflammation. 2010; doi:10.1155/2010/568343.

38 Gerchman F, Tong J, Utzschneider KM, et al. Body mass index is associated with increased creatinine clearance by a mechanism independent of body fat distribution. J Clin Endocrinol Metab. 2009;94:3781–8.

39 Wuerzner G, Pruijm M, Maillard M, et al. Marked association between obesity and glomerular hyperfiltration: a cross-sectional study in an African population. Am J Kidney Dis. 2010;56:303–12.

40 Navaneethan SD, Yehnert H, Moustarah F, Schreiber MJ, Schauer PR, Beddhu S. Weight loss interventions in chronic kidney disease: a systematic review and meta-analysis. Clin J Am Soc Nephrol. 2009;4:1565–74.

41 Foster MC, Hwang SJ, Larson MG, et al. Overweight, obesity, and the development of stage 3 CKD: the Framingham Heart Study. Am J Kidney Dis. 2008;52:39–48.

42 Elsayed EF, Sarnak MJ, Tighiouart H, et al. Waist-to-hip ratio, body mass index, and subsequent kidney disease and death. Am J Kidney Dis. 2008;52:29–38.

43 Griffin KA, Kramer H, Bidani AK. Adverse renal consequences of obesity. Am J Physiol Renal Physiol. 2008;294:F685–96.

44 Ahmed MH, Byrne CD. Bariatric surgery and renal function: a precarious balance between benefit and harm. Nephrol Dial Transplant. 2010.

45 Sugerman H, Windsor A, Bessos M, Kellum J, Reines H, DeMaria E. Effects of surgically induced weight loss on urinary bladder pressure, sagittal abdominal diameter and obesity co-morbidity. Int J Obes Relat Metab Disord. 1998;22:230–5.

46 de Boer IH, Katz R, Fried LF, et al. Obesity and change in estimated GFR among older adults. Am J Kidney Dis. 2009;54:1043–51.

47 Malbrain M, Cheatham M, Kirkpatrick A, et al. Results from the international conference of experts on intra-abdominal

hypertension and abdominal compartment syndrome. II. Intensive Care Med. 2007;33:951–62.

48 Cobb WS, Burns JM, Kercher KW, Matthews BD, James Norton H, Todd Heniford B. Normal intraabdominal pressure in healthy adults. J Surg Res. 2005;129:231–5.

49 De Keulenaer BL, De Waele JJ, Powell B, Malbrain ML. What is normal intra-abdominal pressure and how is it affected by positioning, body mass and positive end-expiratory pressure? Intensive Care Med. 2009;35:969–76.

50 Riserus U, de Faire U, Berglund L, Hellenius ML. Sagittal abdominal diameter as a screening tool in clinical research: cutoffs for cardiometabolic risk. J Obes. 2010;2010; pii:757939.

51 De Waele JJ, De Laet I, Kirkpatrick AW, Hoste E. Intra-abdominal hypertension and abdominal compartment syndrome. Am J Kidney Dis. 2011;57:159–69.

52 Cheatham ML, Malbrain ML. Cardiovascular implications of abdominal compartment syndrome. Acta Clin Belg. 2007;Suppl 1:98–112.

53 Paolini JB, Mancini J, Genestal M, et al. Predictive value of abdominal obesity vs. body mass index for determining risk of intensive care unit mortality. Crit Care Med. 2010;38:1308–14.

54 Berrington de Gonzalez A, Hartge P, Cerhan JR, et al. Body-mass index and mortality among 1.46 million white adults. N Engl J Med. 2010;363:2211–19.

55 Hogue CWJ, Stearns JD, Colantuoni E, et al. The impact of obesity on outcomes after critical illness: a meta-analysis. Intensive Care Med. 2009;35:1152–70.

56 Akinnusi ME, Pineda LA, El Solh AA. Effect of obesity on intensive care morbidity and mortality: a meta-analysis. Crit Care Med. 2008;36:151–8.

57 Kalantar-Zadeh K, Abbott KC, Salahudeen AK, Kilpatrick RD, Horwich TB. Survival advantages of obesity in dialysis patients. Am J Clin Nutr. 2005;81:543–54.

58 Kovesdy CP, Anderson JE, Kalantar-Zadeh K. Paradoxical association between body mass index and mortality in men with CKD not yet on dialysis. Am J Kidney Dis. 2007;49:581–91.

59 Lavie CJ, Milani RV, Ventura HO. Obesity and cardiovascular disease: risk factor, paradox, and impact of weight loss. J Am Coll Cardiol. 2009;53:1925–32.

60 Guenette JA, Jensen D, O'Donnell DE. Respiratory function and the obesity paradox. Curr Opin Clin Nutr Metab Care. 2010;13:618–24.

61 Druml W, Metnitz B, Schaden E, Bauer P, Metnitz PG. Impact of body mass on incidence and prognosis of acute kidney injury requiring renal replacement therapy. Intensive Care Med. 2010;36:1221–8.

Part II   Positive Pressure Ventilation

6

Sedation, Paralysis, and Pain Management of the Critically Ill Obese Patient

Christopher G. Hughes, Lisa Weavind, and Pratik P. Pandharipande
Vanderbilt University School of Medicine, Nashville, TN, USA

KEY POINTS

- Analgesic and sedative medications are often required to provide comfort to critically ill mechanically ventilated patients, but the effects of these medications are altered by obesity and may contribute to worse clinical outcomes, including delirium.
- Targeted sedation, daily spontaneous awakening and breathing trials, delirium monitoring and management, and early physical therapy all decrease morbidity and mortality and should be incorporated into clinical practice.
- Incorporation of analgesics, propofol, and dexmedetomidine into sedation regimens with reduction of benzodiazepine exposure further improves patient outcomes, including rates of cognitive dysfunction.

CONFLICTS OF INTEREST

Dr Pandharipande has received honoraria from Hospira Inc., GlaxoSmithKline, and Orion Pharma.

GENERAL PRINCIPLES

Pain and agitation are extremely common in the intensive care unit (ICU), where they are often underappreciated and inadequately treated [1]. Sedation and analgesia are administered to provide comfort and ensure patient safety because unrelieved or unrecognized pain, anxiety, and delirium contribute to patient distress, evoke the stress response, complicate the management of lifesaving devices, and negatively affect outcome. In order to determine the appropriate treatment strategy, the specific medical problem requiring sedation needs to be

recognized. Routine and objective assessments, with frequent reassessment and adjustment of therapeutic targets, are important to quantify and record sedation, pain, and delirium levels [1].

Unpredictable pharmacokinetics and pharmacodynamics secondary to hemodynamic instability, organ dysfunction, protein binding, and drug interactions lead to the development of complications when sedative and analgesic medications are administered to critically ill obese patients [2]. This is further compounded by the physiological perturbations associated with obesity, which are outlined in detail elsewhere in this book. A few hemodynamic changes worth noting secondary to their profound effects on the provision of sedation and analgesia include increased total body weight (TBW), increased adipose tissue, increased lean body mass (LBM), increased cardiac output, and increased glomerular filtration rate (GFR). Because most sedative agents are administered as continuous infusions, drug accumulation, redistribution, and tachyphylaxis also confound their utilization, and techniques to prevent systemic drug accumulation need to be employed.

PAIN

Existing disease, surgical procedures, trauma, invasive monitors, endotracheal intubation, and nursing interventions are only a few sources of discomfort commonly experienced by patients in the ICU. Inadequately treated pain leads to patient discomfort with resultant tachycardia, increased oxygen consumption, hypercoagulability, immunosuppression, hypermetabolism, and increased

---

Critical Care Management of the Obese Patient, First Edition. Edited by Ali A. El Solh.
© 2012 John Wiley & Sons, Ltd. Published 2012 by John Wiley & Sons, Ltd.

endogenous catecholamine activity [1,2]. Insufficient pain relief can also contribute to deficient sleep, disorientation, anxiety, and long-term effects such as posttraumatic stress disorder (PTSD) [3]. Unfortunately for obese patients, pain is often undertreated secondary to concerns about respiratory depression despite the fact that obese patients likely experience increased pain at baseline (e.g. low back pain) [4] and increased periprocedural pain [5] when compared to lean patients.

Pain assessment

The most valid and reliable indicator of pain is the patient's self-report [6]. Information about pain, including location, quality, and intensity, should be elicited routinely as part of the patient's vital signs. Tools such as the visual analog scale or the numeric rating scale can be utilized to document severity [6]. It is not uncommon for ICU patients to be unable to communicate with caregivers, in which case behavioral and physiologic indicators must be used to assess pain intensity. The FACES scale (Figure 6.1) [7] and Behavioral Pain Scale (Table 6.1) [8] are validated tools for assessing pain, which in themselves

have been associated with lower analgesic and sedative use and decreased time on the ventilator [9].

Pain management

In managing pain, nonpharmacological methods should be attempted first. These include patient repositioning, injury stabilization, removal of noxious or irritating stimuli, and application of heat or cold [1]. Repositioning and additional support, especially to prevent skin breakdown and pressure ulcers, are increasingly important in obese patients [10]. When nonpharmacological approaches are insufficient to provide analgesia, regional or systemic therapy is indicated.

Regional therapy

Regional nerve blockade provides analgesia for specific areas of the body without the systemic effects of intravenous (IV) analgesia. These procedures are useful adjuncts to decrease exposure to the side effects of potent analgesics, especially the enhanced respiratory depressant effects of narcotics in obese patients with obstructive sleep apnea. Difficulty in positioning and identifying

Wong-Baker FACES pain rating scale

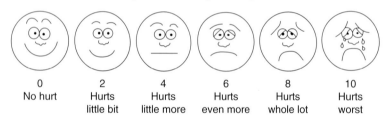

0	2	4	6	8	10
No hurt	Hurts little bit	Hurts little more	Hurts even more	Hurts whole lot	Hurts worst

Figure 6.1 FACES scale. (From [85].)

Table 6.1 The Behavioral Pain Scale. (Modified from [8].)

Item	Description	Score
Facial expression	Relaxed	1
	Partially tightened (e.g. brow lowering)	2
	Fully tightened (e.g. eyelid closing)	3
	Grimacing	4
Upper limbs	No movement	1
	Partially bent	2
	Fully bent with finger flexion	3
	Permanently retracted	4
Compliance with ventilation	Tolerating movement	1
	Coughing but tolerating ventilation for most of the time	2
	Fighting ventilator	3
	Unable to control ventilation	4

anatomical landmarks increases the complexity of these procedures in obese patients, and they should only be performed by specially trained clinicians. Blockade of individual nerves or nerve plexus may provide relief of pain localized to one extremity [11], and placement of peripheral nerve catheters can prolong the benefit of this targeted action. Intercostal blocks can be used to manage pain due to thoracic or upper abdominal trauma or surgery and can improve respiratory mechanics to reduce the risk of pulmonary compromise [12]. Paravertebral blocks are useful for managing pain related to unilateral thoracic or abdominal procedures [13] and traumatic rib fractures [14]. Epidural analgesia has become increasingly popular for the management of pain from thoracic, abdominal, or lower extremity operative procedures [15]. Through a catheter, local anesthetics, opiates, and other pharmaceutical adjuncts such as clonidine can be infused in the epidural space to provide bilateral analgesia in specific dermatomes.

Systemic therapy

Systemic analgesics should be administered as part of a goal-directed sedation and analgesia protocol. Systemic therapies include nonsteroidal antiinflammatory drugs and acetaminophen, but opioids are the most common ICU therapy secondary to their analgesic and sedative properties. Opioids, however, have a number of adverse effects. Respiratory depression is commonly seen, with enhanced effects in patients with obstructive sleep apnea, a common finding in obese patients [16]. Hypotension may result from decreased sympathetic tone or vasodilation from histamine release, especially with morphine. Other side effects include decreased gastrointestinal motility, pruritus, flushing, urinary retention, and delirium. Consequently, nonopioid analgesics should be considered for treatment of low-acuity pain or as adjuncts to decrease opioid exposure in the obese patient to preserve mental status and pulmonary function [17].

The most commonly used opiates in the ICU are morphine, hydromorphone, fentanyl, and remifentanil. Morphine and hydromorphone are typically utilized as intermittent IV injections. Morphine is given in doses of 2–5 mg IV every 5–15 minutes until the pain is controlled, followed by similar doses on a scheduled basis every 1–2 hours. However, 10-fold variation in opioid-induced analgesia has been reported in postoperative morbidly obese patients, with variability unrelated to body surface area [18]. Morphine is characterized by hepatic metabolism and renal excretion, so its effects can be prolonged in patients with renal or hepatic impairment [19].

Increased hepatic blood flow in obese subjects, however, likely increases the hepatic plasma clearance of morphine, and higher GFR may increase renal clearance of morphine metabolites [18]. Hydromorphone is a more potent congener of morphine with similar pharmacokinetic and pharmacodynamic profiles [19]. Its lack of histamine release and decreased incidence of central nervous system side effects make it a useful alternative to morphine, with typical dosing ranges of 0.2–1 mg IV. Both morphine and hydromorphone have intermediate volumes of distribution, but the effect of increased adipose tissue on their pharmacokinetics has not been investigated [18].

Fentanyl is a synthetic opioid with a rapid onset (5–15 minutes) and a short duration of action (30–60 minutes) [19]. Its short half-life allows easy titration as a continuous infusion. In general, loading doses of 25–100 µg are given every 5–10 minutes until the pain is controlled, followed by infusion rates of 25–250 µg/hour. Studies examining fentanyl infusions in obese patients have found that dosing based on TBW may cause overdose since body clearance is correlated with pharmacokinetic mass (similar to LBM) and not TBW [20]. Because it causes less histamine release than morphine and does not undergo renal elimination, fentanyl is the preferred opioid analgesic in hemodynamically unstable patients or those with renal insufficiency [1].

Remifentanil is a derivative of fentanyl that is metabolized by nonspecific blood and tissue esterases [19]. It is utilized primarily as an infusion (0.05–2 µg/kg/hour) and has an elimination half-life of under 10 minutes regardless of infusion duration [21]. The pharmacokinetics of remifentanil are more closely related to LBM than to TBW, and dosing regimens should be based on ideal body weight or LBM [22]. A small prospective study of obese surgical patients demonstrated the rapid development of profound tolerance to remifentanil [23]. Hypotension and bradycardia are the most common side effects of remifentanil administration, and supplemental analgesic medication is usually required at the conclusion of a remifentanil infusion [21].

Traditionally, the selection of an opioid has depended on the likely duration of analgesic infusion and the pharmacology of the specific opioid [1]. In a randomized double-blind study, optimal sedation time, necessity of supplemental sedation, duration of mechanical ventilation, and extubation time favored remifentanil over morphine [24]. Fentanyl and remifentanil displayed equal efficacy in achieving sedation goals with no difference in extubation times [25]. Patients receiving fentanyl required more breakthrough propofol but experienced less pain after extubation compared to patients receiving remifentanil [25]. Concerns about cost, withdrawal, and hyperalgesia after discontinuation of remifentanil have limited the widespread use of this agent [26].

SEDATION AND PARALYSIS

Anxiety and agitation are very common in the ICU and have a variety of causes, including excessive stimulation, pain, dyspnea, delirium, inability to communicate, sleep deprivation, metabolic disturbances, and underlying disorders [1]. Unrelieved anxiety can be a significant source of physical and psychological stress for patients both during an acute event and in the long term, when PTSD may result [3,27]. Left untreated, agitation can become life-threatening if it leads to the removal of lifesaving devices such as endotracheal tubes and intravascular lines; this can be especially problematic in obese patients with difficult airways or difficult IV access.

Sedation assessment and protocols

Many scales are available to assess level of sedation and agitation, including the Ramsay scale [28], Riker sedation-agitation scale [29], motor activity assessment scale [30], and Richmond agitation-sedation scale (RASS) [31]. Their reliability and validity among adult ICU patients allow for targets to be set on these scales for use in goal-directed therapy. However, only the RASS has been shown to detect variations in the level of consciousness over time or in response to changes in sedative and analgesic drug use [31]. The RASS is a 10-point scale with discrete criteria to distinguish levels of agitation and sedation (Table 6.2). Numerous studies have shown that the use of a defined

sedation target for the provision of protocol-based, goal-directed therapy reduces patient discomfort and improves outcome [31–33]. Additionally, daily interruption of sedation [34], as well as linking of these spontaneous awakening trials to daily spontaneous breathing trials [35], has been shown to improve time off mechanical ventilation and shorten ICU stays. Furthermore, the Awakening and Breathing Controlled Trial showed a reduction in mortality at 12 months by incorporating this linked approach [35] without any associated increase in long-term neuropsychological outcomes [36]. An increased rate of self-extubation was witnessed with these protocols, but without a difference in reintubation rates. These protocols did not examine obese patients specifically, and increased vigilance is required when a patient is known or suspected to have a difficult airway to manage. However, the increased volume of distribution and often unknown pharmacokinetics of obese critically ill patients lends further importance to the daily interruption of sedative medications. Patients receiving prolonged sedative infusions may also experience withdrawal symptoms upon removal of the medication [37,38]. Symptoms of depression and PTSD have been positively associated to the days of sedation in the ICU [39]. Similarly, patients who had recall of their ICU stay had less cognitive dysfunction than patients who had no recall of their ICU experience, further emphasizing that excessive sedation (and not the lack of amnesia) may have prolonged neuropsychological and cognitive effects [40].

Pharmacological management

Before administering sedative agents, it is important to search for an underlying cause (e.g. hypoxemia, hypoglycemia, hypotension, drug withdrawal), especially when

Table 6.2 The Richmond sedation-agitation scale. (Adapted from [86].)

Richmond agitation-sedation scale (RASS)		
+4	Combative	Combative, violent, immediate danger to staff
+3	Very agitated	Pulls or removes tubes or catheters; aggressive
+2	Agitated	Frequent nonpurposeful movement; fights ventilator
+1	Restless	Anxious, apprehensive, but movements not aggressive or vigorous
0	Alert and calm	
−1	Drowsy	Not fully alert, but has sustained (>10 sec) awakening (eye opening/contact) to voice
−2	Light sedation	Drowsy, briefly (<10 sec) awakens to voice or physical stimulation
−3	Moderate sedation	Movement or eye opening (but no eye contact) to voice
−4	Deep sedation	No response to voice, but movement or eye opening to physical stimulation
−5	Unarousable	No response to voice or physical stimulation

a previously calm patient becomes anxious or agitated. If pain is present, an analgesic should be the initial therapeutic choice. Once pain has been addressed, propofol, dexmedetomidine, and benzodiazepines are the drugs most often utilized to provide additional sedation.

Analgosedation

The safety and efficacy of analgesia-based sedation with remifentanil has been compared to conventional sedation with hypnotic-based regimens in patients with brain injury [41]. Neurological assessment times and time to extubation were significantly shorter for patients receiving remifentanil than those receiving propofol or midazolam supplemented with morphine or fentanyl. The duration of mechanical ventilation and duration of weaning were significantly shorter in patients receiving remifentanil than midazolam [42]. A randomized multicenter study comparing conventional sedation regimens (propofol or benzodiazepine with as-needed opioid) with an analgesia-based regimen consisting of remifentanil with as-needed propofol displayed shortened duration of mechanical ventilation and ICU length of stay in the analgesia-based group [43]. Another randomized controlled study was performed in a single center that compared the use of an analgesia-based protocol incorporating morphine (intervention group) to sedation with propofol [44]. Patients in the intervention group had shorter times on mechanical ventilation and in the ICU with no adverse events. About 20% of the patients in the "morphine-only" group required rescue with propofol per the protocol; 80% were, however, managed with morphine alone despite being critically ill. The generalizability of this study is limited by the fact that the ICU had 1 : 1 nursing ratios, as well as other personnel to help reassure patients, which may not be available in most other ICUs.

Benzodiazepine-based sedation

Benzodiazepines bind to γ-aminobutyric acid (GABA) receptors in the central nervous system, thereby providing sedation, anxiolysis, hypnosis, muscle relaxation, anticonvulsant activity, and amnesia [45]. Benzodiazepines vary considerably in their pharmacology, and patient-specific factors such as advanced age, drug or alcohol use, and organ dysfunction make their potency, onset, and duration of action even more unpredictable [45]. Diazepam, midazolam, and lorazepam have traditionally been the benzodiazepines most frequently utilized in the ICU. Currently, benzodiazepine sedation in the ICU has been curtailed in favor of other sedation regimens secondary to mounting evidence of increased

morbidity, including increased delirium, time on mechanical ventilation, and ICU length of stay. Benzodiazepines, however, remain the drugs of choice for the treatment of delirium tremens (and other withdrawal syndromes) and seizures.

Propofol-based sedation

Propofol is an IV anesthetic with mechanism of action primarily at the GABA receptor [46]. It has proven utility as a sedating agent in the ICU due to its rapid onset (1–2 minutes) and short duration of action (2–8 minutes). It is typically given as a bolus injection of 40–100 mg IV followed by an infusion of 25–75 µg/kg/minute [47]. Its volume of distribution and clearance both increase with TBW, with similar elimination half-lives in both lean and obese patients, suggesting dosage for maintenance to be based on TBW [48]. Propofol is a respiratory depressant and can also cause significant hypotension by venodilation, vasodilation, and myocardial depression [49]. Propofol has been associated with hypertrigylceridemia when infused for 7 days or greater [1]. Another complication associated with propofol use is the development of propofol infusion syndrome characterized by severe lactic acidosis and rhabdomyolysis [50]. While the majority of reports have been in the pediatric population, a few case reports have been published describing propofol infusion syndrome in adults associated with high-dose (>75 µg/kg/minute) and prolonged (>72 hours) infusions [50]. Obese patients have been reported to be at higher risk of rhabdomyolysis [51]; however, obesity has not been associated with propofol infusion syndrome thus far. Consequently, providers should consider alternative sedative agents for any patient receiving high-dose propofol infusions who develops unexplained metabolic acidosis, arrhythmia, or cardiac failure.

Dexmedetomidine-based sedation

Dexmedetomidine is a selective α_2 receptor agonist with a site of action that includes presynaptic neurons in the locus ceruleus and spinal cord, producing analgesia and sedation without respiratory suppression [52]. The onset of action is within 15 minutes, and peak concentrations are achieved after 1 hour of continuous infusion [52]. Sedation is often initiated with a bolus of 1 µg/kg over 10–20 minutes, followed by an infusion of 0.2–0.7 µg/kg/hour. Several studies have shown safety with doses up to 2 µg/kg/hour, although with increased incidence of bradycardia and hypotension [53]. With volume of distribution and clearance similar to fentanyl [54], it would be plausible to dose dexmedetomidine based on LBM; however, neither TBW or LBM as covariates in a pharmacokinetic model improved predictive performance [55]. Dexmedetomidine is metabolized by the liver, and patients with severe liver disease require lower dosing, whereas there is no need for dose adjustment in those with renal dysfunction [52]. The increased cardiac output of obese patients likely increases hepatic clearance compared to lean patients given dexmedetomidine's high extraction ratio [56], although alterations in cardiac output from critical illness will likely contribute more to its varying pharmacokinetics [57]. Bradycardia is the most common side effect of dexmedetomidine, especially with rapid bolus administration, and a biphasic response in blood pressure may be seen during dexmedetomidine utilization [52]. Dexmedetomidine infusion has been shown to decrease postoperative analgesic and antiemetic therapies after bariatric surgery [58,59].

Comparative studies of sedative regimens

It is important to note that no comparative sedation trials have been performed exclusively on obese patients, and the trials presented next are not specific to obese patients. Propofol has been compared to individual benzodiazepines in several studies and has been shown to reduce mechanical ventilation days [60], increase duration of targeted sedation [61], and be less costly per patient [62]. Dexmedetomidine has also been compared to multiple sedation regimens. In comparison to propofol, patients with dexmedetomidine required less supplemental analgesics [63]. Similarly, utilization of β-blockers, antiemetics, epinephrine, and diuretics after cardiac surgery was reduced with dexmedetomidine sedation [64]. The MENDS [65] and SEDCOM [66] studies demonstrated that patients sedated with dexmedetomidine had a lower likelihood of delirium development and shorter durations of delirium and coma than patients sedated with benzodiazepines. In the SEDCOM study, patients on dexmedetomidine also spent less time on the ventilator and developed less tachycardia and hypertension. The MENDS study further displayed improved survival with dexmedetomidine in septic patients [67], and post hoc analysis demonstrated a significant per-patient reduction in cost associated with dexmedetomidine in the SEDCOM study. Finally, a metaanalysis suggested that sedation with dexmedetomidine decreases ICU length of stay [53].

An empiric protocol (Figure 6.2) for the management of pain and sedation is provided as a reference. Readers are advised to incorporate local culture, patient charac-teristics, and expert opinion from thought leaders in the ICU to determine the best protocol for their ICUs.

Pharmacological paralysis in critical illness

Given the level of evidence supporting lighter sedation paradigms, the utilization of neuromuscular blockade in ICU sedation has decreased considerably. Pharmacological paralysis is now most frequently utilized in patients with open abdomens or with progressive respiratory failure and high peak inspiratory pressures unresponsive to conventional ventilation. Cisatracurium is the recommended paralytic agent for maintenance of paralysis in the ICU secondary to its nonsteroidal benzylisoquinoline structure, lack of histamine release, predominant Hoffman elimination, and independence of hepatic or renal elimination. As a hydrophilic drug, dosing in obese patients should be based on LBM with continuous infusions ranging from 1 to 2 μg/kg/minute [68]. Interestingly, a recent multicenter randomized trial demonstrated that early administration of cisatracurium improved mortality and mechanical ventilation time in patients with severe acute respiratory distress syndrome without increasing muscle weakness [69]. The results and ramifications of this study need to be confirmed and evaluated further.

DELIRIUM

Delirium is an acute fluctuating change in mental status characterized by inattention and altered levels of consciousness that is extremely prevalent in critically ill patients and is associated with morbidity and mortality [70–75]. Obese patients might be at additional risk for developing delirium given their altered response to medications, chronic inflammatory state, and likelihood of obstructive sleep apnea [76]. Delirium can be assessed by health care personnel with the Intensive Care Delirium Screening Checklist [77] and the Confusion Assessment Method for the ICU [78]. A liberation and animation strategy will likely reduce the incidence and duration of brain dysfunction [79], and utilization of dexmedetomidine sedation also decreases the duration of brain organ dysfunction when compared to benzodiazepine sedation [65,66].

Pharmacological therapy to manage delirium should be attempted only after correcting any contributing factors (e.g. pain, anxiety, sleep disturbance, environmental stimuli, medications) or underlying physiological abnormalities (e.g. hypoxia, hypoglycemia, metabolic derangements, shock). Haloperidol [80], olanzapine [81], and quetiapine [82] may prove useful in the treatment of

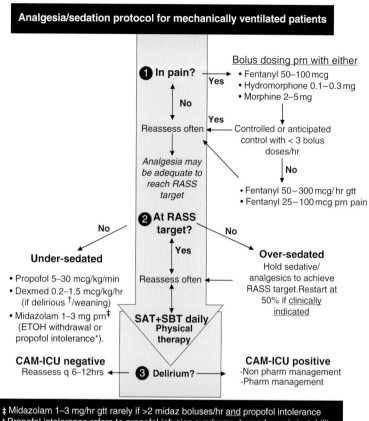

Figure 6.2 Empiric sedation protocol. (With permission from www.icudelirium.org)

delirium; however, larger studies need to be performed before any concrete recommendations can be made regarding the efficacy of typical or atypical antipsychotics in delirium. It should also be recognized that while agents used to treat delirium are intended to improve cognition, they all have psychoactive effects that may further cloud the sensorium and promote a longer overall duration of cognitive impairment. Therefore, until further outcome data confirm the beneficial effects of treatment, these drugs should be used judiciously in the smallest possible dose and for the shortest time necessary.

EARLY MOBILIZATION OF CRITICALLY ILL PATIENTS

Initiating physical therapy early during the patient's ICU stay has been associated with decreased length of stay both in the ICU and in the hospital [83]. Another study examined the effect of combining daily interruption of sedation with physical and occupational therapy on the development of ICU-acquired weakness and delirium in mechanically ventilated patients [84]. It demonstrated that patients who underwent early mobilization had an almost 50% decrease in the duration of delirium in the ICU and hospital and had significant improvement in functional status at hospital discharge.

CONCLUSION

Pain, anxiety, and delirium are common events in critically ill obese patients, and their occurrence is associated with adverse outcomes. Using a systematic management approach that follows the general principles outlined in this chapter can maximize patient comfort while reducing the likelihood of overmedication and its attendant complications.

ACKNOWLEDGEMENT

Dr Hughes is supported by a Foundation for Anesthesia Education and Research Mentored Research Training Grant. Dr Pandharipande is supported by the VA Clinical Science Research and Development Service (VA Career Development Award).

BEST PRACTICE TIPS

1 Identify the cause of pain and anxiety to develop the most appropriate treatment strategy.
2 Establish regular sedation and delirium assessments utilizing validated instruments.
3 Develop protocol-based and goal-directed sedation regimens and delirium-management algorithms.
4 Treat pain first with regional therapies or systemic analgesics and utilize propofol or dexmedetomidine for sedation only if necessary.
5 Perform daily linked spontaneous awakening and breathing trials and incorporate early physical therapy.

REFERENCES

1 Jacobi J, Fraser GL, Coursin DB, Riker RR, Fontaine D, Wittbrodt ET, et al. Clinical practice guidelines for the sustained use of sedatives and analgesics in the critically ill adult. Crit Care Med. 2002 Jan;30(1):119–41.

2 Gehlbach BK, Kress JP. Sedation in the intensive care unit. Curr Opin Crit Care. 2002 Aug;8(4):290–8.

3 Kapfhammer HP, Rothenhausler HB, Krauseneck T, Stoll C, Schelling G. Posttraumatic stress disorder and health-related quality of life in long-term survivors of acute respiratory distress syndrome. Am J Psychiatry. 2004 Jan;161(1):45–52.

4 Melissas J, Volakakis E, Hadjipavlou A. Low-back pain in morbidly obese patients and the effect of weight loss following surgery. Obes Surg. 2003 Jun;13(3):389–93.

5 Acevedo A, Leon J. Ambulatory hernia surgery under local anesthesia is feasible and safe in obese patients. Hernia. 2010 Feb;14(1):57–62.

6 Mularski RA. Pain management in the intensive care unit. Crit Care Clin. 2004 Jul;20(3):381–401, viii.

7 Hicks CL, von Baeyer CL, Spafford PA, van KI, Goodenough B. The Faces Pain Scale-Revised: toward a common metric in pediatric pain measurement. Pain. 2001 Aug;93(2):173–83.

8 Payen JF, Bru O, Bosson JL, Lagrasta A, Novel E, Deschaux I, et al. Assessing pain in critically ill sedated patients by using a behavioral pain scale. Crit Care Med. 2001 Dec;29(12):2258–63.

9 Payen JF, Bosson JL, Chanques G, Mantz J, Labarere J. Pain assessment is associated with decreased duration of mechanical ventilation in the intensive care unit: a post hoc analysis of the DOLOREA study. Anesthesiology. 2009 Dec;111(6):1308–16.

10 Pieracci FM, Barie PS, Pomp A. Critical care of the bariatric patient. Crit Care Med. 2006 Jun;34(6):1796–804.

11 Richman JM, Liu SS, Courpas G, Wong R, Rowlingson AJ, McGready J, et al. Does continuous peripheral nerve block provide superior pain control to opioids? A meta-analysis. Anesth Analg. 2006 Jan;102(1):248–57.

12 Karmakar MK, Ho AM. Acute pain management of patients with multiple fractured ribs. J Trauma. 2003 Mar;54(3):615–25.

13 Richardson J, Sabanathan S, Jones J, Shah RD, Cheema S, Mearns AJ. A prospective, randomized comparison of preoperative and continuous balanced epidural or paravertebral bupivacaine on post-thoracotomy pain, pulmonary function and stress responses. Br J Anaesth. 1999 Sep;83(3):387–92.

14 Mohta M, Verma P, Saxena AK, Sethi AK, Tyagi A, Girotra G. Prospective, randomized comparison of continuous thoracic epidural and thoracic paravertebral infusion in patients with unilateral multiple fractured ribs--a pilot study. J Trauma. 2009 Apr;66(4):1096–101.

15 Block BM, Liu SS, Rowlingson AJ, Cowan AR, Cowan JA, Jr., Wu CL. Efficacy of postoperative epidural analgesia: a meta-analysis. JAMA. 2003 Nov 12;290(18):2455–63.

16 den HC, Schmeck J, Appelboom DJ, de VN. Risks of general anaesthesia in people with obstructive sleep apnoea. BMJ. 2004 Oct 23;329(7472):955–9.

17 King DR, Velmahos GC. Difficulties in managing the surgical patient who is morbidly obese. Crit Care Med. 2010 Sep;38(9 Suppl):S478–82.

18 Lloret LC, Decleves X, Oppert JM, Basdevant A, Clement K, Bardin C, et al. Pharmacology of morphine in obese patients: clinical implications. Clin Pharmacokinet. 2009;48(10):635–51.

19 Horn E, Nesbit SA. Pharmacology and pharmacokinetics of sedatives and analgesics. Gastrointest Endosc Clin N Am. 2004 Apr;14(2):247–68.

20 Shibutani K, Inchiosa MA, Jr., Sawada K, Bairamian M. Pharmacokinetic mass of fentanyl for postoperative analgesia in lean and obese patients. Br J Anaesth. 2005 Sep;95(3):377–83.

21 Battershill AJ, Keating GM. Remifentanil: a review of its analgesic and sedative use in the intensive care unit. Drugs. 2006;66(3):365–85.

22 Egan TD, Huizinga B, Gupta SK, Jaarsma RL, Sperry RJ, Yee JB, et al. Remifentanil pharmacokinetics in obese versus lean patients. Anesthesiology. 1998 Sep;89(3):562–73.

23 Albertin A, La CG, La CL, Bergonzi PC, Deni F, Moizo E. Effect site concentrations of remifentanil maintaining cardiovascular homeostasis in response to surgical stimuli during bispectral index guided propofol anestesia in seriously obese patients. Minerva Anestesiol. 2006 Nov;72(11):915–24.

24 Dahaba AA, Grabner T, Rehak PH, List WF, Metzler H. Remifentanil versus morphine analgesia and sedation for

mechanically ventilated critically ill patients: a randomized double blind study. Anesthesiology. 2004 Sep;101(3):640–6.

25 Muellejans B, Lopez A, Cross MH, Bonome C, Morrison L, Kirkham AJ. Remifentanil versus fentanyl for analgesia based sedation to provide patient comfort in the intensive care unit: a randomized, double-blind controlled trial (ISRCTN43755713). Crit Care. 2004 Feb;8(1):R1–11.

26 Angst MS, Koppert W, Pahl I, Clark DJ, Schmelz M. Short-term infusion of the mu-opioid agonist remifentanil in humans causes hyperalgesia during withdrawal. Pain. 2003 Nov;106(1–2):49–57.

27 Nelson BJ, Weinert CR, Bury CL, Marinelli WA, Gross CR. Intensive care unit drug use and subsequent quality of life in acute lung injury patients. Crit Care Med. 2000 Nov;28(11): 3626–30.

28 Ramsay MA, Savege TM, Simpson BR, Goodwin R. Controlled sedation with alphaxalone-alphadolone. Br Med J. 1974 Jun 22;2(5920):656–9.

29 Riker RR, Picard JT, Fraser GL. Prospective evaluation of the Sedation-Agitation Scale for adult critically ill patients. Crit Care Med. 1999 Jul;27(7):1325–9.

30 Devlin JW, Boleski G, Mlynarek M, Nerenz DR, Peterson E, Jankowski M, et al. Motor Activity Assessment Scale: a valid and reliable sedation scale for use with mechanically ventilated patients in an adult surgical intensive care unit. Crit Care Med. 1999 Jul;27(7):1271–5.

31 Ely EW, Truman B, Shintani A, Thomason JW, Wheeler AP, Gordon S, et al. Monitoring sedation status over time in ICU patients: reliability and validity of the Richmond Agitation-Sedation Scale (RASS). JAMA. 2003 Jun 11;289(22):2983–91.

32 Brattebo G, Hofoss D, Flaatten H, Muri AK, Gjerde S, Plsek PE. Effect of a scoring system and protocol for sedation on duration of patients' need for ventilator support in a surgical intensive care unit. Qual Saf Health Care. 2004 Jun;13(3): 203–5.

33 Brook AD, Ahrens TS, Schaiff R, Prentice D, Sherman G, Shannon W, et al. Effect of a nursing-implemented sedation protocol on the duration of mechanical ventilation. Crit Care Med. 1999 Dec;27(12):2609–15.

34 Kress JP, Pohlman AS, O'Connor MF, Hall JB. Daily interruption of sedative infusions in critically ill patients undergoing mechanical ventilation. N Engl J Med. 2000 May 18;342(20): 1471–7.

35 Girard TD, Kress JP, Fuchs BD, Thomason JW, Schweickert WD, Pun BT, et al. Efficacy and safety of a paired sedation and ventilator weaning protocol for mechanically ventilated patients in intensive care (Awakening and Breathing Controlled trial): a randomised controlled trial. Lancet. 2008 Jan 12;371(9607):126–34.

36 Jackson JC, Girard TD, Gordon SM, Thompson JL, Shintani AK, Thomason JW, et al. Long-Term Cognitive and Psychological Outcomes in the Awakening and Breathing Controlled Trial. Am J Respir Crit Care Med. 2010 Mar; doi:10.1164/rccm.200903-0442OC.

37 Jacobi J, Fraser GL, Coursin DB, Riker RR, Fontaine D, Wittbrodt ET, et al. Clinical practice guidelines for the sustained use of sedatives and analgesics in the critically ill adult. Crit Care Med. 2002 Jan;30(1):119–41.

38 Gehlbach BK, Kress JP. Sedation in the intensive care unit. Curr Opin Crit Care. 2002;8:290–8.

39 Nelson BJ, Weinert CR, Bury CL, Marinelli WA, Gross CR. Intensive care unit drug use and subsequent quality of life in acute lung injury patients. Crit Care Med. 2000 Nov;28(11): 3626–30.

40 Larson MJ, Weaver LK, Hopkins RO. Cognitive sequelae in acute respiratory distress syndrome patients with and without recall of the intensive care unit. J Int Neuropsychol Soc. 2007 Jul;13(4):595–605.

41 Karabinis A, Mandragos K, Stergiopoulos S, Komnos A, Soukup J, Speelberg B, et al. Safety and efficacy of analgesia-based sedation with remifentanil versus standard hypnotic-based regimens in intensive care unit patients with brain injuries: a randomised, controlled trial (ISRCTN50308308). Crit Care. 2004 Aug;8(4):R268–80.

42 Breen D, Karabinis A, Malbrain M, Morais R, Albrecht S, Jarnvig IL, et al. Decreased duration of mechanical ventilation when comparing analgesia-based sedation using remifentanil with standard hypnotic-based sedation for up to 10 days in intensive care unit patients: a randomised trial (ISRCTN47583497). Crit Care. 2005 Jun;9(3):R200–10.

43 Rozendaal FW, Spronk PE, Snellen FF, Schoen A, van Zanten AR, Foudraine NA, et al. Remifentanil-propofol analgo-sedation shortens duration of ventilation and length of ICU stay compared to a conventional regimen: a centre randomised, cross-over, open-label study in the Netherlands. Intensive Care Med. 2009 Feb;35(2):291–8.

44 Strom T, Martinussen T, Toft P. A protocol of no sedation for critically ill patients receiving mechanical ventilation: a randomised trial. Lancet. 2010 Feb 6;375(9713):475–80.

45 Young C, Knudsen N, Hilton A, Reves JG. Sedation in the intensive care unit. Crit Care Med. 2000 Mar;28(3):854–66.

46 Trapani G, Altomare C, Liso G, Sanna E, Biggio G. Propofol in anesthesia. Mechanism of action, structure-activity relationships, and drug delivery. Curr Med Chem. 2000 Feb;7(2):249–71.

47 Barr J, Egan TD, Sandoval NF, Zomorodi K, Cohane C, Gambus PL, et al. Propofol dosing regimens for ICU sedation based upon an integrated pharmacokinetic-pharmacodynamic model. Anesthesiology. 2001 Aug;95(2):324–33.

48 Lemmens HJ. Perioperative pharmacology in morbid obesity. Curr Opin Anaesthesiol. 2010 Aug;23(4):485–91.

49 Bentley GN, Gent JP, Goodchild CS. Vascular effects of propofol: smooth muscle relaxation in isolated veins and arteries. J Pharm Pharmacol. 1989 Nov;41(11):797–8.

50 Vasile B, Rasulo F, Candiani A, Latronico N. The pathophysiology of propofol infusion syndrome: a simple name for a complex syndrome. Intensive Care Med. 2003 Sep;29(9): 1417–25.

51 Mognol P, Vignes S, Chosidow D, Marmuse JP. Rhabdomyolysis after laparoscopic bariatric surgery. Obes Surg. 2004 Jan;14(1):91–4.

52 Maze M, Scarfini C, Cavaliere F. New agents for sedation in the intensive care unit. Crit Care Clin. 2001 Oct;17(4): 881–97.

53 Tan JA, Ho KM. Use of dexmedetomidine as a sedative and analgesic agent in critically ill adult patients: a meta-analysis. Intensive Care Med. 2010 Apr; doi:10.1016/j.jcrc.2009.05.015.

54 Dyck JB, Maze M, Haack C, Vuorilehto L, Shafer SL. The pharmacokinetics and hemodynamic effects of intravenous and intramuscular dexmedetomidine hydrochloride in adult human volunteers. Anesthesiology. 1993 May;78(5):813–20.

55 Dyck JB, Maze M, Haack C, Azarnoff DL, Vuorilehto L, Shafer SL. Computer-controlled infusion of intravenous dexmedetomidine hydrochloride in adult human volunteers. Anesthesiology. 1993 May;78(5):821–8.

56 Dutta S, Lal R, Karol MD, Cohen T, Ebert T. Influence of cardiac output on dexmedetomidine pharmacokinetics. J Pharm Sci. 2000 Apr;89(4):519–27.

57 Iirola T, Laitio R, Kentala E, Aantaa R, Kurvinen JP, Scheinin M, et al. Highly variable pharmacokinetics of dexmedetomidine during intensive care: a case report. J Med Case Reports. 2010;4:73.

58 Bakhamees HS, El-Halafawy YM, El-Kerdawy HM, Gouda NM, Altemyatt S. Effects of dexmedetomidine in morbidly obese patients undergoing laparoscopic gastric bypass. Middle East J Anesthesiol. 2007 Oct;19(3):537–51.

59 Tufanogullari B, White PF, Peixoto MP, Kianpour D, Lacour T, Griffin J, et al. Dexmedetomidine infusion during laparoscopic bariatric surgery: the effect on recovery outcome variables. Anesth Analg. 2008 Jun;106(6):1741–8.

60 Carson SS, Kress JP, Rodgers JE, Vinayak A, Campbell-Bright S, Levitt J, et al. A randomized trial of intermittent lorazepam versus propofol with daily interruption in mechanically ventilated patients. Crit Care Med. 2006 May;34(5):1326–32.

61 Walder B, Elia N, Henzi I, Romand JR, Tramer MR. A lack of evidence of superiority of propofol versus midazolam for sedation in mechanically ventilated critically ill patients: a qualitative and quantitative systematic review. Anesth Analg. 2001 Apr;92(4):975–83.

62 Barrientos-Vega R, Mar Sanchez-Soria M, Morales-Garcia C, Robas-Gomez A, Cuena-Boy R, yensa-Rincon A. Prolonged sedation of critically ill patients with midazolam or propofol: impact on weaning and costs. Crit Care Med 1997 Jan;25(1):33–40.

63 Venn RM, Grounds RM. Comparison between dexmedetomidine and propofol for sedation in the intensive care unit: patient and clinician perceptions. Br J Anaesth. 2001 Nov;87(5):684–90.

64 Herr DL, Sum-Ping ST, England M. ICU sedation after coronary artery bypass graft surgery: dexmedetomidine-based versus propofol-based sedation regimens. J Cardiothorac Vasc Anesth. 2003 Oct;17(5):576–84.

65 Pandharipande PP, Pun BT, Herr DL, Maze M, Girard TD, Miller RR, et al. Effect of sedation with dexmedetomidine vs lorazepam on acute brain dysfunction in mechanically ventilated patients: the MENDS randomized controlled trial. JAMA. 2007 Dec 12;298(22):2644–53.

66 Riker RR, Shehabi Y, Bokesch PM, Ceraso D, Wisemandle W, Koura F, et al. Dexmedetomidine vs midazolam for sedation of critically ill patients: a randomized trial. JAMA. 2009 Feb 4;301(5):489–99.

67 Pandharipande PP, Sanders RD, Girard TD, McGrane S, Thompson JL, Shintani AK, et al. Effect of dexmedetomidine versus lorazepam on outcome in patients with sepsis: an a priori-designed analysis of the MENDS randomized controlled trial. Crit Care. 2010 Mar 16;14(2):R38.

68 Leykin Y, Pellis T, Lucca M, Lomangino G, Marzano B, Gullo A. The effects of cisatracurium on morbidly obese women. Anesth Analg. 2004 Oct;99(4):1090–4, table.

69 Papazian L, Forel JM, Gacouin A, Penot-Ragon C, Perrin G, Loundou A, et al. Neuromuscular blockers in early acute respiratory distress syndrome. N Engl J Med. 2010 Sep 16;363(12):1107–16.

70 Ely EW, Shintani A, Truman B, Speroff T, Gordon SM, Harrell FE, Jr., et al. Delirium as a predictor of mortality in mechanically ventilated patients in the intensive care unit. JAMA. 2004 Apr 14;291(14):1753–62.

71 Shehabi Y, Riker RR, Bokesch PM, Wisemandle W, Shintani A, Ely EW. Delirium duration and mortality in lightly sedated, mechanically ventilated intensive care patients. Crit Care Med. 2010 Dec;38(12):2311–18.

72 Lin SM, Liu CY, Wang CH, Lin HC, Huang CD, Huang PY, et al. The impact of delirium on the survival of mechanically ventilated patients. Crit Care Med. 2004 Nov;32(11):2254–9.

73 Milbrandt EB, Deppen S, Harrison PL, Shintani AK, Speroff T, Stiles RA, et al. Costs associated with delirium in mechanically ventilated patients. Crit Care Med. 2004 Apr;32(4):955–62.

74 Pisani MA, Kong SY, Kasl SV, Murphy TE, Araujo KL, Van Ness PH. Days of delirium are associated with 1-year mortality in an older intensive care unit population. Am J Respir Crit Care Med. 2009 Dec 1;180(11):1092–7.

75 Pun BT, Ely EW. The importance of diagnosing and managing ICU delirium. Chest. 2007 Aug;132(2):624–36.

76 Munoz X, Marti S, Sumalla J, Bosch J, Sampol G. Acute delirium as a manifestation of obstructive sleep apnea syndrome. Am J Respir Crit Care Med. 1998 Oct;158(4):1306–7.

77 Bergeron N, Dubois MJ, Dumont M, Dial S, Skrobik Y. Intensive Care Delirium Screening Checklist: evaluation of a new screening tool. Intensive Care Med. 2001 May;27(5):859–64.

78 Ely EW, Inouye SK, Bernard GR, Gordon S, Francis J, May L, et al. Delirium in mechanically ventilated patients: validity and reliability of the confusion assessment method for the intensive care unit (CAM-ICU). JAMA. 2001 Dec 5;286(21):2703–10.

79 King MS, Render ML, Ely EW, Watson PL. Liberation and animation: strategies to minimize brain dysfunction in

critically ill patients. Semin Respir Crit Care Med. 2010 Feb;31(1):87–96.

80 Milbrandt EB, Kersten A, Kong L, Weissfeld LA, Clermont G, Fink MP, et al. Haloperidol use is associated with lower hospital mortality in mechanically ventilated patients. Crit Care Med. 2005 Jan;33(1):226–9.

81 Skrobik YK, Bergeron N, Dumont M, Gottfried SB. Olanzapine vs haloperidol: treating delirium in a critical care setting. Intensive Care Med. 2004 Mar;30(3): 444–9.

82 Devlin JW, Roberts RJ, Fong JJ, Skrobik Y, Riker RR, Hill NS, et al. Efficacy and safety of quetiapine in critically ill patients with delirium: a prospective, multicenter, randomized, double-blind, placebo-controlled pilot study. Crit Care Med. 2010 Feb;38(2):419–27.

83 Morris PE, Goad A, Thompson C, Taylor K, Harry B, Passmore L, et al. Early intensive care unit mobility therapy in the treatment of acute respiratory failure. Crit Care Med. 2008 Aug;36(8):2238–43.

84 Schweickert WD, Pohlman MC, Pohlman AS, Nigos C, Pawlik AJ, Esbrook CL, et al. Early physical and occupational therapy in mechanically ventilated, critically ill patients: a randomised controlled trial. Lancet. 2009 May 30;373 (9678):1874–82.

85 Wong DL, Hockenberry-Eaton M, Wilson D, et al. Wong's Essentials of Pediatric Nursing, 6 edn. St Louis, Mosby. 2001. P. 1301.

86 Sessler CN, et al. The Richmond Agitation-Sedation Scale: validity and reliability in adult intensive care unit patients. Am J Respir Crit Care Med. 2002;166:1338–44.

7 Upper Airway Management in the Morbidly Obese Patient

Michael Tielborg and Anthony Passannante

University of North Carolina, Chapel Hill, NC, USA

KEY POINTS

- Difficult laryngoscopy and difficult mask ventilation are not as cleanly correlated with elevated BMI as once generally believed. Other patient factors play a significant role in determining how challenging these essential tasks might be.
- Proper preinduction positioning improves preoxygenation and ease of mask ventilation and laryngoscopy in morbidly obese patients.
- Effective coupling of a well-planned assortment of modern airway equipment with a comprehensive set of difficult airway management skills can result in very low morbidity and mortality secondary to airway management in morbidly obese patients.

INTRODUCTION

Caring for a morbidly obese patient presents physicians with a host of challenges, and one of the most daunting is safe and efficient airway management. The physiological changes associated with excess body weight are responsible for both derangements in pulmonary mechanics and increased oxygen consumption. Obesity increases the volume of soft tissue surrounding the pharyngeal airway, while at the same time decreasing lung volumes [1]. These mechanical and anatomical changes in the upper airway can easily lead to airway obstruction when the patient's respiratory drive, airway reflexes, and resting pharyngeal muscle tone are abolished on the induction of anesthesia. Morbidly obese patients will have a reduced time until the onset of hypoxia if ventilation by facemask is difficult or impossible, due to reduced functional residual capacity and increased oxygen consumption. This

justifies a conservative approach to airway management in the morbidly obese, but we must acknowledge that endotracheal intubation, failure of which may lead to death and hypoxic brain damage if ventilation is not ensured, is no longer as difficult as it used to be. This is thanks to technological advances, widespread application of indirect visualization devices, improved airway management algorithms, and skilled practitioners [2]. In addition, the widespread availability and implementation of supraglottic ventilation devices such as the laryngeal mask airway (LMA) have made it easier to ventilate many patients when facemask ventilation is difficult or impossible, and to establish a reliable means of ventilation when the attempt at endotracheal intubation fails.

While technological improvements in airway management have provided anesthesiology clinicians with a wider variety of options, and likely increased perioperative safety, recent investigations have called into question the longstanding assumption that obesity and sleep apnea are de facto indicators of difficult airway management. In addition to providing a review of this literature, the following chapter provides a strategy for anticipating, preparing, and executing an effective upper airway management plan for the morbidly obese, a plan that utilizes basic clinical strategies, pharmacological adjuncts, and the latest in technological advances.

PREPROCEDURE EVALUATION

It is ideal for patients with morbid obesity to have an anesthesiology consultation well in advance of their scheduled procedure. This allows for a full physical examination, assessment of comorbid conditions, and review

---

Critical Care Management of the Obese Patient, First Edition. Edited by Ali A. El Solh.
© 2012 John Wiley & Sons, Ltd. Published 2012 by John Wiley & Sons, Ltd.

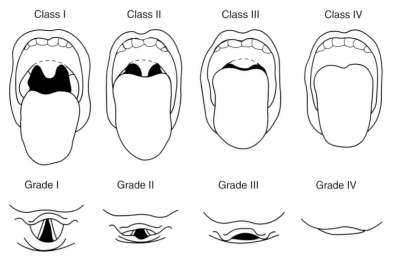

Figure 7.1 Top: Pictorial classification of the pharyngeal structures as seen when conducting the tests (note: class III, soft palate visible; class IV, soft palate not visible). Bottom: Laryngoscopic views obtained by modifying the drawings used by Cormack and Lehane in their original classification. Adapted from [5–7].

of old medical records. A history of prior difficult intubation, difficult mask ventilation, or difficult extubation may thus be identified. A complete anesthetic record will also document the Cormack–Lehane view obtained on direct laryngoscopy (Cormack–Lehane and Mallampati class) (see Figure 7.1). The preanesthetic visit also affords an opportunity to refer the patient for evaluation of presumptive obstructive sleep apnea (OSA). A recent practice advisory published by the American Society of Anesthesiologists (ASA) provides an assessment tool for gauging the likelihood that a given individual has OSA based on a constellation of physical and historical characteristics [3]. Alternatively, a simple questionnaire (Snoring, Tiredness, Observed apnea, and high blood Pressure) combined with Body mass index (BMI), Age, Neck circumference, and Gender – called the STOP-BANG assessment – is very sensitive in identifying patients with moderate to severe OSA [4]. Finally, the preoperative evaluation is an opportunity to educate the patient about their trip to the surgical suite. Some individuals will benefit from counseling about the procedures involved with airway management, particularly if awake fiberoptic intubation (AFOI) is anticipated.

AIRWAY EXAMINATION

While the preprocedure evaluation has numerous objectives, the overarching principle is to identify factors that work independently or synergistically with other patient characteristics to increase anesthetic risk. One obvious focus has been on airway assessment, with conventional wisdom generally dictating that morbid obesity and OSA were more likely to be associated with a "difficult airway." Recent investigations, however, reveal a more nuanced and not entirely consistent picture. Siyam and Benhamou reported an association with sleep apnea syndrome and difficult intubation [8], while in the same year Brodsky et al. reported no specific association with obesity alone and difficult laryngoscopy [9]. Neligan et al. reported findings consistent with the Brodsky study in 2009, failing to identify a correlation between OSA and difficult intubation while at the same time identifying high Mallampati class and male gender as difficult laryngoscopy predictors [10]. Ezri et al. also found no association with difficult laryngoscopy and obesity, but did identify an association with high Mallampati class, OSA, and abnormal front dentition [11]. A large retrospective study published by Lundstrom et al. also failed to show a strong correlation between elevated BMI and failed laryngoscopy [12]. See Table 7.1 for a list of factors associated with difficult laryngoscopy.

The relationship between obesity and difficult mask ventilation (as opposed to difficult laryngoscopy) is also not completely straightforward. The presence of a beard, BMI > 26, lack of teeth, age > 55, and a history of snoring were identified as risk factors for difficult mask ventilation [13]. A large, retrospective study endorsed several of the above predictors, with limited jaw protrusion and

Table 7.1 Factors associated with difficult laryngoscopy.

Retrognathia
Macroglossia
Prominent incisors
Inability to protrude the mandible
Cervical hump (fat pad) limiting neck extension
Prior facial or airway surgery
Head and neck radiation
Head, neck, and mediastinal masses
Thermal and chemical burns
Head, neck, or facial trauma
Cervical collar or other cervical spine immobilizers
Chipped front teeth (question of prior difficult intubations)
Pregnancy
Preeclampsia
Congenital diseases (Treacher Collins, Goldenhar, Trisomy 21, etc.)

Table 7.2 Factors associated with difficult mask ventilation.

Presence of a beard
BMI > 26 kg/m^2
Edentulous
Age > 55
History of snoring
Mallampati class III or IV
Male gender
Airway masses
Changes associated with neck radiation

thick neck anatomy as additional risk factors for grade 3 or 4 mask ventilation. In short, certain characteristics associated with elevated BMI such as OSA, high Mallampati class, and thick neck circumference may be associated with both difficult mask ventilation and laryngoscopy. See Table 7.2 for a list of factors associated with difficult mask ventilation.

While no one would suggest that an elevated BMI makes mask ventilation or endotracheal intubation easier, there is a wide spectrum of likely level of difficulty and risk. At one end lies a female patient with a Mallampati I airway exam and a BMI of 40 without evidence of OSA, at the other end would lie a 55-year-old male with a BMI of 65, a Mallampati IV airway exam, obvious OSA, and a 24 inch neck circumference. Standard direct laryngoscopy is a reasonable approach for the first patient, while extreme care is indicated for the second patient. If there is significant concern regarding the ability to mask ventilate

the patient (multiple risk factors associated with difficult mask ventilation, documented history of very difficult or impossible mask ventilation), the patient should have their airway secured awake, in most cases with an oral or nasal fiberoptic intubation.

PREPARING THE OPERATING ROOM

An essential component of operating room (OR) preparation is having drugs in the proper dosages close at hand. Many agents have altered volumes of distribution in morbidly obese patients and require dosage adjustments based on presumed lean body mass versus total body weight (TBW) [14], [15]. The pharmacokinetics of opioids is more complex. Fentanyl, the most commonly used lipophilic opioid in current clinical practice, requires an adjustment in dosing from TBW. Shibutani et al. introduced the concept of "pharmacokinetic mass," which more accurately guides the dosing of fentanyl downward from what might be administered by TBW [16]. An important factor to keep in mind as one considers the entire anesthetic from induction to emergence is that nondepolarizing neuromuscular blockers are generally effective when dosed on ideal body weight rather than TBW. To dose these medications based on TBW may mean prolonged time to recovery and difficulty with timely emergence and safe extubation at the end of the case.

Communication with the surgical team regarding their preferences for endotracheal tube (ETT) type, placement, and position should be done in advance. Prior communication with the OR nursing staff is also an essential component of caring for the morbidly obese patient. In addition, establishing the availability of anesthesia technician support or other skilled assistance in advance will help ensure the smooth execution of the task at hand. Management of the difficult airway has advanced significantly over the past decade, and a modern operating suite must have easy access to fiberoptic bronchoscopy, some type of indirect visualization device such as a videolaryngoscope or a Glidescope (trademark), and intubating and nonintubating LMAs. It is typical to concentrate equipment for difficult airway management in easily portable carts. The exact contents of the cart should be planned by the anesthesiology clinicians who will be using it, and the carts must be well-stocked and well-maintained.

Even when direct laryngoscopy is the primary plan for securing the airway, quick access to a difficult airway

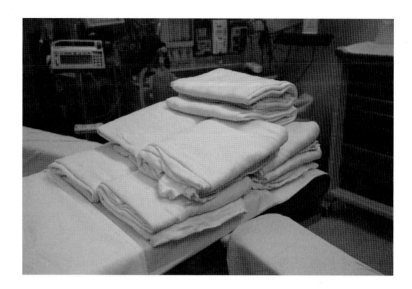

Figure 7.2 Blanket ramp. Blankets are folded with a gap in the center to facilitate removal after induction.

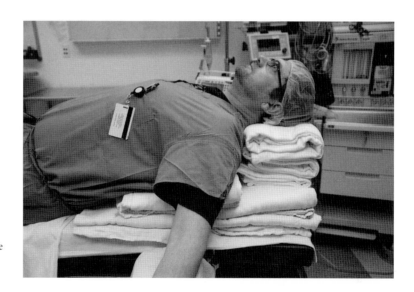

Figure 7.3 Blanket ramp. The subject is positioned so that the chin is above the chest and external auditory meatus more closely aligned in a horizontal line with the sternum.

cart in case of failure should be ensured. Airway adjuncts such as oral airways, nasal trumpets, bougies, LMAs, and surgical airway kits should be immediately available.

Preparing the OR table is the final step in readying the OR for the morbidly obese patient. A ramp created from folded blankets, a foam wedge, or by adjusting the configuration of the bed itself to create a sniffing position when the patient is supine will help optimize the view obtained when performing laryngoscopy (see Figures 7.2–7.5) [14,17]. Proper positioning will minimize the number of

difficult glottic exposures during direct laryngoscopy encountered by the anesthesiology clinican.

Many patients will benefit from a modest dose of benzodiazapine before proceeding to the OR. Whenever a patient arrives from the emergency department, has received a neuraxial or peripheral nerve block placed for postoperative pain, or has come from an inpatient bed, it is prudent to confirm that other central nervous system (CNS) depressants or opioids have not been given recently. A quick survey assessing what medications were taken prior to arrival in holding may avert an unintended overdose.

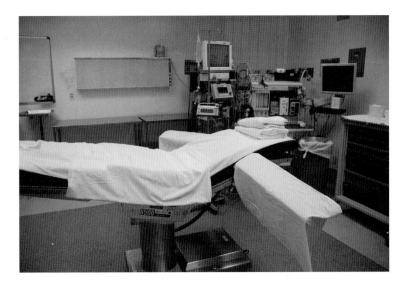

Figure 7.4 Bed ramp.

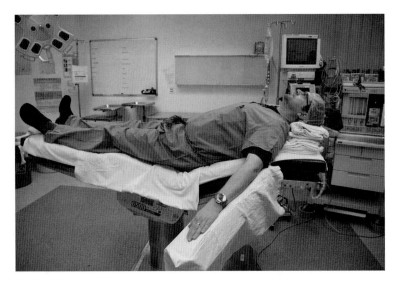

Figure 7.5 Bed ramp – an alternative to the use of blankets or a foam wedge. With the patient supine on the table, head 3–5 inches off the end of bed, the patient is first placed in Trendelenburg. The back is then raised, and the headpiece of the bed extended. The patient's head will then move to the appropriate position. The legs are flexed, creating a modified beach chair position. The position can be adjusted to optimize positioning. In addition, the arm boards will be more useful as the patient's shoulders remain level with the OR table.

Finally, before proceeding back to the operating suite, it is often helpful to arrange lifting assistance in advance and confirm that the bed being used will accommodate the anticipated weight. Many patients find the simple transfer from the gurney to the OR table challenging, and a shifting pannus can actually pull a person from a narrow table even when it appears that they are safely positioned.

IN THE OPERATING ROOM

Once the patient is safely and comfortably positioned, monitors are applied, and adequate intravenous access is assured, the patient may be preoxygenated and deni-trogenated prior to induction. Preoxygenation in a reclined, rather than supine, position has been reported to improve preinduction oxygenation [18]. This means the application of the mask with an adequate seal, demonstration of exhaled carbon dioxide, and an approach to equilibrium of inhaled and exhaled oxygen concentration. This technique will ensure the maximum amount of apneic time before desaturation begins to occur. The patient should be placed in a ramped position, with the chin above the chest, in a "sniffing" pose. Many practitioners will often employ a rapid sequence induction using a fast-acting sedative hypnotic agent in combination with succinylcholine, as these patients tend to quickly desaturate secondary to decreased functional residual capacity and increased oxygen consumption. A recent dose ranging study for succinylcholine in this population suggested that a dose of 1 mg/kg based on TBW provided satisfactory muscle relaxation [19]. When succinylcholine is contraindicated, a bolus dose of the ultra short-acting narcotic remifentanil in combination with propofol has been reported to provide satisfactory intubating conditions comparable to propofol and succinylcholine [20]. It should be noted that in the referenced trial, the subjects were lean and without substantial comorbidities, and experienced a significant degree of hypotension. Yet another alternative would be to use propofol, remifentanil, and low-dose rocuronium to achieve satisfactory intubating conditions similar to what might be obtained with propofol and succinylcholine alone [21]. The use of a video laryngoscope may improve the view beyond what might be expected with standard laryngoscopy [22].

The principles espoused in the ASA Difficult Airway management algorithm still apply. If an attempt at endotracheal intubation fails, something should be changed before another attempt (head position, operator, laryngoscope blade, direct laryngoscope for a videolaryngoscope). Each attempt at laryngoscopy can be expected to increase airway swelling, so the total number of attempts must be limited to avoid turning a "cannot intubate" scenario into a "cannot ventilate" scenario. If mask ventilation becomes difficult, a LMA can be inserted, and it may be possible to secure the airway through the LMA. If attempts to secure the airway are unsuccessful, spontaneous ventilation should be reestablished and the patient allowed to awaken.

If there is a question regarding how successful a standard induction will be, it may be possible to perform an "awake look" using a combination of midazolam and a single bolus dose of remifentanil [23]. With this technique, the patient is positioned in the standard

fashion, preoxygenated, and a dose of 1–2 µg/kg of remifentanil is given. After approximately 90 seconds, it is possible to instruct the patient to open his or her mouth, and perform laryngoscopy in the usual fashion. If a reasonable view is obtained, the ETT may be placed, or induction may proceed while holding the view obtained. While this technique has not been validated in the morbidly obese population, it is an airway management option available in obese patients with unrestricted mouth opening.

AWAKE FIBEROPTIC INTUBATION (AFOI)

It is not uncommon for the preoperative physical examination of the morbidly obese patient to raise questions about whether or not the airway can be safely and swiftly secured using standard laryngoscopy. Under these conditions, AFOI might be the preferred option. As mentioned above, clear and concise communication with the OR nursing teams as well as anesthesia technician support will help set the stage for a smooth and safe procedure. In special circumstances, it may be reasonable to ask the operating surgeon to stand by while the airway is being secured in the event that a surgical airway is required.

In holding

After preparation of the OR, other preparatory steps may be undertaken. Many practitioners utilize glycopyrrolate as an antisialagogue. This medication should be used cautiously in patients who have known or suspected coronary artery disease, obstructive cardiac lesions, stenotic valves, or other conditions under which cardiac performance may suffer with tachycardia.

Topicalization of the airway is necessary to blunt the noxious stimulation of awake airway manipulation. The glossopharyngeal nerve provides sensory innervation of the posterior third of the tongue, the tonsillar pillars, and the oropharynx. The larynx is innervated by the superior and inferior laryngeal nerves, which are branches of the vagus. The application of local anesthetic to the mucous membranes will do much to accomplish effective anesthesia of the airway and can be achieved by several methods, including aeresolization by nebulizer, lidocaine jelly "lollipops," or directly spraying the mucous membranes with an atomizer. Benzocaine spray may also be used, but may result in methemoglobinemia [24]. While the toxic dose of local anesthetic applied to the airway will vary with the method of application, concentration of drug, total dose given, and the size of the patient, it is prudent be mindful of the quantity of local anesthetic administered by any route. A superior laryngeal nerve block may also be applied by injecting 2 cc of local anesthetic close to the cornu of the hyoid bone bilaterally. Because of accumulation of adipose tissue around the neck, identification of appropriate landmarks may be difficult or impossible in some patients. Ultrasound has been used to identify the hyoid bone and subglottic structures in lean subjects [25], and may prove useful in the management of obese patients as well.

In the OR

In anticipation of AFOI, the operating table should be configured with the back elevated in a beach chair configuration to ensure comfort while monitors are applied and supplemental oxygen is administered. Drugs for induction and muscle relaxation should be immediately available. Additional topicalization may be applied at this time, while intravenous sedation is started. While adequate topicalization of the tracheal mucosa below the vocal cords can be accomplished with nebulization, it may at times be necessary to inject local anesthetic through the cricothyroid membrane with a small-gauge needle.

The selective α-2 agonist dexmedetomidine has been used successfully as an adjunct to AFOI [26]. A loading dose of 1 μg/kg, given over 10 minutes, with an infusion of 0.7 μg/kg/hour, is generally sufficient. Smaller doses should be considered for patients over the age of 65. Side effects of dexmedetomidine include bradycardia, hypertension, hypotension, dizziness, and nausea. Rarely, sinus arrest has been reported. This medication provides excellent sedation with minimal impact on respiratory drive. The intraoperative use of this medication will also augment other anesthetics and reduce the need for both intraoperative and postoperative opioids [27].

Benzodiazepines, particularly midazolam, are also useful in this scenario. While midazolam has predictable activity at clinically effective doses and may be reversed with flumazenil in overdose, it works synergistically with other CNS depressants, increasing the potential for respiratory embarrassment.

The short-acting narcotic remifentanil has also been employed to sedate patients undergoing AFOI [28]. This medication, while having a significant impact on respiratory drive at higher doses, may be used both as a bolus [29] and as an infusion while the ETT is being secured. It is also useful when applying airway devices, such as nasal trumpets or oral airways, which are noxious when positioned. A bolus dose of 25–100 μg may be given intravenously before the infusion is started, generally at 0.05–0.1 μg/kg/minute, based on ideal body weight [30]. Smaller doses should be used in older patients, or in patients who have received other CNS or respiratory depressants. Chest-wall rigidity can occur at higher bolus doses. The advantages of remifentanil include its exceedingly short half-life and context-sensitive half-time, and its reversability with naloxone.

Ketamine has also been used in conjunction with other agents for this indication [31]. This medication has been associated with dysphoria and increased airway secretions at higher doses, two side effects that limit its usefulness as a sole agent.

Alternative methods

On occasion, AFOI of the airway is either unsuccessful, or simply not an option because of patient factors such as a bleeding or obstructed airway. Under these circumstances, alternatives must be considered.

When the airway is bloody or obscured by other material, making the use of video equipment impossible, it may be reasonable to attempt a retrograde wire technique. With this method, a needle is placed just into the trachea at the level of the cricothyroid membrane. A wire or catheter is then fed cephalad through the needle until it emerges from the mouth or nose. The ETT or ETT exchanger can then be guided into the trachea in a Seldinger-type fashion. When the tip of the tube reaches the level of the wire's insertion site, the wire may be removed and the ETT advanced. A recent case report documents a retrograde technique utilizing a gum elastic bougie in a morbidly obese trauma patient with head and facial injuries [32].

Occasionally, awake tracheostomy is the only feasible option for successfully managing what would otherwise be an impossible airway. Under these conditions, careful coordination between the surgical and anesthetic teams is essential. Transportation of these patients even from the intensive care unit (ICU) or the emergency department can be perilous. Preoperative sedating medications should be used with caution. Once the patient is positioned on the bed in the OR, judicious use of sedatives and opioids may be employed as the skin superficial to the tracheostomy site is anesthetized. Once the tracheostomy is secured and end-title carbon dioxide is observed, induction agents and muscle relaxants can be given safely.

EXTUBATION

When the plan is to extubate the patient in the OR at the end of the procedure, it is wise to have available the same equipment for airway management that was present at the beginning of the case. Some practitioners will place nasal and oral airways prior to emergence. Full reversal of neuromuscular blockade is essential to ensure adequate airway protection and adequate ventilation once the ETT is removed. The patient should be awake and following commands prior to extubation, with unambiguous demonstration of purposeful movement. Once the ETT has been removed, a few minutes of observation in the OR prior to transfer to the recovery room is prudent. In some circumstances, particularly when airway swelling or difficult ETT replacement is anticipated, extubation over a tube exchanger may be advantageous. In the event the patient fails the extubation attempt, an ETT can be reinserted over the in situ tube exchanger.

In the postanesthesia care unit, careful communication with the recovery room nurses will minimize complications. While adequate control of postoperative pain is essential, significant respiratory depression must be avoided. When patients receive neuraxial analgesic techniques, peripheral nerve blocks, or infiltration of the surgical site with local anesthetic, opioid requirements will be altered, and may be dynamic as those measures dissipate. The use of other analgesics, including NSAIDS, acetaminophen, pregabalin, and dexmedetomidine, may reduce the need for postoperative opioids.

CONCLUSION

While caring for individuals with morbid obesity presents a constellation of medical challenges, the safe and smooth management of the airway can reliably be achieved with careful preprocedure evaluation, meticulous attention to detail in positioning the patient, a cautious and stepwise approach to airway management, and the intelligent application of now widely available airway management techniques and tools. Indirect visualization devices such as video laryngoscopes provide an additional degree of flexibility and safety by allowing much easier access to anterior glottic openings than is possible with standard direct laryngoscopy. For patients who require it (limited mouth opening, very difficult or impossible mask ventilation, need for maintenance of spontaneous ventilation), fiberoptic intubation via either a nasal or an oral route is a safe and widely practiced option. Given the epidemic of obesity worldwide, a consistent and reliable process for taking care of these individuals should be part of every medical center's armamentarium.

BEST PRACTICE TIPS

1 Preanesthetic evaluation may help risk-stratify patients with elevated BMI before they present to the operating suite. This evaluation provides an important opportunity to educate patients about special airway maneuvers that may be needed to optimize their safe care.

2 Proper OR preparation is essential. Clear communication with OR staff, anesthesia technician support, and the surgical team is critical. Assurance that the OR table will accommodate the patient's weight prior to transfer is mandatory.

3 Proper positioning of the patient in a "ramped" configuration prior to induction improves oxygenation, conditions for mask ventilation, and intubating conditions.

4 Ideal pharmacological adjuncts to AFOI include those medications that have minimal adverse effects on respiratory drive, such as dexmedetomidine, or have pharmacological antagonists, such as short-acting opioids and benzodiazepines.

5 Prior to extubation of the morbidly obese patient, return of muscle strength, adequate airway reflexes, and purposeful movement must be confirmed.

REFERENCES

1 Isono S. Obstructive sleep apnea of obese adults: pathophysiology and perioperative airway management. Anesthesiology. 2009 Apr;110(4):908–21.

2 Amathieu R, Combes X, Abdi W, Housseini LE, Rezzoug A, Dinca A, et al. An algorithm for difficult airway management, modified for modern optical devices (Airtraq laryngoscope; LMA CTrach): a 2-year prospective validation in patients for elective abdominal, gynecologic, and thyroid surgery. Anesthesiology. 2011 Jan;114(1):25–33.

3 Gross JB, Bachenberg KL, Benumof JL, Caplan RA, Connis RT, Cote CJ, et al. Practice guidelines for the perioperative management of patients with obstructive sleep apnea: a report by the American Society of Anesthesiologists Task Force on Perioperative Management of patients with obstructive sleep apnea. Anesthesiology. 2006 May;104(5):1081–93; quiz 117–18.

4 Chung F, Yegneswaran B, Liao P, Chung SA, Vairavanathan S, Islam S, et al. STOP questionnaire: a tool to screen patients for obstructive sleep apnea. Anesthesiology. 2008 May;108(5): 812–21.

5 Mallampati SR. Clinical signs to predict difficult tracheal intubation (hypothesis). Can Anaesth Soc J. 1983;30:316–17.

6 Mallampati SR, Gatt SP, Gugino LD, et al. A clinical sign to predict difficult tracheal intubation: a prospective study. Can Anaesth Soc J. 1985;32:429–34.

7 Cormack RS, Lehane J. Difficlut tracheal intubation in obstetrics. Anaesthesia. 1984;39:1105–11.

8 Siyam MA, Benhamou D. Difficult endotracheal intubation in patients with sleep apnea syndrome. Anesth Analg. 2002 Oct;95(4):1098–102, table of contents.

9 Brodsky JB, Lemmens HJ, Brock-Utne JG, Vierra M, Saidman LJ. Morbid obesity and tracheal intubation. Anesth Analg. 2002 Mar;94(3):732–6; table of contents.

10 Neligan PJ, Porter S, Max B, Malhotra G, Greenblatt EP, Ochroch EA. Obstructive sleep apnea is not a risk factor for difficult intubation in morbidly obese patients. Anesth Analg. 2009 Oct;109(4):1182–6.

11 Ezri T, Medalion B, Weisenberg M, Szmuk P, Warters RD, Charuzi I. Increased body mass index per se is not a predictor of difficult laryngoscopy. Can J Anaesth. 2003 Feb;50(2):179–83.

12 Lundstrom LH, Moller AM, Rosenstock C, Astrup G, Wetterslev J. High body mass index is a weak predictor for difficult and failed tracheal intubation: a cohort study of 91,332 consecutive patients scheduled for direct laryngoscopy registered in the Danish Anesthesia Database. Anesthesiology. 2009 Feb;110(2):266–74.

13 Langeron O, Masso E, Huraux C, Guggiari M, Bianchi A, Coriat P, et al. Prediction of difficult mask ventilation. Anesthesiology. 2000 May;92(5):1229–36.

14 Ogunnaike BO, Jones SB, Jones DB, Provost D, Whitten CW. Anesthetic considerations for bariatric surgery. Anesth Analg. 2002 Dec;95(6):1793–805.

15 Servin F, Farinotti R, Haberer JP, Desmonts JM. Propofol infusion for maintenance of anesthesia in morbidly obese patients receiving nitrous oxide: a clinical and pharmacokinetic study. Anesthesiology. 1993 Apr;78(4):657–65.

16 Shibutani K, Inchiosa MA, Jr., Sawada K, Bairamian M. Pharmacokinetic mass of fentanyl for postoperative analgesia in lean and obese patients. Br J Anaesth. 2005 Sep;95(3):377–83.

17 Rao SL, Kunselman AR, Schuler HG, DesHarnais S. Laryngoscopy and tracheal intubation in the head-elevated position in obese patients: a randomized, controlled, equivalence trial. Anesth Analg. 2008 Dec;107(6):1912–18.

18 Dixon BJ, Dixon JB, Carden JR, Burn AJ, Schachter LM, Playfair JM, et al. Preoxygenation is more effective in the 25 degrees head-up position than in the supine position in severely obese patients: a randomized controlled study. Anesthesiology. 2005 Jun;102(6):1110–5; disc. 5A.

19 Lemmens HJ, Brodsky JB. The dose of succinylcholine in morbid obesity. Anesth Analg. 2006 Feb;102(2):438–42.

20 McNeil IA, Culbert B, Russell I. Comparison of intubating conditions following propofol and succinylcholine with propofol and remifentanil 2 micrograms kg-1 or 4 micrograms kg-1. Br J Anaesth. 2000 Oct;85(4):623–5.

21 Siddik-Sayyid SM, Taha SK, Kanazi GE, Chehade JM, Zbeidy RA, Al Alami AA, et al. Excellent intubating conditions with remifentanil-propofol and either low-dose rocuronium or succinylcholine. Can J Anaesth. 2009 Jul;56(7):483–8.

22 Maassen R, Lee R, van Zundert A, Cooper R. The videolaryngoscope is less traumatic than the classic laryngoscope for a difficult airway in an obese patient. J Anesth. 2009;23(3):445–8.

23 Johnson KB, Swenson JD, Egan TD, Jarrett R, Johnson M. Midazolam and remifentanil by bolus injection for intensely stimulating procedures of brief duration: experience with awake laryngoscopy. Anesth Analg. 2002 May;94(5):1241–3, table of contents.

24 Sachdeva R, Pugeda JG, Casale LR, Meizlish JL, Zarich SW. Benzocaine-induced methemoglobinemia: a potentially fatal complication of transesophageal echocardiography. Tex Heart Inst J. 2003;30(4):308–10.

25 Singh M, Chin KJ, Chan VW, Wong DT, Prasad GA, Yu E. Use of sonography for airway assessment: an observational study. J Ultrasound Med. Jan;29(1):79–85.

26 Bergese SD, Khabiri B, Roberts WD, Howie MB, McSweeney TD, Gerhardt MA. Dexmedetomidine for conscious sedation in difficult awake fiberoptic intubation cases. J Clin Anesth. 2007 Mar;19(2):141–4.

27 Hofer RE, Sprung J, Sarr MG, Wedel DJ. Anesthesia for a patient with morbid obesity using dexmedetomidine without narcotics. Can J Anaesth. 2005 Feb;52(2):176–80.

28 Machata AM, Gonano C, Holzer A, Andel D, Spiss CK, Zimpfer M, et al. Awake nasotracheal fiberoptic intubation: patient comfort, intubating conditions, and hemodynamic stability during conscious sedation with remifentanil. Anesth Analg. 2003 Sep;97(3):904–8.

29 Egan TD, Kern SE, Muir KT, White J. Remifentanil by bolus injection: a safety, pharmacokinetic, pharmacodynamic, and age effect investigation in human volunteers. Br J Anaesth. 2004 Mar;92(3):335–43.

30 Egan TD, Huizinga B, Gupta SK, Jaarsma RL, Sperry RJ, Yee JB, et al. Remifentanil pharmacokinetics in obese versus lean patients. Anesthesiology. 1998 Sep;89(3):562–73.

31 Scher CS, Gitlin MC. Dexmedetomidine and low-dose ketamine provide adequate sedation for awake fiberoptic intubation. Can J Anaesth. 2003 Jun–Jul;50(6):607–10.

32 Marciniak D, Smith CE. Emergent retrograde tracheal intubation with a gum-elastic bougie in a trauma patient. Anesth Analg. 2007 Dec;105(6):1720–1, table of contents.

8 Mechanical Ventilation of the Obese Patient

Mohammed Mogri and M. Jeffery Mador

State University of New York at Buffalo, Buffalo, NY, USA

KEY POINTS

- Noninvasive ventilation is useful in selected obese patients presenting with acute hypercapnic respiratory failure.
- Tidal volume should be calculated based on ideal body weight of the patient.
- Obese patients requiring mechanical ventilation do not have a higher mortality compared to normal-weight patients.

INTRODUCTION

As the prevalence of obesity continues to increase worldwide, intensivists are encountering more and more obese patients in their intensive care units (ICUs). The prevalence of obesity ranges from 9 to 26% in medical and surgical ICUs [1]. The care of obese patients is made more challenging by common accompanying comorbidities including hypertension, asthma, diabetes mellitus, and heart failure [2]. In addition to presenting with the usual common etiologies of respiratory failure present in the nonobese patient, like septic shock, trauma, and so on, obese patients are more prone to acute or chronic respiratory failure in the absence of any cardiopulmonary disease.

Obesity-related hypoventilation can cause acute respiratory failure in a subgroup of obese patients [3]. Most obese patients can maintain adequate ventilation and eucapnia during the awake state but a minor proportion of obese patients can develop hypercapnic respiratory failure, a condition known as the obesity hypoventilation syndrome (OHS). Ninety per cent of patients with OHS also have obstructive sleep apnea (OSA) [4].

It is important to promptly identify OSA and obesity-related hypoventilation in obese patients presenting to the ICU with respiratory failure as the management strategies for these patients are different. The failure to implement these standard practices may lead to difficulties with weaning from the ventilator, prolonged length of stay, and increased morbidity [5].

In this chapter, we present an overview of mechanical ventilation strategies in the obese patient and the pathophysiological principles that determine their use.

PATHOPHYSIOLOGY

Obesity causes a number of changes in pulmonary function. The most consistently reported effect is a decrease in functional residual capacity (FRC). There is an exponential relationship between body mass index (BMI) and FRC; FRC decreases with increasing BMI [6]. The FRC in the severely obese can be so low that the closing capacity exceeds the FRC and airway closure occurs within tidal breaths. Compliance of the total respiratory system is decreased in obese patients [7]. A significant proportion of the decrease in the total respiratory compliance is a result of decreased lung compliance from atelectasis, closure of the dependent airways, and increased blood volume [8]. Chest-wall compliance likely remains unchanged [7,8]. Obesity, when compared to normal-weight patients, produces a parallel rightward shift of the chest-wall pressure–volume curve without affecting the compliance. These changes result in an inspiratory threshold load and an increase in the work of breathing. Forced expiratory volume in 1 second (FEV1) and forced vital capacity (FVC) tend to decrease with increasing BMI but their ratio is usually well preserved or even increased [9]. Tidal volumes are often reduced in severe obesity, and breathing follows a rapid, shallow pattern [10].

Obese patients have a restrictive disease pattern on pulmonary function testing post extubation. These patients are also noted to have a decrease in peak expiratory flow rate (PEFR) and FEV1, which is likely a result of both a decreased FRC and small-airway collapse [11]. To complicate matters, the prevalence of OSA among obese patients exceeds 30%, reaching as high as 50–98% in the morbidly obese (defined as a BMI > 35) population [12]. OHS can commonly accompany OSA [13]. These comorbidities, along with the lingering effects of sedatives which accumulate in the adipose tissue in the obese patient, increase the likelihood of postextubation respiratory failure [14].

Mechanical ventilation in the obese patient leads to atelectasis, alterations in respiratory mechanics, and hypoxemia [15]. The amount of atelectasis is inversely correlated with body weight. Computerized tomography studies have shown atelectasis of 10% of the total lung volume in obese patients after induction of anesthesia and paralysis [16]. The degree of atelectasis is more prominent in the basal portions of the lungs in the pleural recess. This effect is more prominent in the supine position due to the push on the diaphragm by abdominal contents [7]. The increase in atelectasis results in increased chest-wall and lung elastance. Atelectasis also leads to reductions in arterial oxygenation, which may be marked, as has been observed by many investigators. The increases in dead-space ventilation, intrapulmonary shunt, and ventilation perfusion mismatch are the main reasons for the derangement in gas exchange.

MECHANICAL VENTILATION

Noninvasive ventilation

Continuous positive airway pressure (CPAP) increases intrathoracic pressure and in doing so minimizes airway and alveolar collapse, prevents atelectasis, and maintains FRC. In obese patients it can decrease the work of breathing by counteracting the inspiratory threshold load and by pushing the FRC upwards towards the steeper portion of the compliance curve [17–19]. CPAP, when used with pressure support ventilation, is called expiratory positive airway pressure (EPAP) during noninvasive ventilation (NIV) and positive end expiratory pressure (PEEP) during invasive ventilation. Bilevel positive airway pressure (BiPAP) provides pressure support ventilation added to EPAP. The patient's spontaneous inspiratory effort triggers the respiratory device, which provides a flow of gas until a predefined pressure level is reached. Once the pre-

set level is attained, the patient can continue to inhale based on their own effort until the flow decreases below a threshold level (usually 25% of the maximum flow). BiPAP improves patient ventilator synchrony, improves alveolar ventilation, and unloads the respiratory muscles in the morbidly obese [18,19]. Depending on the ventilatory drive, an obese patient can utilize BiPAP primarily to increase ventilation or to reduce his work of breathing, or both.

NIV is commonly instituted in patients with chronic obstructive pulmonary disease (COPD) exacerbations and acute pulmonary edema. Multiple controlled trials have demonstrated that therapy with NIV avoids intubation [20,21] and, in the case of COPD patients, reduces mortality as well [1,22,23]. The benefit of NIV is less clear in patients with hypoxic respiratory failure because of the heterogeneity amongst the patients in various trials [24]. Obese patients with OSA and OHS may first be discovered on presentation with acute combined hypoxic and hypercarbic respiratory failure. In a retrospective survey of 50 morbidly obese patients with respiratory failure requiring mechanical ventilation, almost two thirds of the patients started on NIV avoided subsequent intubation. However, patients who failed a trial of NIV and who were eventually intubated had a higher mortality when compared to patients intubated immediately on presentation or to patients with successful NIV use. Patients with NIV failure were younger with a higher BMI compared to patients with successful use of NIV or patients who were intubated directly. Failure of NIV was likely a marker of worse underlying disease and not an adverse event in itself [25]. In another prospective trial, obese patients with OSA and congestive heart failure who presented with hypercarbic respiratory failure were successfully treated with nasal CPAP. None of the patients in this trial required intubation [26].

NIV is a safe means of treating respiratory failure in the obese patient, provided there are no contraindications to its use. Of course, patients requiring emergent intubations should not have intubation delayed by a trial of NIV. Relative contraindications to NIV use include altered sensorium, inability to protect the airway or clear secretions, high risk of aspiration, and recent facial trauma or facial surgery. Patients who are tried on NIV should be monitored closely in a supervised setting. Response to NIV therapy is usually evident within the first 2 hours. Patients who fail to improve or show worsening of their respiratory status should be promptly intubated. There is no standardized method to determine initial NIV mode or settings. BiPAP has been the most commonly used mode of NIV. Conventionally, EPAP pressures are kept at 5 cm H_2O to minimize any potential CO_2 rebreathing. If the patient has a known diagnosis of sleep apnea, it is reasonable to set the EPAP at the same level as the outpatient CPAP pressure requirements. IPAP should be set to provide a pressure support of at least 6 cm of H_2O and titrated as tolerated by the patient while monitoring the response in terms of decrease in respiratory rate, increase in minute ventilation, and improvement in acidosis and $PaCO_2$.

Invasive ventilation

Mode

There are currently no available data on the optimal ventilator mode in the ICU for the obese patient. The literature on ventilator modes is derived from anesthesiology experience during laparoscopic and nonlaparoscopic surgeries in obese patients. While these provide data on improvement in physiological parameters in the short term on otherwise healthy patients, they do not compare outcomes important to ICU patients.

Conventionally, volume-controlled ventilation (VCV) has been used in the operating room. Due to the previously mentioned alterations in lung volumes and compliance, this mode may not provide the same benefits as it does in the nonobese. Obese patients have decreased respiratory system compliance. In theory, pressure-controlled ventilation (PCV) can provide protection against the high pressures needed to deliver a given tidal volume in VCV. In a patient population with BMI > 35 undergoing laparoscopic surgery, PCV with a pressure limit of 35 cm H_2O, target tidal volume of 10 ml/kg of ideal body weight (IBW), was compared with VCV with the same target tidal volume. With constant minute ventilation, it was noted that PCV had equal airway pressures and hemodynamic effects with a higher $PaCO_2$ at 15 minutes. Oxygenation was similar in both arms [27]. In another study, VCV with a tidal volume of 8 ml/kg IBW was compared with PCV with a plateau pressure limit of 40 cm H_2O. PCV ventilation resulted in higher PaO_2, oxygen saturations and $PaO_2 : FiO_2$ ratios compared to VCV with similar plateau pressures and hemodynamics. This improvement in oxygenation was felt to be due to improved ventilation perfusion matching in the PCV group [28].

In patients who can breathe spontaneously, pressure support has been shown to be superior to PCV in providing higher oxygenation index and postoperative lung function [29]. Spontaneous breathing during pressure support results in recruitment of the posteriorly located juxtadiaphramatic alveoli secondary to more pronounced excursion of the posterior body of the diaphragm. This leads to decreased atelectasis, decreased dead-space ventilation, and improved lung compliance. The drawback of pressure support is that heavily sedated patients may have a blunted respiratory drive and this can lead to a decreased minute ventilation and respiratory acidosis.

The above studies were done intraoperatively and the different modes were used for less than 1 hour. Until further studies are done with longer durations of ventilator use and variable clinical scenarios, for example septic shock with a high minute ventilation requirement, the selection of ventilator mode should depend upon institutional experience.

In a secondary analysis of the landmark ARDSnet trial, the benefit of low-tidal-volume strategy (6 ml/kg of IBW) in patients with acute lung injury (ALI) was found to be similar amongst normal, overweight, and obese patients. The primary trial did however exclude patients who were morbidly obese with a weight : height ratio (kg/cm) of ≥1 [30]. VCV with a plateau pressure threshold of 30 cm H_2O may be a reasonable initial ventilator mode strategy. If this threshold is not adequate, higher plateau pressures can be accepted in obese patients since a high plateau pressure usually does not indicate a true increase in transpulmonary pressure, which is the distending pressure across the lungs and the pressure gradient responsible for ventilator-induced lung injury. It is thought that the extraalveolar pressure imposed by the pressure of the abdominal contents on the chest cavity partially mitigates the intraalveolar distention caused by the positive pressure ventilation.

PEEP and recruitment maneuvers

In mechanically ventilated obese patients, application of PEEP increases lung volumes and opens atelectatic lung regions. In obese patients, the elastance of the total respiratory system significantly decreases with PEEP because of a similar reduction in chest-wall and lung elastance [15].

In surgical patients during general anesthesia, Pelosi showed that in the morbidly obese (mean BMI > 50) a PEEP of 10 cm H_2O recruited collapsed alveoli and this in turn translated into a significant increase in PaO_2 and a decrease in the alveolar–arterial oxygen difference [15]. Later studies done with a similar level of PEEP but on less obese patients failed to show this effect [31,32]. While the difference in BMI may have led to the conflicting results between studies, it is possible the level of PEEP used was not optimal. In a recent study on obese patients using electrical impedance tomography, investigators found that the optimal PEEP in their study population was 15 cm H_2O. A recruitment maneuver at this level of PEEP led to further improvement in the $PaO_2:FiO_2$, ratio suggesting that there was additional lung tissue that could only be recruited at such high levels of PEEP [33].

The failure of PEEP alone in improving lung recruitment and hypoxemia has led to the use of recruitment maneuvers preceding the use of PEEP by investigators. This is in keeping with the concept of "opening the lung and keeping it open" by alveolar recruitment achieved by a high-inspiratory-pressure maneuver and minimizing alveolar derecruitment by applying PEEP. Multiple studies using different inspiratory pressures and duration ranges for a recruitment maneuver that was followed by the application of 8–10 cm H_2O of PEEP have shown improvement in oxygenation in the short term [16,32,34]. Oxygenation parameters in these studies were studied for a maximum duration of 2 hours after intervention. Almarakbi and colleagues showed that lung recruitment repeated every 10 minutes along with PEEP in mechanically ventilated anesthetized patients resulted in more significant and sustained improvement in oxygenation [31]. However, this strategy, while useful during anesthesia for a surgical procedure, is not practical in the critical care setting.

Currently there are no specific published data on PEEP usage in mechanically ventilated obese ICU patients. The above data were derived from obese patients undergoing laparoscopic and nonlaparoscopic surgeries. Hence, caution needs to be used in extrapolating the data to patients who require longer durations of ventilatory support and who may have coexisting acute or chronic pulmonary diseases. It is reasonable to apply a higher than conventional level of PEEP in an obese patient or to attempt to measure optimal PEEP in patients in the ICU who are difficult to oxygenate. There are various ways of estimating the optimal PEEP. Esophageal pressure measurement to estimate the intrapleural pressure and subsequently determine the optimal level of PEEP required is cumbersome and not routinely performed. A more widely used method is based on using the pressure–volume curve and setting the at PEEP slightly greater than the lower inflection point. Alternatively, the clinical provider can increase or decrease PEEP with a fixed FiO_2 while monitoring the improvement in the oxygenation. Currently there is not enough evidence to advocate routine use of recruitment maneuvers. Further studies need to be done in obese patients to analyse the effects of these strategies on clinically relevant long-term outcomes including duration of mechanical ventilation, ICU and hospital length of stay, and mortality.

Tidal volume

Tidal volume in obese patients must be estimated using IBW. The rationale for this is that when patients gain weight the lungs do not increase in size. There is a tendency to overestimate the tidal volume requirements in obese patients [35,36]. Reports of use of high tidal volumes in obese surgical patients have shown mixed results [37]. The use of high tidal volumes in the obese was historically employed in an attempt to recruit more alveoli and hence improve oxygenation during mechanical ventilation. Recent studies have shown no improvement in oxygenation using this strategy in obese mechanically ventilated patient in the short term [37,38]. However, high tidal volumes did cause significantly higher peak and plateau pressures. Even though this cyclic overdistention of the alveoli may be of little or no consequence in the normal lung in the short term, it has been well shown to cause increased mortality in the diseased lung when applied over a longer period of time [39]. In a secondary analysis of the landmark ARDSnet study, the mortality benefit from a low-tidal-volume strategy was found to be similar in overweight and obese patients with ALI [30] compared to those with a normal body weight. This analysis supports the use of low tidal volumes of 6 cc/kg IBW in obese patients with ALI. In obese patients without ALI, conventional tidal volumes of 6–10 cc/kg IBW may be used.

Positioning

Obese patients have a cranial shift of the diaphragm which results in a significant decrease in the FRC during mechanical ventilation [40]. The reduction of FRC is closely related to BMI. However, the decrease in FRC is also related to other interacting factors like the shape of the chest-wall structures, and the volume and distribution of blood. Placing patients in the reverse Trendelenburg position (RTP, 30–45°) may reduce the effect of the increased intraabdominal pressure by pushing the abdominal contents down via gravity and allowing for increased movement of the diaphragm [7].

The safe apnea period is increased in patients placed in the RTP, due to the increase in FRC, and is considered the optimal position for placement of an airway in morbidly obese patients [41]. Marked improvement in oxygenation and respiratory system compliance was noted when obese patients were placed in RTP during general anesthesia [7,32]. These results were explained on the basis of an increase in FRC as a result of recruitment of collapsed alveoli and an increase in the size of the alveoli. Interestingly, in one study PEEP and RTP had comparable improvement in oxygenation but RTP resulted in much lower peak pressures [7] and hence may be more useful as a lung protective ventilation strategy.

In addition to the above, RTP has been shown to decrease aspiration of gastric contents in mechanically ventilated patients [42]. Obese patients have a higher volume of gastric contents at a lower pH and may be at increased risk of complications from aspiration [43]. While the efficacy of position in the prevention of ventilator-associated pneumonia has shown contradictory results, a recent metaanalysis demonstrated that mechanically ventilated patients positioned at 45° in RTP have a significantly lower incidence of clinically diagnosed ventilator-associated pneumonias compared to patients positioned supinely [44]. Hence, unless otherwise contraindicated, mechanically ventilated obese patients should be placed in RTP at 30–45°.

LIBERATION FROM MECHANICAL VENTILATION

There are no specific guidelines for liberating an obese patient off mechanical ventilation. General guidelines for liberation from mechanical ventilation apply to this patient population. Using a weaning protocol may be useful. Liberation from mechanical ventilation is a two-step process involving first testing for readiness for extubation and second doing a spontaneous breathing trial. Patients should be considered ready for extubation once they have an unaltered sensorium, improvement or resolution of the underlying disease, hemodynamic stability off vasopressors, and adequate oxygenation with low FiO_2 requirements (≤ 0.4) and PEEP (≤ 5)[45]. Weaning is most commonly performed using T-tube trials or pressure-support ventilation. It is acceptable to perform one spontaneous breathing trial per day of 30–120 minutes' duration [46]. Patients who tolerate the spontaneous breathing trial should be extubated and those who fail the spontaneous breathing trial should be returned to mechanical ventilation.

Patients who require reintubation have been noted to have a significantly higher mortality rate than those who are successfully extubated on the first attempt [47]. After adjusting for the severity of illness and coexisting conditions, extubation failure is an independent predictor of death [48]. Whether extubation failure is truly an independent predictor of adverse outcomes or merely reflects patients who are more severely ill despite similar severity-of-illness scores remains to be delineated. This observation makes any strategy which decreases reintubation rates an attractive option to pursue, provided it does not delay liberation from mechanical ventilation.

Noninvasive ventilation has been used post extubation to improve the chances of successful liberation and to decrease reintubation rates. In postoperative obese patients, use of BiPAP (with an IPAP of $8\,cm\,H_2O$ and EPAP of $4\,cm\,H_2O$) for 24 hours resulted in significant improvement in physiological parameters and oxygenation compared to patients receiving just oxygen therapy. The benefit was seen at day one and persisted after BiPAP was discontinued [11].

A multicenter randomized controlled trial showed that instituting NIV in patients with postextubation respiratory failure did not decrease reintubation rates and the delay in reintubation in the NIV group may have explained the increased mortality in these patients [48]. Similarly, use of NIV in 93 patients with both accidental and elective extubation failed to reduce the rates of reintubation [49]. It was however noted that the NIV arm had more patients with accidental extubations and this may have led to inaccurate results. Patients who were reintubated had a significantly higher mortality [49].

The above studies instituted NIV ventilation after the onset of respiratory failure. In a different multicenter randomized control trial, high-risk patients were assigned to BiPAP therapy post extubation versus standard therapy. Patients received at least 8 hours per day of BiPAP therapy for the first 48 hours. IPAP was set at $10\,cm$ of H_2O above the EPAP pressure. Results showed a reduced rate of reintubation in the high-risk group with use of NIV versus standard therapy. The need for reintubation was associated with a higher ICU mortality [50].

In the only study done in obese ICU patients, NIV immediately post extubation with BiPAP was shown to be effective in preventing respiratory failure. Using a standard protocol, patients who were successfully liberated from mechanical ventilation were started on 48 hours of BiPAP therapy immediately after extubation. The inspiratory airway pressure was started at $12\,cm\,H_2O$ and titrated to achieve a respiratory rate < 25 breaths per minute and oxygen saturations $> 90\%$. EPAP was held constant at $4\,cm\,H_2O$. NIV resulted in a 16% absolute reduction in the rate of respiratory failure post extubation in the morbidly obese compared to conventional medical therapy [51].

PROGNOSIS

Obesity in critically ill patients is not associated with increased mortality but is linked to a prolonged duration of mechanical ventilation and ICU length of stay [1]. Survival of severely obese patients with ALI does not differ from normal-weight individuals [30,35]. There is no difference in mortality between severely obese and nonobese patients who require mechanical ventilation [30,36]. However, in comparison to normal-weight patients, obese patients have increased morbidity including increased incidence of difficult intubation, postextubation stridor, increase in duration of mechanical ventilation, and increased ICU and hospital length of stay [1,35]. Severely obese patients are more likely to be discharged to a rehabilitation center or a skilled nursing facility compared to normal-weight patients.

> **BEST PRACTICE TIPS**
>
> 1 FRC is decreased significantly in obese patients and interventions should be targeted to improve FRC and hence improve recruitment of atelectatic lung units.
> 2 Noninvasive ventilation is a safe means of treating acute hypercapnic respiratory failure in the obese patient, provided there are no contraindications to its use.
> 3 Current data support the use of VCV in obese patients with hypoxic respiratory failure. Obese patients with ALI receive similar benefits from low-tidal-volume strategy (6 ml/kg of IBW) to their normal-weight counterparts.
> 4 Tidal volume should be calculated based on the IBW of the patient.
> 5 Mechanically ventilated obese patients should be placed on higher than conventional levels of PEEP and in RTP at 30–45°.
> 6 Reintubation rates may be decreased in the obese patient by using noninvasive ventilation immediately post extubation.

REFERENCES

1 Akinnusi ME, Pineda LA, El Solh AA. Effects of obesity on intensive care morbidity and mortality: a meta-analysis. Crit Care Med. 2008;36:151–8.

2 El Solh A, Sikka P, Bozkanat E, et al. Morbid obesity in the medical ICU. Chest. 2001;120:1989–97.

3 Malhotra A, Hillman D. Obesity and the lung: 3. Obesity, respiration and intensive care. Thorax. 2008;63:925–31.

4 Mokhlesi B, Tulaimat A. Recent advances in obesity hypoventilation syndrome. Chest. 2007;132(4):1322–36.

5 Perez de Llano LA, Golpe R, Ortiz Piquer M, et al. Short-term and long-term effects of nasal intermittent positive pressure ventilation in patients with obesity-hypoventilation syndrome. Chest. 2005;128:587–94.

6 Jones RL, Nzekwu MMU. The effects of body mass index on lung volumes. Chest. 2006;130:827–33.

7 Pelosi P, Croci M, Ravagnan I et al. The effects of body mass index on lung volumes, respiratory mechanics, and gas exchange during general anesthesia. Anesth Analg. 1998; 87:654–60.

8 Hedenstierna G, Santesson J. Breathing mechanics, dead space and gas exchange in the extremely obese, breathing spontaneously and during anaesthesia with intermittent positive pressure ventilation. Acta Anaesthesiol Scand. 1976(20):248–54.

9 Sin DD, Jones RL, Man SF. Obesity is a risk factor for dyspnea but not for airflow obstruction. Arch Intern Med. 2002;162:1477–81.

10 Sampson MG, Grassino AE. Load compensation in obese patients during quiet tidal breathing. J Appl Physiol. 1983 Oct;55(4):1269–76.

11 Joris JL, Sottiaux TM, Chiche JD, et al. Effects of bi-level positive airway pressure (BiPAP) nasal ventilation on the postoperative pulmonary restrictive syndrome in obese patients undergoing gastroplasty. Chest. 1997:111;665–70.

12 Pillar G, Shehadeh N. Abdominal fat and sleep apnea: the chicken or the egg? Diabetes Care. 2008 Feb;31(Suppl 2): S303–9.

13 Kaw R, Hernandez AV, Walker E, et al. Determinants of hypercapnia in obese patients with hypercapnia: a systematic review and meta-analysis of cohort studies. Chest. 2009;136(3):787–96.

14 Reves JG, Fragen RJ, Vinik HR, et al. Midazolam: pharmacology and uses. Anesthesiology. 1985;62:310–24.

15 Pelosi P, Ravagnan I, Giurati G, et al. Positive end-expiratory pressure improves respiratory function in obese but not in normal subjects during anesthesia and paralysis. Anesthesiology. 1999;91:1221–31.

16 Reinius H, Jonsson L, Gustafsson S et al. Prevention of atelectasis in morbidly obese patients during general anesthesia and paralysis. Anesthesiology. 2009;111:979–87.

17 O'Donoghue, P Catcheside, A Jordan, et al. Effects of CPAP on intrinsic PEEP, inspiratory effort, and lung volume in severe stable COPD. Thorax. 2002;57:533–9.

18 Pankow W, Hijjeh N, Schüttler F, et al. Influence of noninvasive positive pressure ventilation on inspiratory muscle activity in obese subjects. Eur Respir J. 1997;10:2847–52.

19 Jaber S, Chanques G, Jung B, et al. Postoperative noninvasive ventilation. Anesthesiology. 2010;112:453–61.

20 Peter JV, Moran JL, Phillips-Hughes J, et al. Noninvasive ventilation in acute respiratory failure: a meta-analysis update. Crit Care Med. 2002;30:555–62.

21 Weng CL, Zhao YT, Liu QH, et al. Meta-analysis: noninvasive ventilation in acute cardiogenic pulmonary edema. Ann Intern Med. 2010;152:590–600.

22 Liesching T, Kwok H, Hill NS. Acute applications of noninvasive positive pressure ventilation. Chest. 2003;124(2): 699–713.

23 Ram FS, Picot J, Lightowler J, et al. Non-invasive positive pressure ventilation for treatment of respiratory failure due to exacerbations of chronic obstructive pulmonary disease. Cochrane Database Syst Rev. 2004;CD004104.

24 Keenan SP, Sinuff T, Cook DJ, et al. Does noninvasive positive pressure ventilation improve outcome in acute hypoxemic respiratory failure? A systemic review. Crit Care Med. 2004;32(12).

25 Duarte AG, Justino E, Bigler T, et al. Outcomes of morbidly obese patients requiring mechanical ventilation for acute respiratory failure. Crit Care Med. 2007;(35);732–7.

26 Shivaram U, Cash ME, Beal A. Nasal continuous positive airway pressure in decompensated hypercapnic respiratory failure as a complication of sleep apnea. Chest. 1993;104:770–4.

27 De Baerdemaeker LE, Van der Herten C, Gillardin JM, et al. Comparison of volume-controlled and pressure controlled ventilation during laparoscopic gastric banding in morbidly obese patients. Obes Surg. 2008;18(6):680–5.

28 Cadi P, Guenoun T, Journois D, et al. Pressure-controlled ventilation improves oxygenation during laparoscopic obesity surgery compared with volume-controlled ventilation. Br J Anaesth. 2008;100(5)709–16.

29 Zoremba M, Kalmus G, Dette F, et al. Effects of intra-operative pressure support vs pressure controlled ventilation on oxygenation and lung function in moderately obese adults. Anaesthesia. 2010;65 (2):124–9.

30 O'Brien JM Jr, Welsh CH, Fish RH, et al. Excess body weight is not independently associated with outcome in mechanically ventilated patients with acute lung injury. Ann Intern Med. 2004;140(5):338–45.

31 Almarakbi WA, Fawzi HM, Alhashemi JA. Effects of fourintraoperative ventilatory strategies on respiratory compliance and gas exchange during laparoscopic gastric banding in obese patients. Br J Anaesth. 2009;102(6):862–8.

32 Valenza F, Vagginelli F, Tiby A, et al. Effects of the beach chair position, positive end-expiratory pressure, and pneumoperitoneum on respiratory function in morbidly obese patients during anesthesia and paralysis. Anesthesiology. 2007; 107(5):725–32.

33 Erlandsson K, Odenstedt H, Lundin S, et al. Positive end-expiratory pressure optimization using electric impedance tomography in morbidly obese patients during laparoscopic gastric bypass surgery. Acta Anaesthesiol Scand. 2006; 50:833–9.

34 Chalhoub V, Yazigi A, Sleilaty G, et al. Effect of vital capacity manoeuvres on arterial oxygenation in morbidly obese patients undergoing open bariatric surgery European Journal of Anaesthesiology. 2007;24:283–8.

35 Morris AE, Stapleton RD, Rubenfeld GD, et al. The association between body mass index and clinical outcomes in acute lung injury. Chest. 2007 Feb;131:342–8.

36 Frat JP, Gissot V, Ragot S, et al. Impact of obesity in mechanically ventilated patients: a prospective study. Intensive Care Med. 2008;34(11):1991–8.

37 Bardoczky GI, Yernault J-C, Houben J-J, et al. Large tidal volume ventilation does not improve oxygenation in morbidly obese patients during anesthesia. Anesth Analg. 1995;81:385–8.

38 Sprung J, Whalley DG, Falcone T, et al. The effects of tidal volume and respiratory rate on oxygenation and respiratory mechanics during laparoscopy in morbidly obese patients. Anesth Analg. 2003;97:268.

39 The Acute Respiratory Distress Syndrome Network. Ventilation with lower tidal volumes as compared with traditional tidal volumes for acute lung injury and the acute respiratory distress syndrome. N Engl J Med. 2000 May;342(18):1301–8.

40 Pelosi P, Croci M, Ravagnan I, et al. Respiratory system mechanics in sedated, paralyzed, morbidly obese patients. J Appl Physiol. 1997;82:811–8.

41 Perilli V, Sollazzi L, Bozza P, et al. The effects of the reverse Tredelenburg position on the respiratory mechanics and blood gases in morbidly obese patients during bariatric surgery. Anesth Analg. 2000;91:1520–5.

42 Torres A, Serra-Batlles J, Ros E, et al. Pulmonary aspiration of gastric contents in patients receiving mechanical ventilation: the effect of body position. Ann Intern Med. 1992;116(7):540–3.

43 Vaughan RW, Bauer S, Wise L, et al. Volume and pH of gastric juice in obese patients. Anesthesiol. 1975;43:686–9.

44 Alexiou VG, Lerodiakonou V, Dimopoulos G, et al. Impact of patient position on the incidence of ventilator-associated pneumonia: a meta-analysis of randomized controlled trials. J Crit Care. 2009 Dec;24(4):515–22.

45 MacIntyre NR, Cook DJ, Ely EW Jr, et al. Evidence-based guidelines for weaning and discontinuing ventilatory support: a collective task force facilitated by the American College of Chest Physicians; the American Association for Respiratory Care; and the American College of Critical Care Medicine. Chest. 2001;120:375S.

46 Esteban A, Alia I, Tobin MJ, et al. Effect of spontaneous breathing trial duration on outcome of attempts to discontinue mechanical ventilation. Spanish Lung Failure Collaborative Group. Am J Respir Crit Care Med. 1999; 159(2):512–18.

47 Epstein SK, Ciubotaru RL, Wong JB. Effect of failed extubation on the outcome of mechanical ventilation. Chest. 1997;112:186–92.

48 Esteban A, Frutos-Vivar F, Ferguson ND, et al. Noninvasive positive-pressure ventilation for respiratory failure after extubation. N Engl J Med. 2004;350:2452–60.

49 Jiang JS, Kao SJ, Wang SN. Effect of early application of biphasic positive airway pressure on the outcome of extubation in ventilator weaning. Respirology. 1999;4:161–5.

50 Nava S, Gregoretti C, Fanfulla F, et al. Noninvasive ventilation to prevent respiratory failure after extubation in high-risk patients. Crit Care Med. 2005;33(11):2465–70.

51 El-Sohl AA, Aquilina A, Pineda L, et al. Noninvasive ventilation for prevention of post-extubation respiratory failure in obese patients. Eur Respir J. 2006;28:588–95.

9 Management of Acute Lung Injury in the Obese Patient

Hallie C. Prescott and James M. O'Brien Jr

The Ohio State University Medical Center, Columbus, OH, USA

KEY POINTS

- Mortality appears to be similar between obese and nonobese acute lung injury patients.
- Evidence-based therapy for acute lung injury includes lung-protective ventilation, conservative fluid management, and strict transfusion thresholds.
- While obesity alters respiratory physiology and may modulate immunity, evidence for body mass index-specific treatment of ALI is lacking.

INTRODUCTION

Acute lung injury (ALI) is a syndrome defined by the sudden onset of bilateral infiltrates on chest radiograph, $PaO_2 : FIO_2$ (P/F) ratio < 300, and pulmonary capillary wedge pressure $< 18\,mm\,Hg$ (or no signs of left atrial hypertension) [1]. Acute respiratory distress syndrome (ARDS) is a more severe form of ALI with P/F < 200 [1]. The mortality rate for ALI is 30–40% [2] and increases to 37–50% in patients with ARDS [3,4]. While these definitions are used widely in research and clinical practice, the diagnosis of ALI can be challenging because it requires identifying a constellation of clinical findings, rather than relying on a laboratory value or test result [2]. The diagnosis may be further complicated in obese patients because of the relatively poor quality of chest radiographs in this population [5], although a recent observational study of critically ill patients did not show an increased incidence of bilateral infiltrates in obese patients [4].

PATHOPHYSIOLOGY AND PROGNOSIS OF ARDS IN OBESE PATIENTS

In ALI and ARDS, the immune system, the coagulation system, and the reparative pathways within the lungs become dysregulated, resulting in activation of cytokines, oxidants, coagulation factors, and proteases that contribute to lung injury [6]. Greater derangements in the concentrations of proinflammatory cytokines, coagulation factors, and other biomarkers are associated with higher mortality [7–9].

On histological examination, the lungs from ALI/ARDS patients demonstrate inflammation, alveolar hyaline membrane formation, decreased surfactant, and regional atelectasis that lead to low respiratory compliance and high airway pressures during mechanical ventilation [6,10]. Because respiratory compliance is already lower in obese patients than in nonobese patients, achieving low-pressure ventilation may be particularly difficult [10].

Healthy obese patients have higher levels of proinflammatory cytokines than nonobese patients [11]. This suggests that obese patients may be predisposed to developing ALI, or developing more severe lung injury compared to nonobese patients. A recent observational study reported an association between obesity and the development of ARDS in critically ill patients at risk for ARDS [4]. The authors hypothesize that this association may be due to the altered inflammatory response, initial injurious ventilator settings, a greater propensity for pulmonary infections, or an increased risk of aspiration [4].

While healthy obese patients have greater concentrations of proinflammatory cytokines than nonobese patients [11], and proinflammatory cytokines are associated with increased mortality in ALI [7,8], obesity has not been clearly associated with worse mortality in ALI patients [12–14]. In fact, one retrospective analysis demonstrates decreased mortality in ALI patients with higher body mass index (BMI), despite initial ventilation with higher tidal volumes [12].

To further evaluate the relationship of obesity, inflammation, and mortality in ALI patients, Stapleton et al. analysed plasma biomarkers of patients in the ARDS Network database [15]. They found lower levels of surfactant protein D (a biomarker of epithelial injury) and the inflammatory cytokines interleukin-6 and interleukin-8 in obese ALI patients, leading to the hypothesis that obesity may attenuate the inflammatory response in critical illnesses such as ALI [15]. Alternatively, obese patients may tolerate mechanical ventilation better than nonobese patients. Fat deposition around the ribs and diaphragm has the potential of decreasing chest-wall compliance, which could increase pleural pressure and decrease transpulmonary pressures [10,16]. This decrease in transpulmonary pressure may allow obese patients to tolerate high plateau pressures better than normal-weight patients [10]. Another reason obese ALI patients may have lower inflammatory markers than nonobese patients is that the diagnostic criteria for ALI may be more sensitive in obese patients, leading to the inclusion of obese patients with less severe pathological lung damage. Further studies are needed to evaluate the relationship between obesity, inflammation, and immunity in critical illness.

STANDARD MANAGEMENT OF ALI AND ARDS IN OBESE PATIENTS

Due to a lack of data supporting BMI-specific care, obese ALI patients should be treated similarly to normal-weight patients with this condition. Altered respiratory mechanics and inflammatory response change the physiology of ALI in obese patients, but the impact of obesity on response to treatment is unclear. No large clinical trials have enrolled only obese patients or stratified randomization by BMI to determine a modification of the therapeutic effect based on obesity or to support differing treatment of obese patients with ALI. Standard therapy includes lung-protective ventilation with a tidal volume of ≤ 6 ml/kg ideal body weight (IBW), plateau pressure of ≤ 30 cm H_2O, moderate levels of positive end expiratory pressure (PEEP) (shown in Table 9.1), and a conservative fluid strategy [17–19].

Lung-protective ventilation

Ventilation with low tidal volumes (≤ 6 ml/kg IBW) and low plateau pressures (≤ 30 cm H_2O) decreases ventilator-associated lung injury and mortality [17]. Although obese patients may tolerate high plateau pressures better than normal-weight patients, retrospective evaluation of the ARDS Network data with analysis of subjects by BMI suggests that obese patients with ALI still benefit from lung-protective ventilation [14]. Tidal volume must be calculated based on height and gender since nonsystemic selection of tidal volume may result in larger than ideal volumes in obese patients [4,13–14]. Even when tidal volume is calculated appropriately, obese patients may have higher plateau pressures than normal BMI controls, likely due to worse respiratory compliance [20]. Initial plateau pressures are closely associated with mortality [21], and mortality decreases linearly with plateau pressure [22], so it is important to reassess plateau pressure over time and adjust tidal volume as needed.

Positive end expiratory pressure

The ventilation strategy used in the landmark ARDS Network trial is the standard against which newer protective ventilation strategies are compared [17,23]. In the

Table 9.1 PEEP strategies used in ARDS Network [17], ALVEOLI [25], LOVS [23], and EXPRESS [26] trials.

		0.3	0.4	0.5	0.6	0.7	0.8	0.9	1
	Fraction of inspired oxygen (FIO$_2$)								
Standard lung-protective ventilation	ARDS Network PEEP range (cm H$_2$O)	5	5–8	8–10	10	10–14	14	14–28	18–24
Lung-open ventilation strategies	ALVEOLI PEEP range (cm H$_2$O)	5–14	14–16	16–20	20	20	20–22	22	22–24
	LOVS PEEP range (cm H$_2$O)	5–10	10–18	14–20	20	20	20–22	20–22	20–24
	EXPRESS PEEP range (cm H$_2$O)	PEEP as high as possible without raising maximum inspiratory pressure > 28–30 cm H$_2$O							

original trial, PEEP was set at moderate levels according to a specified PEEP/FIO$_2$ algorithm shown in Table 9.1 [17]. One concern about low-tidal-volume ventilation is the development of atelectrauma, injury from repetitive opening and closing of alveoli [23,24]. Three recent studies (ALVEOLI [25], LOVS[23], and EXPRESS[26]) evaluated the benefit "lung-open" ventilation strategies using higher levels of PEEP in ALI patients receiving low-tidal-volume ventilation. The specific PEEP strategies are shown in Table 9.1. These studies showed improved oxygenation with high PEEP without any effect on mortality [23,25,26]. Two of the studies also reported decreased use of rescue therapies in patients receiving higher PEEP [23,26]. A metaanalysis pooling the data from these trials revealed decreased hospital mortality among the subgroup with ARDS [27]. These trials suggest that high PEEP is a safe practice that improves oxygenation and may be associated with a survival benefit in patients with more severe lung injury. Theoretically, high PEEP may be particularly helpful in obese patients who have a greater potential for atelectasis due to their increased body mass and elevated intraabdominal pressures [28], but outcome data is lacking.

Restrictive fluid strategy

Fluid retention and elevated hydrostatic pressures have been associated with worse outcomes in patients with ALI [29]. In the absence of shock, a conservative fluid-management strategy targeting a central venous pressure (CVP) < 4 mm Hg can decrease length of mechanical ventilation and length of stay (LOS) in patients with ALI [19]. In patients with a tenuous hemodynamic status, using albumin in conjunction with furosemide can improve fluid balance and oxygenation while maintaining hemodynamic stability [30,31]. These strategies may be particularly relevant for obese patients who are less tolerant of fluid loading than normal-weight controls [32].

Restrictive transfusion strategy

Blood-product transfusion is associated with the development of pulmonary edema, impaired gas exchange, transfusion-associated cardiopulmonary overload, and transfusion-associated lung injury [33,34]. Furthermore, in patients with ALI, red-blood-cell transfusion has been associated with higher mortality [35]. Available data supports a transfusion threshold of 7 g/dl in critically ill patients [36], but more liberal transfusion thresholds remain common in clinical practice [37]. Adherence to conservative transfusion thresholds is particularly important in ALI patients given the association of transfusion and mortality in this population. Fresh frozen plasma and platelets are associated with similar complications, so should also be used judiciously [33].

Corticosteroids

The role of corticosteroids in critically ill patients is the subject of much debate. Two randomized controlled trials (RCTs) showed increased oxygenation with corticosteroids in ARDS patients with persistent respiratory failure [38,39]. While neither study showed a significant mortality benefit [38,39], one had a nonsignificant trend toward improved mortality in subjects randomized to steroids betweens days 7 and 13 after diagnosis of ARDS and a significantly higher mortality in subjects randomized after 14 days [39]. These finding suggest the possibility of a window of efficacy for corticosteroids. A more recent RCT showed an oxygenation benefit in ALI patients randomized to corticosteroid therapy within 72 hours of diagnosis [40]. A metaanalysis revealed an overall decrease in the relative risk of mortality with steroid treatment of 0.62 (p = 0.01), as well as decreased length of mechanical ventilation, ICU LOS, organ dysfunction, and improved oxygenation, without an increase in infection or neuromuscular weakness [41]. In recent studies of ALI patients, 42–52% of patients received corticosteroids, although the indication for this therapy was not reported [23,26]. Clinicians must weigh the risks of adverse effects of corticosteroids (e.g. immune suppression, increased neuromuscular weakness) with the possible benefits of their administration (e.g. increased oxygenation and compliance). The optimal timing, dosage, duration, and need for adjustment based on body weight remain unknown.

Neuromuscular blockade

Neuromuscular blockade (NMB) improves oxygenation in ALI, likely through several mechanisms, such as increased patient–ventilator synchrony, decreased oxygen consumption, and decreased pulmonary inflammatory response [42,43]. However, because these drugs have been associated with ICU-acquired weakness and require deep sedation, many authorities recommend minimizing their use [44,45]. A recent trial evaluating NMB in patients with ARDS showed a mortality benefit in patients with P/F < 120[46]. The mechanism of action and optimal timing for this treatment remain unknown [44]. In recent studies of patients with ALI, 44–53% of patients received NMB [23,26].

In theory, the use of NMB is not associated with any additional risks in obese patients since the elimination of these medications is independent of BMI [47]. However, since heavy sedation is needed during NMB, and the volume of distribution of benzodiazepines is greater in obese patients, there is potential for delayed elimination of benzodiazepines [48]. Physicians should be cognizant of the differing pharmacokinetics of benzodiazepines in obese patients to avoid prolonged sedation.

Ventilator liberation

Using intermittent boluses of sedating medications rather than continuous infusions can prevent oversedation and reduce length of ventilation [49]. When continuous infusions are necessary, daily interruption and evaluation for ventilator liberation can significantly reduce length of mechanical ventilation, ICU LOS, and mortality [50]. Ultimately, however, the decision to extubate a patient after passing a spontaneous breathing trial falls to the physician, and may be affected by the physician's perception of the chance of success and the consequences of failed extubation. In healthy patients, obesity is weakly correlated with difficulty of endotracheal intubation [51]. In critically ill patients, obesity is associated with a greater incidence of difficult intubations and postextubation strider [52]. In addition, sleep apnea is common in obese patients, can be aggravated by sedating medications used in the ICU, and may increase the risk of failed extubation [53]. These risks may sway physicians against extubation and contribute to prolonged mechanical ventilation in obese patients. A recent survey confirmed that intensivists are more likely to pursue early tracheostomy in obese patients [54], potentially due to concerns about extubation failure and difficult reintubation.

While obesity was associated with prolonged duration of mechanical ventilation in a recent metaanalysis, this association was not seen in all included studies [55]. Several smaller studies report equivalent ventilation lengths in obese and nonobese patients [14,56,57], suggesting that comparable outcomes may be possible between obese and nonobese patients. The differences in ventilation length in the various studies may be due to treatment effect rather than disease severity. Protocolized ventilator liberation strategies may prevent physician biases from unnecessarily delaying extubation in this population. In the only study of ALI patients reporting an association between obesity and decreased mortality, obese patients had a relatively high tracheostomy rate [12]. While robust outcome data on early tracheostomy in obese and nonobese patients requiring mechanical ventilation are lacking, one metaanalysis showed an association between early tracheostomy and decreased ventilator length [58]. The optimal timing and patient population for early tracheostomy remain unknown.

RESCUE THERAPIES FOR REFRACTORY HYPOXEMIA IN OBESE PATIENTS

Despite treatment with lung-protective ventilation and conservative fluid practices, some patients with ALI will develop severe and prolonged hypoxemia. In one recent trial, about 7% of patients with ALI had a $PaO_2 < 60 \, mm \, Hg$ for at least 1 hour while breathing FIO_2 1.0 [23]. When treating patients with such profound hypoxemia, clinicians often employ therapies aimed at improving oxygenation, even if they have limited supporting evidence [59]. These experimental therapies designed to improve gas exchange are often referred to as "rescue" therapies, although this terminology is criticized because of their uncertain benefit [59]. Without data to guide the choice of rescue therapy or clear guidelines defining "failure" of conventional treatment [60], the initiation and selection of rescue therapies is likely driven by available resources, expert recommendations, and institutional preferences [18]. One recent trial reported that rescue therapies, defined as inhaled nitric oxide, prone positioning, alternative ventilation strategies, and/or ECMO, were used in 12% of ALI patients receiving low-tidal-volume and low-pressure ventilation [23]. Another trial reported using prone positioning in 19% and inhaled nitric oxide in 26% of ALI patients treated with a lung-protective ventilation strategy [26].

Ventilatory rescue therapies, nonventilatory rescue therapies, and suggested triggers for their use are listed in Figure 9.1. While alternative ventilator modes may improve oxygenation, there is little outcome data to support their use. Recent metaanalyses of inhaled nitric oxide and aerosolized prostacyclins in ALI patients have not been favorable [61,62].

Prone positioning

Several mechanisms have been proposed to explain how prone positioning might improve oxygenation, such as enhancing ventilation/perfusion (V/Q) matching, recruiting alveoli, and reducing atelectasis from the gravitational effect of the heart and decreasing left-to-right shunting [63]. While prone positioning has not

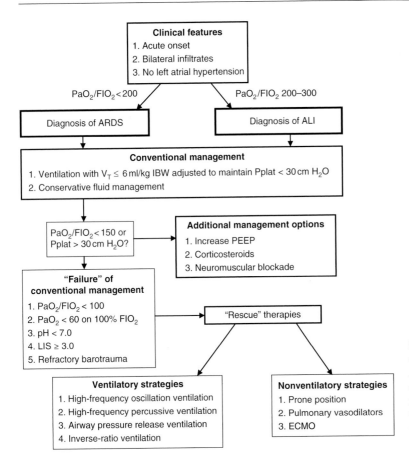

Figure 9.1 Algorithm for management of ALI and ARDS. ALI, acute lung injury; ARDS, acute respiratory distress syndrome; ECMO, extracorporeal membrane oxygenation; IBW, ideal body weight; LIS, lung injury score; PEEP, positive end expiratory pressure; Pplat, plateau pressure; V_T, tidal volume.

been clearly associated with a mortality benefit, two studies have demonstrated nonsignificant trends towards decreased mortality in patients with severe hypoxia (P/F < 100) [64,65]. Furthermore, in healthy obese patients, prone positioning improves residual capacity, lung compliance, and oxygenation [66], so it may be a particularly beneficial intervention in obese ALI patients (although it might be technically difficult to perform).

Extracorporeal membrane oxygenation

Extracorporeal membrane oxygenation (ECMO) is typically viewed as the therapy of last resort in patients who cannot be oxygenated adequately by other means [67]. Early studies did not provide compelling evidence for widespread use. CESAR, a multicenter RTC evaluating the use of ECMO, showed a mortality benefit in the treatment group [68]. However, this study is criticized because of differences in the management of the intervention and control subjects [67]. The treatment arm received

protocolized care with low-tidal-volume ventilation at a single academic medical center, while subjects in the control group received variable treatment at > 100 different hospitals [68]. Despite the methodological flaws of the CESAR trial, it likely increased awareness and acceptance of the use of ECMO as a therapy for refractory ARDS.

The novel H1N1 influenza A pandemic in 2009–2010 led to an increased volume of young, otherwise healthy patients with severe respiratory failure [69]. Obesity was a common comorbidity in patients requiring ICU admission for H1N1 infection [70]. ECMO use increased dramatically in response to the epidemic, with 68 patients receiving ECMO in Australia and New Zealand during a two-month period [69]. Half the patients treated with ECMO had a BMI > 30 [69]. ICU and hospital survival for patients receiving ECMO was 75%, similar to the outcomes achieved in the CESAR trial [71]. Despite its increased use and greater publicity, ECMO remains controversial because of inconclusive data, high cost, high risk, and limited availability [67,72].

CONCLUSION

ALI is a common condition with high mortality. Obesity has been associated with an increased incidence of ARDS in at-risk patients, although it is unclear whether this is due to a greater propensity for lung injury, a difference in treatment, or an increased sensitivity of the diagnostic criteria in obese patients. Once diagnosed with ALI, patients seem to have a similar mortality to normal-weight patients, although they are more likely to receive higher initial tidal volumes. Regardless of BMI, conventional treatment of ALI should focus on minimizing further lung injury through lung-protective ventilation and conservative fluid-management strategies. In the event of severe hypoxemia, additional therapies such as higher PEEP, corticosteroids, NMB, and prone positioning can be considered.

BEST PRACTICE TIPS

1 Lung-protective ventilation including lower tidal volumes (e.g. 6 ml/kg IBW) and plateau pressure limits (e.g. < 30 cm H_2O) should be standard of care for ALI patients, regardless of BMI.

2 Tidal volumes should be calculated based on height and gender. Patients with higher BMIs may be at risk of exposure to larger, and potentially injurious, tidal volumes if such calculations are not performed.

3 For obese patients with ARDS, consider increasing PEEP or using prone positioning since these interventions improve respiratory physiology in obese patients and improve oxygenation in ALI patients.

4 Schedule daily sedation interruption and evaluation for ventilator liberation. Due to an expanded volume of distribution, obese patients may be at particular risk of oversedation when continuous infusions of sedatives are used.

5 Once hemodynamically stable, ALI patients should have fluid management and diuresis targeted to reduce CVP < 4 mm Hg.

REFERENCES

1 Bernard GR, Artigas A, Brigham KL, Carlet J, Falke K, Hudson L, et al. The American-European Consensus Conference on ARDS. Definitions, mechanisms, relevant outcomes, and clinical trial coordination. Am J Respir Crit Care Med. 1994 Mar;149(3 Pt 1):818–24.

2 Rubenfeld GD, Herridge MS. Epidemiology and outcomes of acute lung injury. Chest. 2007 Feb;131(2):554–62.

3 Zilberberg MD, Luippold RS, Sulsky S, Shorr AF. Prolonged acute mechanical ventilation, hospital resource utilization, and mortality in the United States. Crit Care Med. 2008 Mar;36(3):724–30.

4 Gong MN, Bajwa EK, Thompson BT, Christiani DC. Body mass index is associated with the development of acute respiratory distress syndrome. Thorax. 2010 Jan;65(1):44–50.

5 Uppot RN, Sahani DV, Hahn PF, Kalra MK, Saini SS, Mueller PR. Effect of obesity on image quality: fifteen-year longitudinal study for evaluation of dictated radiology reports. Radiology. 2006 Aug;240(2):435–9.

6 Ware LB. Pathophysiology of acute lung injury and the acute respiratory distress syndrome. Semin Respir Crit Care Med. 2006 Aug;27(4):337–49.

7 Meduri GU, Headley S, Kohler G, Stentz F, Tolley E, Umberger R, et al. Persistent elevation of inflammatory cytokines predicts a poor outcome in ARDS. Plasma IL-1 beta and IL-6 levels are consistent and efficient predictors of outcome over time. Chest. 1995 Apr;107(4):1062–73.

8 Parsons PE, Eisner MD, Thompson BT, Matthay MA, Ancukiewicz M, Bernard GR, et al. Lower tidal volume ventilation and plasma cytokine markers of inflammation in patients with acute lung injury. Crit Care Med. 2005 Jan; 33(1):1–6; disc. 230–2.

9 Ware LB, Conner ER, Matthay MA. von Willebrand factor antigen is an independent marker of poor outcome in patients with early acute lung injury. Crit Care Med. 2001 Dec;29(12):2325–31.

10 Ashburn DD, DeAntonio A, Reed MJ. Pulmonary system and obesity. Crit Care Clin. 2010 Oct;26(4):597–602.

11 Ferrante AW, Jr. Obesity-induced inflammation: a metabolic dialogue in the language of inflammation. J Intern Med. 2007 Oct;262(4):408–14.

12 O'Brien JM, Jr., Phillips GS, Ali NA, Lucarelli M, Marsh CB, Lemeshow S. Body mass index is independently associated with hospital mortality in mechanically ventilated adults with acute lung injury. Crit Care Med. 2006 Mar;34(3): 738–44.

13 Morris AE, Stapleton RD, Rubenfeld GD, Hudson LD, Caldwell E, Steinberg KP. The association between body mass index and clinical outcomes in acute lung injury. Chest. 2007 Feb;131(2):342–8.

14 O'Brien JM, Jr., Welsh CH, Fish RH, Ancukiewicz M, Kramer AM. Excess body weight is not independently associated with outcome in mechanically ventilated patients with acute lung injury. Ann Intern Med. 2004 Mar 2;140(5):338–45.

15 Stapleton RD, Dixon AE, Parsons PE, Ware LB, Suratt BT. The association between body mass index and plasma cytokine levels in patients with acute lung injury. Chest. 2010 Sep;138(3):568–77.

16 Hess DR, Bigatello LM. The chest wall in acute lung injury/acute respiratory distress syndrome. Curr Opin Crit Care. 2008 Feb;14(1):94–102.

17 The Acute Respiratory Distress Syndrome Network. Ventilation with lower tidal volumes as compared with traditional tidal volumes for acute lung injury and the acute respiratory distress syndrome. N Engl J Med. 2000 May 4;342(18):1301–8.

18 Esan A, Hess DR, Raoof S, George L, Sessler CN. Severe hypoxemic respiratory failure: Part 1. Ventilatory strategies. Chest. 2010 May;137(5):1203–16.

19 Wiedemann HP, Wheeler AP, Bernard GR, Thompson BT, Hayden D, deBoisblanc B, et al. Comparison of two fluid-management strategies in acute lung injury. N Engl J Med. 2006 Jun 15;354(24):2564–75.

20 Pelosi P, Croci M, Ravagnan I, Cerisara M, Vicardi P, Lissoni A, et al. Respiratory system mechanics in sedated, paralyzed, morbidly obese patients. J Appl Physiol. 1997 Mar;82(3):811–18.

21 Checkley W, Brower R, Korpak A, Thompson BT. Effects of a clinical trial on mechanical ventilation practices in patients with acute lung injury. Am J Respir Crit Care Med. 2008 Jun 1;177(11):1215–22.

22 Brower RG, Matthay M, Schoenfeld D. Meta-analysis of acute lung injury and acute respiratory distress syndrome trials. Am J Respir Crit Care Med. 2002 Dec 1;166(11):1515–17.

23 Meade MO, Cook DJ, Guyatt GH, Slutsky AS, Arabi YM, Cooper DJ, et al. Ventilation strategy using low tidal volumes, recruitment maneuvers, and high positive end-expiratory pressure for acute lung injury and acute respiratory distress syndrome: a randomized controlled trial. JAMA. 2008 Feb 13;299(6):637–45.

24 Slutsky AS. Lung injury caused by mechanical ventilation. Chest. 1999 Jul;116(1 Suppl):9S–15S.

25 Brower RG, Lanken PN, MacIntyre N, Matthay MA, Morris A, Ancukiewicz M, et al. Higher versus lower positive end-expiratory pressures in patients with the acute respiratory distress syndrome. N Engl J Med. 2004 Jul 22;351(4):327–36.

26 Mercat A, Richard JC, Vielle B, Jaber S, Osman D, Diehl JL, et al. Positive end-expiratory pressure setting in adults with acute lung injury and acute respiratory distress syndrome: a randomized controlled trial. JAMA. 2008 Feb 13;299(6):646–55.

27 Briel M, Meade M, Mercat A, Brower RG, Talmor D, Walter SD, et al. Higher vs lower positive end-expiratory pressure in patients with acute lung injury and acute respiratory distress syndrome: systematic review and meta-analysis. JAMA. 2010 Mar 3;303(9):865–73.

28 Pelosi P, Ravagnan I, Giurati G, Panigada M, Bottino N, Tredici S, et al. Positive end-expiratory pressure improves respiratory function in obese but not in normal subjects during anesthesia and paralysis. Anesthesiology. 1999 Nov;91(5):1221–31.

29 Simmons RS, Berdine GG, Seidenfeld JJ, Prihoda TJ, Harris GD, Smith JD, et al. Fluid balance and the adult respiratory distress syndrome. Am Rev Respir Dis. 1987 Apr;135(4):924–9.

30 Martin GS, Mangialardi RJ, Wheeler AP, Dupont WD, Morris JA, Bernard GR. Albumin and furosemide therapy in hypoproteinemic patients with acute lung injury. Crit Care Med. 2002 Oct;30(10):2175–82.

31 Martin GS, Moss M, Wheeler AP, Mealer M, Morris JA, Bernard GR. A randomized, controlled trial of furosemide with or without albumin in hypoproteinemic patients with acute lung injury. Crit Care Med. 2005 Aug;33(8):1681–7.

32 Alpert MA, Lambert CR, Panayiotou H, Terry BE, Cohen MV, Massey CV, et al. Relation of duration of morbid obesity to left ventricular mass, systolic function, and diastolic filling, and effect of weight loss. Am J Cardiol. 1995 Dec 1;76(16):1194–7.

33 Gajic O, Rana R, Winters JL, Yilmaz M, Mendez JL, Rickman OB, et al. Transfusion-related acute lung injury in the critically ill: prospective nested case–control study. Am J Respir Crit Care Med. 2007 Nov 1;176(9):886–91.

34 Gong MN, Thompson BT, Williams P, Pothier L, Boyce PD, Christiani DC. Clinical predictors of and mortality in acute respiratory distress syndrome: potential role of red cell transfusion. Crit Care Med. 2005 Jun;33(6):1191–8.

35 Netzer G, Shah CV, Iwashyna TJ, Lanken PN, Finkel B, Fuchs B, et al. Association of RBC transfusion with mortality in patients with acute lung injury. Chest. 2007 Oct;132(4):1116–23.

36 Hebert PC, Wells G, Blajchman MA, Marshall J, Martin C, Pagliarello G, et al. A multicenter, randomized, controlled clinical trial of transfusion requirements in critical care. Transfusion Requirements in Critical Care Investigators, Canadian Critical Care Trials Group. N Engl J Med. 1999 Feb 11;340(6):409–17.

37 Corwin HL, Gettinger A, Pearl RG, Fink MP, Levy MM, Abraham E, et al. The CRIT Study: Anemia and blood transfusion in the critically ill: current clinical practice in the United States. Crit Care Med. 2004 Jan;32(1):39–52.

38 Meduri GU, Headley AS, Golden E, Carson SJ, Umberger RA, Kelso T, et al. Effect of prolonged methylprednisolone therapy in unresolving acute respiratory distress syndrome: a randomized controlled trial. JAMA. 1998 Jul 8;280(2):159–65.

39 Steinberg KP, Hudson LD, Goodman RB, Hough CL, Lanken PN, Hyzy R, et al. Efficacy and safety of corticosteroids for persistent acute respiratory distress syndrome. N Engl J Med. 2006 Apr 20;354(16):1671–84.

40 Meduri GU, Golden E, Freire AX, Taylor E, Zaman M, Carson SJ, et al. Methylprednisolone infusion in early severe ARDS: results of a randomized controlled trial. Chest. 2007 Apr;131(4):954–63.

41 Tang BM, Craig JC, Eslick GD, Seppelt I, McLean AS. Use of corticosteroids in acute lung injury and acute respiratory distress syndrome: a systematic review and meta-analysis. Crit Care Med. 2009 May;37(5):1594–603.

42 Gainnier M, Roch A, Forel JM, Thirion X, Arnal JM, Donati S, et al. Effect of neuromuscular blocking agents on gas exchange in patients presenting with acute respiratory distress syndrome. Crit Care Med. 2004 Jan;32(1):113–19.

43 Forel JM, Roch A, Marin V, Michelet P, Demory D, Blache JL, et al. Neuromuscular blocking agents decrease inflammatory response in patients presenting with acute respiratory distress syndrome. Crit Care Med. 2006 Nov;34(11):2749–57.

44 Slutsky AS. Neuromuscular Blocking Agents in ARDS. New England Journal of Medicine. 2010;363(12):1176–80.

45 Dellinger RP, Levy MM, Carlet JM, Bion J, Parker MM, Jaeschke R, et al. Surviving Sepsis Campaign: international guidelines for management of severe sepsis and septic shock: 2008. Crit Care Med. 2008 Jan;36(1):296–327.

46 Papazian L, Forel JM, Gacouin A, Penot-Ragon C, Perrin G, Loundou A, et al. Neuromuscular blockers in early acute respiratory distress syndrome. N Engl J Med. 2010 Sep 16;363(12):1107–16.

47 Varin F, Ducharme J, Theoret Y, Besner JG, Bevan DR, Donati F. Influence of extreme obesity on the body disposition and neuromuscular blocking effect of atracurium. Clin Pharmacol Ther. 1990 Jul;48(1):18–25.

48 Casati A, Putzu M. Anesthesia in the obese patient: pharmacokinetic considerations. J Clin Anesth. 2005 Mar;17(2):134–45.

49 Strom T, Martinussen T, Toft P. A protocol of no sedation for critically ill patients receiving mechanical ventilation: a randomised trial. Lancet. 2010 Feb 6;375(9713):475–80.

50 Girard TD, Kress JP, Fuchs BD, Thomason JW, Schweickert WD, Pun BT, et al. Efficacy and safety of a paired sedation and ventilator weaning protocol for mechanically ventilated patients in intensive care (Awakening and Breathing Controlled trial): a randomised controlled trial. Lancet. 2008 Jan 12;371(9607):126–34.

51 Lundstrom LH, Moller AM, Rosenstock C, Astrup G, Wetterslev J. High body mass index is a weak predictor for difficult and failed tracheal intubation: a cohort study of 91,332 consecutive patients scheduled for direct laryngoscopy registered in the Danish Anesthesia Database. Anesthesiology. 2009 Feb;110(2):266–74.

52 Frat JP, Gissot V, Ragot S, Desachy A, Runge I, Lebert C, et al. Impact of obesity in mechanically ventilated patients: a prospective study. Intensive Care Med. 2008 Nov;34(11):1991–8.

53 Miehsler W. Mortality, morbidity and special issues of obese ICU patients. Wien Med Wochenschr. 2010 Mar;160(5–6): 124–8.

54 O'Brien JM, Jr., Aberegg SK, Ali NA, Diette GB, Lemeshow S. Results from the National Sepsis Practice Survey: use of drotrecogin alpha (activated) and other therapeutic decisions. J Crit Care. 2010 Jun 18.

55 Akinnusi ME, Pineda LA, El Solh AA. Effect of obesity on intensive care morbidity and mortality: a meta-analysis. Crit Care Med. 2008 Jan;36(1):151–8.

56 Peake SL, Moran JL, Ghelani DR, Lloyd AJ, Walker MJ. The effect of obesity on 12-month survival following admission to intensive care: a prospective study. Crit Care Med. 2006 Dec;34(12):2929–39.

57 Ray DE, Matchett SC, Baker K, Wasser T, Young MJ. The effect of body mass index on patient outcomes in a medical ICU. Chest. 2005 Jun;127(6):2125–31.

58 Griffiths J, Barber VS, Morgan L, Young JD. Systematic review and meta-analysis of studies of the timing of

tracheostomy in adult patients undergoing artificial ventilation. BMJ. 2005 May 28;330(7502):1243.

59 Diaz JV, Brower R, Calfee CS, Matthay MA. Therapeutic strategies for severe acute lung injury. Crit Care Med. 2010 Aug;38(8):1644–50.

60 Hubmayr RD, Farmer JC. Should we "rescue" patients with 2009 influenza A(H1N1) and lung injury from conventional mechanical ventilation? Chest. 2010 Apr;137(4):745–7.

61 Afshari A, Brok J, Moller AM, Wetterslev J. Inhaled nitric oxide for acute respiratory distress syndrome (ARDS) and acute lung injury in children and adults. Cochrane Database Syst Rev. 2010(7):CD002787.

62 Afshari A, Brok J, Moller AM, Wetterslev J. Aerosolized prostacyclin for acute lung injury (ALI) and acute respiratory distress syndrome (ARDS). Cochrane Database Syst Rev. 2010(8):CD007733.

63 Girard TD, Bernard GR. Mechanical ventilation in ARDS: a state-of-the-art review. Chest. 2007 Mar;131(3):921–9.

64 Gattinoni L, Tognoni G, Pesenti A, Taccone P, Mascheroni D, Labarta V, et al. Effect of prone positioning on the survival of patients with acute respiratory failure. N Engl J Med. 2001 Aug 23;345(8):568–73.

65 Taccone P, Pesenti A, Latini R, Polli F, Vagginelli F, Mietto C, et al. Prone positioning in patients with moderate and severe acute respiratory distress syndrome: a randomized controlled trial. JAMA. 2009 Nov 11;302(18):1977–84.

66 Pelosi P, Croci M, Calappi E, Mulazzi D, Cerisara M, Vercesi P, et al. Prone positioning improves pulmonary function in obese patients during general anesthesia. Anesth Analg. 1996 Sep;83(3):578–83.

67 Raoof S, Goulet K, Esan A, Hess DR, Sessler CN. Severe hypoxemic respiratory failure: Part 2. Nonventilatory strategies. Chest. 2010 Jun;137(6):1437–48.

68 Peek GJ, Mugford M, Tiruvoipati R, Wilson A, Allen E, Thalanany MM, et al. Efficacy and economic assessment of conventional ventilatory support versus extracorporeal membrane oxygenation for severe adult respiratory failure (CESAR): a multicentre randomised controlled trial. Lancet. 2009 Oct 17;374(9698):1351–63.

69 Davies A, Jones D, Bailey M, Beca J, Bellomo R, Blackwell N, et al. Extracorporeal Membrane Oxygenation for 2009 Influenza A(H1N1) Acute Respiratory Distress Syndrome. JAMA. 2009 Nov 4;302(17):1888–95.

70 Diaz E, Rodriguez A, Martin-Loeches I, Lorente L, Del Mar Martin M, Pozo JC, et al. Impact of obesity in patients infected with new influenza A (H1N1)v. Chest. 2010 Aug 5.

71 Davies A, Jones D, Gattas D. Extracorporeal membrane oxygenation for ARDS due to 2009 influenza A (H1N1): Reply. JAMA. 2010 March 10, 2010;303(10):942.

72 Schuerer DJ, Kolovos NS, Boyd KV, Coopersmith CM. Extracorporeal membrane oxygenation: current clinical practice, coding, and reimbursement. Chest. 2008 Jul;134(1): 179–84.

Part III

Management of Obesity Complications in Critical Care

10 Management of Infectious Complications in the Critically Ill Obese Patient

Kristin Turza Campbell, Laura H. Rosenberger, Amani D. Politano, Tjasa Hranjec, and Robert G. Sawyer

University of Virginia Health System, Charlottesville, VA, USA

KEY POINTS

- Obese patients are prone to an exaggerated physiological response to inflammation associated with infection.
- Blood-stream, catheter-related, and surgical-site infection rates appear to be consistently higher in critically ill obese patients. The data regarding urinary-tract infections and pneumonia are less consistent.
- While aggressive prevention of infection in obese patients is a cornerstone of management, it is unknown how or if the treatment of infected obese patients should differ from that of nonobese patients.

INCIDENCE AND CLINICAL EVIDENCE

The United States Centers for Disease Control and Prevention (CDC) estimates the annual incidence of all health care-associated infections to be 1.7 million, including urinary-tract infections (UTIs) (32%), surgical-site infections (SSIs) (22%), pneumonia (15%), and blood-stream infections (14%) [1]. Such infections burden the health care industry annually, costing up to $45 billion [2]. Financial benefit has been demonstrated with preventative measures, and 70% of nosocomial infections are preventable [2].

A range of infections afflict critically ill obese patients. Local infections include SSIs, catheter-related blood-stream infections (CRBSIs), UTIs, pneumonia, *Clostridium diffi-cile*-associated colitis (CDAC), intraabdominal infections, and infections of the central nervous system, pleura, skin/

soft tissue, upper gastrointestinal tract, and vagina. Truly systemic infections (indicated by blood-stream infection and multiorgan system (MOS) failure) may incur from local infections or may result from a primary, disseminated event. Sepsis remains the number one cause of death in noncoronary artery disease intensive care units (ICUs) worldwide, with a growing body of evidence suggesting that the increase in morbidity associated with severe obesity in critically ill patients results in increased resource utilization, adding further to the cost of care [3,4].

There is a relative paucity of information regarding the pathophysiology and treatment of obese critically ill patients, especially with infection. Obesity as an exclusion criterion in landmark trials is partly responsible for this paucity. However, clinical evidence suggests that obese patients suffer more infections than nonobese. Obese patients in the surgical/trauma ICUs of two separate institutions had higher incidence of blood-stream infections ($p = 0.009$) and CRBSIs ($p < 0.001$) than normal-weight patients [5,6]. The rate of overall infections in obese trauma ICU patients is twice the number of non-obese (61 vs 34%), including a twofold increase in the relative risk of urinary tract, blood stream, and respiratory infections from more catheter and ventilator support days [6]. After adjusting for sociodemographic variables, obesity remains an independent risk factor for nosocomial infection in trauma patients. Specifically, pulmonary and wound infections were seen to be the main areas of increased risk in obese patients ($p < 0.01$) [7]. Namba et al. [8] reported that in patients with a $BMI > 35 \, kg/m^2$, the risk of postoperative infection was 6.7 times higher when

---

Critical Care Management of the Obese Patient, First Edition. Edited by Ali A. El Solh.
© 2012 John Wiley & Sons, Ltd. Published 2012 by John Wiley & Sons, Ltd.

undergoing total knee athroplasty and 4.2 times higher when undergoing total hip athroplasty when compared with patients with a BMI <35 kg/m². In another study of 574 women undergoing elective and nonelective caesarean sections, Myles et al. [9] found BMI≥30 kg/m² to be associated with significantly increased risk of postoperative infectious complications including endomyometritis, UTIs, septic pelvic thrombophlebitis, and pneumonia. The results showed the relative risk for postoperative infectious morbidity to be 1.6 (95% confidence interval (CI) 1.2, 2.0) in obese patients undergoing an elective caesarean and 3.0 (95% CI 1.6, 5.8) in obese patients undergoing nonelective caesarean.

Obesity places patients at higher risk for SSIs [10]. One of the reasons for this increased infection is the association between obesity and colonization of nares with *S. aureus*, which is considered a risk factor for surgical-wound infections [11]. Among colorectal surgery patients, SSIs are independently associated with increased BMI and intraoperative hypotension [12]. In a recent study carried out by Merkow et al. [13], the impact of BMI on short-term outcomes after colectomy was assessed in 3202 patients using prospectively collected data from the American College of Surgeons National Surgical Quality Improvement Project database. The results showed that morbid obesity (BMI > 35 kg/m²) was a strong risk factor for wound complications. When compared with patients with a normal BMI, morbidly obese patients were 2.6 times more likely to incur an SSI, superficial or deep, and 3.5 times more likely to experience wound dehiscence. In cardiothoracic patients, obesity was determined to be an independent predictor of SSIs, along with vascular disease, diabetes mellitus, and operative time [14,15]. Sternal-wound infections following coronary artery bypass surgery (CABG) are serious complications associated with increased mortality [16]. In the UK, BMI > 30 kg/m² is an independent risk factor for sternal-wound infection (OR 2.0 (95% CI 1.3–2.9); p < 0.001) [17]. Several similar studies have also identified a BMI > 30 kg/m² as a significant risk factor for deep and superficial sternal-wound infections post CABG [18,19]. In addition, morbidly obese patients were 4.17 (p < 0.001) times more likely to develop harvest-site infections compared with normal-weight patients [20].

Obese patients spend more days with catheters and ventilators, which increases the risk of ICU-acquired infection [21]. In the medical ICU, obese patients have a significantly longer duration of mechanical ventilation (7.7 vs 4.6 days), higher rate of central venous catheter (CVC) (88 vs 45%) and pulmonary artery catheter (18 vs

8%) placement, and a longer duration of catheterization [22]. Yet the difference in catheter-related bacteremia or pneumonia has varied between studies, with no clear evidence of incremental incidence between obese and nonobese. An evaluation of nosocomial infection rates in the context of glycemic control showed that the incidence of all infections (pneumonia mostly) did not differ by BMI either before or after controlling for insulin infusion need [23]. Other studies observed no difference in pneumonia and UTI rates between obese and nonobese patients [5,14,15], and no increased incidence of SSIs [5].

By the same token, investigations of infection-related mortality rate yield inconsistent results.

Obesity presents a unique challenge in transplant patients with respect to infectious complications. Morbidly obese kidney transplant patients have a higher incidence of postsurgical complications, including infectious complications (p = 0.002) [24]. For a renal transplant patient to have a BMI > 30 is an independent risk factor for SSI, and SSI significantly increases the risk of graft loss (HR 2.19, 95% CI 1.35–3.5) [25]. Another study shows that obesity in renal transplantation is a risk factor for recipient delayed graft function (p < 0.001) and decreased graft survival overall (p = 0.001) [26]. In pancreas transplants, obesity is associated with increased intraabdominal infection, gangrene, and necrotizing fasciitis, as well as overall postoperative complications (including infectious complications) (81 vs 40%, p < 0.001) [27]. Viral infections in pancreas transplant recipients are most commonly related to cytomegalovirus (CMV) infection [28]. Severely obese liver transplant patients demonstrated a higher rate of wound infection (p = 0.0001) and death from multisystem organ failure (p = 0.0001), though long-term mortality and total complications in obese and nonobese patients were no different [29].

Obese heart and lung transplant patients are likewise at high risk for infectious complications. Obese lung transplant patients are at a threefold increased mortality risk according to one study, as well as at higher risk of developing bronchiolitis obliterans [30]. Two studies showed similar results, one demonstrating that adjusted death rates were 15% higher for overweight lung transplant recipients than normal-weight patients [31], and the other that the risk of death increased in obese patients (HR 1.16; 95% CI 1.04–1.28, p = 0.005) [32]. *Pseudomonas aeruginosa* is an example of an infection that can be prevalent and difficult to manage in these patients [33]. Obese heart transplant patients demonstrate increased mortality rates [34,35], as well as increased incidence of primary graft failure [32].

Because of the immunosuppression required for prevention of organ rejection, transplant patients are prone to opportunistic infections. In obese and nonobese lung transplant patients, invasive fungal disease (aspergillus, candida, mucor) was seen in 16% and CMV in 3% [36]. Invasive fungal disease was significantly associated with all-cause mortality in this group [33]. Similarly, liver transplant patients with fungal infections tend to have Candida species, while viral infections tend to include CMV and human herpes virus 6 [37]. CMV is the most common viral pathogen negatively impacting liver transplant outcomes, and it has been shown to predispose obese and nonobese liver transplant patients to organ rejection, accelerated hepatitis C recurrence, and reduced overall patient and graft survival [38].

Gastric bypass patients are another unique group with respect to postoperative infectious concerns. Infectious problems are consistently higher in open surgery than laparoscopic, especially wound infections and pneumonia [39]. Wound infection in open surgery patients has been reported as high as 20%, with *S. aureus* (39%), α-hemolytic streptococcus (26%), and enterococcus (16%) being the predominant isolates [40]. Epidural analgesia and antibiotic prophylaxis given after surgical incision increase the odds ratio of developing a wound infection in bypass patients [37]. In laparoscopic gastric bypass, peritoneal contamination is not infrequent, with routine intraabdominal cultures showing a 22.7% positivity rate for streptococci or anaerobes [41]. Some concern exists that bypass surgery increases patient susceptibility to gastric *Helicobacter pylori* infection, but this was not substantiated in an animal model [42]. Preoperative *H. pylori* testing also does not appear to decrease the risk of postoperative anastomotic ulcer or pouch gastritis [43]. One unique consideration in gastric banding is port site infection, as the port constitutes a foreign object within the soft tissue, allowing for band inflation. Port infection frequently necessitates its removal, but fortunately, the incidence of infection is low (5.3% in one gastric band series) [44].

Cellular mechanisms for increased infections in excessive obesity

Obesity is a chronic inflammatory state. Inflammation in obesity predisposes obese mice to an exaggerated response to endotoxemia and sepsis. Circulating cell adhesion, which is an early rate-limiting factor in the inflammatory response in sepsis, is increased in the cerebral microvasculature of obese mice compared with their lean counterparts [45]. This increased adhesive response is accompanied by an increase in the expression of the adhesion molecule P-selectin in various microvascular beds of obese compared with lean septic mice. The functional relevance of these findings is highlighted by the fact that the obese animals exhibit more signs of sickness behavior, and increased blood–brain barrier dysfunction.

Adipocytes secrete cytokines including IL-1, IL-6, and TNF-α, and basal concentrations of the latter two, are higher in obesity [46,47]. TNF-α is detrimental to microvasculature by inducing oxidative stress and decreasing endothelial barrier function [48,49]. Adipose tissue also secretes cytokine-like substances (adipokines), including leptin, resistin, and adiponectin, implicated in the proinflammatory obesity phenotype. Adiponectin is potently immunosuppressive [50], while leptin activates polymorphonuclear neutrophils [51], exerts proliferative and antiapoptotic activities on T lymphocytes, and causes production of reactive oxygen species and immune cell recruitment by engaging endothelial cell receptors [44,52,53]. Resistin similarly increases TNF-α, IL-6, and MCP-1 production and has correlated with a prolonged inflammatory state and disease severity in infected patients [54]. Other adipokines have been linked to sepsis and septic shock, but not necessarily in obese subjects. Further research is needed to understand the interaction between these active molecules and sepsis in obesity.

UNIQUE PHYSIOLOGICAL AND PATHOPHYSIOLOGICAL CONSIDERATIONS

Managing infectious complications in critically ill obese patients requires an understanding of the unique physiology and pathophysiology pertaining to these patients. This includes differences in monitoring, physiology, and inflammation related to weight.

Cutaneous physiology of healing

The reduction in tissue oxygenation that occurs in obese patients increases SSI risk. Intraoperative subcutaneous oxygen partial pressure at the incision site is lower in obese patients than nonobese patients (36 vs 57 mm Hg, p = 0.002) [55]. The intraoperative and immediately postoperative period has been termed the "decisive period" when low tissue oxygenation may result in SSI [42,56]. As the partial pressure of tissue oxygen decreases, so too does oxidative neutrophil killing [57]. A relative hypoperfusion of subcutaneous tissue in obese patients predisposes them to ischemic tissue necrosis, as fat cell size increases without increases in accompanying circulatory flow [42,58,59].

Access-related anatomy

Skin organisms migrating into insertion sites of cutaneously positioned catheters are the most common infection route [60]. Infections associated with CVCs include local infections, CRBSIs, and septic thrombophlebitis. The site of CVC insertion influences infection risk. Subclavian vein CVCs tend to have fewer infections, since they are accessible for hygiene maintenance in patients with large neck and groin size. Though the internal jugular (IJ) location has a lower bacterial colonization rate than femoral sites [44,51], subclavian sites are preferable and femoral sites should generally be avoided altogether. Logistical considerations of catheter placement and fixation are also more complex in obese individuals. Identifying candidate veins (central or peripheral) is more difficult, resulting in a greater number of damaging skin punctures during placement and a longer duration of line usage.

Urinary-tract infections

UTIs are commonly associated with urinary catheters. Endogenous infection sources include colonization at the meatus, rectum, or vagina, and exogenous sources include contaminated hands and insertion equipment. Catheters left in place for a long duration (≥ 30 days) are more likely to be coated with biofilm harboring sessile organisms that are not eradicated by antibiotics. Catheter removal is the preferred approach. Due to hygiene and mobility concerns, hospital staff may be less likely to remove catheters, thus increasing UTI incidence.

Pulmonary infections

Obesity alters lung function mechanics. Total respiratory system and chest-wall compliance are significantly lower in obese patients (80 and 92% of predicted values, respectively) [61]. Obese patients are more likely to suffer atelectasis from low functional residual capacity. With decreased compliance and increased resistance, mechanical ventilation often results in high airway pressures, alveolar overdistension, barotrauma, and higher infection rates from increased ventilator days [53]. A positive association between obesity and respiratory infections has been suggested from a cohort study of more than 100 000

participants of two large US health surveys [62]. The risk of pneumonia was nearly twofold higher among individuals who gained 40 pounds or more during adulthood. A similar increase in frequency of nosocomial pneumonia was reported in critically ill morbidly obese patients [17]. Whether the increased rate of respiratory infections observed in cohort studies is simply a reflection of comorbid conditions associated with obesity or actually results from a disturbance in the noncellular components of innate immunity will require further investigations [63].

MANAGEMENT STRATEGIES

Aggressive prevention of infection by a multidisciplinary team is the cornerstone of optimal management of critically ill obese patients.

SSI management

Obese patients are prone to insulin resistance and hyperglycemia, and maintaining euglycemia pre-, intra-, and postoperatively decreases SSI incidence [64–66]. Maintaining normothermia intra- and postoperatively in obese surgical patients may also reduce the risk of SSI [67] as hypothermia reduces antibody production and phagocytosis. Hypothermia-associated vasoconstriction decreases tissue oxygen partial pressure, thereby lowering infection resistance [68,69]. For surgical patients, preoperative antibiotics lower infection rates, if dosed and timed appropriately (given within 1 hour prior to incision) [42,70]. Preoperative antibiotic dosing should be adjusted to ensure therapeutic levels are obtained.

Although no preventative measures specific to obese patients have been proposed, standard measures should be followed to minimize the risk of CRBSI, UTI, and pneumonia. Therefore, interventions applicable to all patients will be presented.

Catheter-related blood stream infections

Evidence-based interventions demonstrate benefit in prevention of CRBSI. Ideally, prevention is accomplished by avoiding line placement altogether. Proper handwashing and use of full barrier precautions during line insertion is critical. Barrier equipment includes long-sleeve sterile gowns, sterile gloves, mask, surgical cap, and sterile drapes, and decreases infection rates from 3.6 to 0.6% (p < 0.05) [71]. Proper skin cleansing, especially with chlorhexidine, has been shown to decrease CRBSI compared to povidone-iodine solutions (RR 0.49, 95%

CI 0.28–0.88) [72]. Femoral insertion sites should be avoided and subclavian lines attempted. Appropriate insertion-site care should be performed daily. Transparent, semipermeable polyurethane dressings are ideal and allow visualization by staff and showering by patients without barrier disruption. The function and purpose of every indwelling catheter must be reassessed daily by the critical care team. A linear increase in CRBSI exists for each day a catheter remains in place. Reassessment will ensure early catheter removal [73,74]. Teflon or polyurethane catheters should be used if possible.

Urinary-catheter infections

UTI prevention is best accomplished by avoiding catheters. Proper hand sanitization and use of sterile gowns, gloves, and periurethral antiseptic solution decreases infection. Infection rates decrease from maintenance of a closed drainage system following aseptic insertion [75]. If possible, external catheters should be used in males. The presence and utility of urinary catheters should be reassessed daily to decreases infection rates [79].

Pneumonia

For mechanically ventilated obese patients, ventilator tidal volume should be calculated from ideal (not actual) body weight to minimize the risk of alveolar overdistension, barotrauma, and pneumonia. Positive end-expiratory pressure (PEEP) helps in preventing atelectasis by averting alveolar closure [53]. To aid in ventilator weaning, placing the patient in reverse Trendelenburg position may increase tidal volume and lower respiratory rate [53]. The critical care teams must reassess daily ventilator weaning to minimize ventilator days and risk of pneumonia. Adequate pain control, including epidural catheters or patient-controlled analgesia (PCA), is vital to prevent atelectasis. Sedation holiday should be performed daily when possible. Aggressive chest physiotherapy and pulmonary toilet is vital as well.

Antibiotics

Appropriately selected and dosed antibiotics are fundamental to infection treatment. Empirical broad-spectrum antibiotics should be started when there is high suspicion of infection to cover potential pathogens, considering the pattern of local flora. This is generally a combination, such as vancomycin and piperacillin-tazobactam, and may include an additional agent, such as an aminoglycoside or

appropriate fluoroquinolone, if pseudomonas infection is suspected. Microbial cultures must be sent from all potential infection sites to tailor antibiotics. Once culture results are complete, antibiotics should be deescalated by selecting narrow-spectrum antibiotics targeting isolated organisms. Deescalation has not been shown to increase recurrent pneumonias or mortality [76].

General recommendations on antibiotic dosing in obese patients include the following. Vancomycin should be dosed at 15 mg/kg every 12 hours for treatment of pneumonia, bacteremia, graft infections, or endocarditis, with adjustments made for plasma peaks and troughs. Aminoglycosides should be dosed based on obese dosing weight (ODW), since obese patients have increased V_d [56]. Preoperative β-lactam drugs, specifically cefazolin, should be dosed at 2 g in individuals over 80 kg to decrease postoperative infections [58]. Definitive evidence is lacking with respect to dosing alterations in fluoroquinolones. One study showed the tissue penetration of ciprofloxacin to be lower in obese patients, thereby suggesting the value of higher dosing [77], though a trovafloxacin study found no dosing changes to be necessary [78]. Little consistent data exists from which to recommend alterations in linezolid dosing as well. One linezolid study showed no statistically significant difference in drug pharmacokinetics in obese patients, indicating that no dose adjustments are needed [79]. Another rather limited study with a small sample size demonstrated that linezolid dosed at 600 mg every 12 hours for cellulitis yielded a peak concentration lower than that in normal-weight patients [80].

CONCLUSION

The obesity epidemic affecting ICUs has raised concerns about managing this unique patient population suffering from infectious complications. Laboratory studies indicate exaggeration of inflammatory response in obese subjects compared to lean. The exact mechanism for this exaggeration is unknown. Available clinical studies in critically ill obese patients have largely indicated increased morbidity but do not specifically address the issue of obesity and infection. Clinical studies also suffer from non-homogeneity of patients due to comorbid conditions such as hypertension, hypercholesterolemia, diabetes mellitus, coronary artery disease, and so on. Larger clinical studies with carefully selected patients should be undertaken to understand the pathophysiology of obesity in sepsis and septic shock to enable us to manage these patients efficiently in the ICU. It is necessary to undertake clinical as well as laboratory studies that focus on the influence of obesity on infections, in view of the fact that more than 30% of the US population is obese.

BEST PRACTICE TIPS

1 Prior to placement, carefully assess the purpose and need of every vascular catheter placed into an obese patient, diligently avoiding unnecessary placement, as these catheters are very frequently associated with infectious complications of all sorts.

2 The critical care team must reassess the need and function of every vascular or urinary catheter on daily rounds and remove them as early as possible to decrease infection risk.

3 Proper hand sanitation, sterile barrier precautions, and cutaneous antisepsis should be utilized during placement of all catheters and lines.

4 For mechanically ventilated patients, reassess progress toward extubation daily to minimize days on the ventilator, ensure an appropriate tidal volume is being delivered based on ideal (not actual) body weight, and use PEEP to recruit alveoli.

5 Aggressive chest physiotherapy and early ambulation will help the patient normalize physiologically.

REFERENCES

1 CDC Estimates of Healthcare-Associated Infections. Centers for Disease Control and Prevention. 2010.

2 Scott RD. The Direct Medical Costs of Healthcare-Associated Infections in U.S. Hospitals and the Benefits of Prevention. Centers for Disease Control and Infection, Division of Healthcare Quality Promotion. 2009.

3 Angus D, Linde-Zwirble WT, Lidicker J, et al. Epidemiology of severe sepsis in the United States: analysis of incidence, outcome, and associated costs of care. Crit Care Med. 2001;29(7):1303–10.

4 Vachharajani V. Influence of obesity on sepsis. Pathophysiology. 2008;15(2):123–34.

5 Dossett L, Dageforde LA, Swenson BR, et al. Obesity and site-specific nosocomial infection risk in the intensive care unit. Surg Infect (Larchmt). 2009;10(2):137–42.

6 Bochicchio G, Joshi M, Bochicchio K, et al. Impact of obesity in the critically ill trauma patient: a prospective study. J Am Coll Surg. 2006;203(4):533–8.

7 Serrano PE, Khuder SA, Fath JJ. Obesity as a risk factor for nosocomial infections in trauma patients. J Am Coll Surg. 2010;211(1):61–66.

8 Namba RS, Paxton L, Fithian DC, Stone ML. Obesity and perioperative morbidity in total hip and total knee arthroplasty patients. J Arthroplasty. 2005;20:46–50.

9 Myles TD, Gooch J, Santolaya J. Obesity as an independent risk factor for infectious morbidity in patients who undergo cesarean delivery. Obstet Gynecol. 2002;100:959–64.

10 Anaya D, Dellinger EP. The obese surgical patient: a susceptible host for infection. Surg Infect (Larchmt). 2006;7(5):473–80.

11 Herwaldt LA, Cullen JJ, French P, Hu J, Pfaller MA, Wenzel RP, Perl TM. Preoperative risk factors for nasal carriage of Staphylococcus aureus. Infect Control Hosp Epidemiol. 2004;25(6):481–4.

12 Smith R, Bohl JK, McElearney ST, Friel CM, Barclay MM, Sawyer RG, Foley EF. Wound infection after elective colorectal resection. Ann Surg. 2004;239(5):599–605.

13 Merkow RP, Bilimoria KY, McCarter MD, Bentrem DJ. Effect of body mass index on short-term outcomes after colectomy for cancer. J Am Coll Surg. 2009;208:53–61.

14 Russo P, Spelman DW. A new surgical-site infection risk index using risk factors identified by multivariate analysis for patients undergoing coronary artery bypass graft surgery. Infect Control Hosp Epidemiol. 2002;23(7):372–6.

15 Harrington G, Russo P, Spelman D, et al. Surgical-site infection rates and risk factor analysis in coronary artery bypass graft surgery. Infect Control Hosp Epidemiol. 2004;25(6):472–6.

16 Ridderstolpe L, Gill H, Granfeldt H, Ahlfeldt H, Rutberg H. Superficial and deep sternal wound complications: incidence, risk factors and mortality. Eur J Cardiothorac Surg. 2001;20:1168–75.

17 Lu JC, Grayson AD, Jha P, Srinivasan AK, Fabri BM. Risk factors for sternal wound infection and mid-term survival following coronary artery bypass surgery. Eur J Cardiothorac Surg. 2003;23:943–9.

18 Crabtree TD, Codd JE, Fraser VJ, Bailey MS, Olsen MA, Damiano RJ Jr. Multivariate analysis of risk factors for deep and superficial sternal infection after coronary artery bypass grafting at a tertiary care medical center. Semin Thorac Cardiovasc Surg. 2004;16:53–61.

19 Parisian Mediastinitis Study Group. Risk factors for deep sternal wound infection after sternotomy: a prospective, multicenter study. J Thorac Cardiovasc Surg. 1996;111:1200–7.

20 Kuduvalli M, Grayson AD, Oo AY, Fabri BM, Rashid A. The effect of obesity on mid-term survival following coronary artery bypass surgery. Eur J Cardiothorac Surg. 2003;23:368–73.

21 Frat J, Gissot V, Ragot S, et al. Impact of obesity in mechanically ventilated patients: a prospective study. Intensive Care Med. 2008;34(11):1991–8.

22 El Solh A, Sikka P, Bozkanat E, et al. Morbid obesity in the medical ICU. Chest. 2001;120(6):1989–97.

23 Pieracci F, Hydo L, Eachempati S, et al. Higher body mass index predicts need for insulin but not hyperglycemia, nosocomial infection, or death in critically ill surgical patients. Surg Infect (Larchmt). 2008;9(2):121–30.

24 Ditonno P, Lucarelli G, Impedovo SV, Spilotros M, Grandaliano G, Selvaggi FP, Bettocchi C, Battaglia M. Obesity in kidney transplantation affects renal function but not graft survival and patient survival. Transplant Proc. 2011;43(1):367–72.

25 Lynch RJ, Ranney DN, Shijie C, Lee DS, Samala N, Englesbe MJ. Obesity, surgical site infection, and outcome following renal transplantation. Ann Surg. 2009;250(6):1014–20.

26 Gore JL, Pham PT, Danovitch GM, Wilkinson AH, Rosenthal JT, Lipshutz GS, Singer JS. Obesity and outcome following renal transplantation. Am J Transplant. 2006;6(2):357–63.

27 Hanish SI, Petersen RP, Collins BH, Tuttle-Newhall J, Marroquin CE, Kuo PC, Butterly DW, Smith SR, Desai DM. Obesity predicts increased overall complications following pancreas transplantation. Transplant Proc. 2005;37(8):3564–6.

28 Fridell JA, Mangus RS, Taber TE, Goble ML, Milgrom ML, Good J, Vetor R, Powelson JA. Growth of a nation part II: impact of recipient obesity on whole-organ pancreas transplantation. Clin Transplant. 2011 Mar 3 [Epub ahead of print].

29 Sawyer RG, Pelletier SJ, Pruett TL. Increased early morbidity and mortality with acceptable long-term function in severely obese patients undergoing liver transplantation. Clin Transplant. 1999;13(1 Pt 2):126–30.

30 Kanasky WF, Anton SD, Rodriguez JR, Perri MG, Szwed T, Baz MA. Impact of body weight on long-term survival after lung transplantation. Chest. 2002;121(2):401–6.

31 Lederer DJ, Wilt JS, D'Ovidio F, Bacchetta MD, Shah L, Ravichandran S, Lenoir J, Klein B, Sonett JR, Arcasoy SM. Obesity and underweight are associated with an increased risk of death after lunch transplantation. Am J Respir Crit Care Med. 2009;180(9):887–95.

32 Allen JG, Arnaoutakis GJ, Weiss ES, Merlo CA, Conte JV, Shah AS. The impact of recipient body mass index on survival after lung transplantation. J Heart Lung Transplant. 2010;29(9):1026–33.

33 Lease ED, Zaas DW. Complex bacterial infections pre- and posttransplant. Semin Respir Crit Care Med. 2010;31(2):234–42.

34 Russo MJ, Hong KN, Davies RR, Chen JM, Mancini DM, Oz MC, Rose EA, Gelijins A, Naka Y. The effect of body mass index on survival following heart transplantation: do outcomes support consensus guidelines? Ann Surg. 2010;251(1):144–52.

35 Guisado Rasco A, Sobrino Marquez JM, Nevado Portero J, Romero Rodriguez N, Ballesteros Prada S, Lage Galle E. Impact of overweight on survival and primary graft failure after heart transplantation. Transplant Proc. 2010;42(8):3178–80.

36 Arthurs SK, Eid AJ, Deziel PJ, Marshall WF, Cassivi SD, Walker RC, Razonable RR. The impact of invasive fungal diseases after lung transplantation. Clin Transplant. 2010;24(3):341–8.

37 Saner FH, Akkiz H, Canbay A. Infectious complications in the early postoperative period in liver transplant patients. Minerva Gastroenterol Dietol. 2010;56(3):355–65.

38 Lee SO, Razonable RR. Current concepts on cytomegalovirus infection after liver transplantation. World J Hepatol. 2010;2(9):325–36.

39 Nguyen NT, Hinojosa M, Fayad C, Varela E, Wilson SE. Use and outcomes of laparoscopic versus open gastric bypass at academic medical centers. J Am Coll Surg. 2007;205(2):248–55.

40 Cristou NV, Jarand J, Sylvestre JL, McLean AP. Analysis of the incidence and risk factors for wound infections in open bariatric surgery. Obes Surg. 2004;14(1):16–22.

41 Williams MD, Champion JK. Experience with routine intraabdominal cultures during laparoscopic gastric bypass with implications for antibiotic prophylaxis. Surg Endosc. 2004;18(5):755–6.

42 Stenstrom B, Loseth K, Bevanger L, Sturegard E, Wadstrom T, Chen D. Gastric bypass surgery does not increase susceptibility to Helicobacter pylori infection in the stomach of rat or mouse. Inflammopharmacology. 2005;13(1–3):229–34.

43 Papasavas PK, Gagne DJ, Donnelly PE, Salgado J, Urbandt JE, Burton KK, Caushaj PF. Prevalence of Helicobacter pylori infection and value of preoperative testing and treatment in patients undergoing laparoscopic Roux-en-Y gastric bypass. Surg Obes Relat Dis. 2008;4(3):383–8.

44 Bueter M, Maroske J, Thalheimer A, Gasser M, Stingl T, Heimbucher J, Meyer D, Fuchs KH, Fein M. Short- and long-term results of laparoscopic gastric banding for morbid obesity. Langenbecks Arch Surg. 2008;393(2):199–205.

45 V Vachharajani, S. Vital, J. Russell, L.K. Scott, D.N. Granger, Glucocorticoids inhibit the cerebral microvascular dysfunction associated with sepsis in obese mice, Microcirculation. 2006;13:477–87.

46 Ronti T, Lupattelli G, Mannarino E. The endocrine function of adipose tissue: an update. Clin Endocrinol (Oxf). 2006;64(4):355–65.

47 Singer G, Granger DN. Inflammatory responses underlying the microvascular dysfunction associated with obesity and insulin resistance. Microcirculation. 2007;14(4–5):375–87.

48 Goetz AM, Wagener MM, Miller JM. Risk of infection due to central venous catheters: effect of site of placement and catheter type. Infect Control Hosp Epidemiol. 1998;19:842–5.

49 Aggarwal B, Natarajan K. Tumor necrosis factors: developments during the last decade. Eur Cytokine Netw. 1996;7(2):93–124.

50 Wolf AM, Wolf D, Rumpold H, Enrich B, Tilq H. Adiponectin induces the anti-inflammatory cytokines IL-10 and IL-1RA in human leukocytes. Biochem Biophys Res Commun. 2004;323(2):630–5.

51 Zarkesh-Esfahani H, Pockley AG, Wu Z, Hellewell PG, Weetman AP, Ross RJ. Leptin indirectly activates human neutrophils via induction of TNF-alpha. J Immunol. 2004;172(3):1809–14.

52 Pacifico L, Di RL, Anania C, et al. Increased T-helper interferon-gamma-secreting cells in obese children. Eur J Endocrinol. 2006;154:691–7.

53 Lord G, Matarese G, Howard JK, et al. Leptin modulates the T-cell immune response and reverses starvation-induced immunosuppression. Nature. 1998;394:897–901.

54 Sundén-Cullberg J, Nyström T, Lee ML, et al. Pronounced elevation of resistin correlates with severity of disease in

severe sepsis and septic shock. Crit Care Med. 2007;35(6): 1536–42.

55 Kabon B, Nagele A, Reddy D, et al. Obesity decreases perioperative tissue oxygenation. Anesthesiology. 2004;100(2):274–80.

56 Miles A. The value and duration of defense reactions of the skin of the skin to the primary lodgement of bacteria. Br J Exp Pathol. 1957;38:79.

57 Babior B. Oxygen-dependent microbial killing by phagocytes. N Engl J Med. 1978;298:659–68.

58 Jansson P, Larsson A, Smith U, et al. Glycerol production in subcutaneous adipose tissue in lean and obese humans. J Clin Invest. 1992;89(5):1610–17.

59 Di Girolamo M, Skinner NS, Hanley HG, et al. Relationship of adipose tissue blood flow to fat cell size and number. Am J Physiol. 1971;220(4):932–7.

60 O'Grady N, Alexander M, Dellinger EP, et al. Guidelines for the prevention of intravascular catheter-related infections. Centers for Disease Control and Infection, MMWR Recomm Rep. 2002;51(RR-10):1–29.

61 Koenig SM. Pulmonary complications of obesity. Am J Med Sci. 2001;321:249–79.

62 Baik I, Curhan GC, Rimm EB, Bendich A, Willett WC, Fawzi WW. A prospective study of age and lifestyle factors in relation to community-acquired pneumonia in US men and women. Arch Intern Med. 2000;160(20):3082–8.

63 El Solh A, Porhomayon J, Szarpa K. Proinflammatory and phagocytic functions of alveolar macrophages in obesity. Obesity Research and Clinical Practice. 2009;3(4):203–7.

64 Hranjec T, Swenson BR, Sawyer RG. Surgical site infection prevention: how we do it. Surg Infect (Larchmt). 2010;11(3):1–6.

65 Latham R, Lancaster AD, Covington JF, et al. The association of diabetes and glucose control with surgical-site infections among cardiothoracic surgery patients. Infect Control Hosp Epidemiol. 2001;22(10):607–12.

66 Furnary A, Zerr KJ, Grunkemeier GL, et al. Continuous intravenous insulin infusion reduces the incidence of deep sternal wound infection in diabetic patients after cardiac surgical procedures. Ann Thorac Surg. 1999;67(2):352–60.

67 Kurz A, Sessler DI, Lenhardt RA. Study of wound infections and temperature group. Perioperative normothermia to reduce the incidence of surgical-wound infection and shorten hospitalization. N Engl J Med. 1996;334:1209–15.

68 Chang N, Mathes SJ. Comparison of the effect of bacterial inoculation in musculocutaneous and random pattern flaps. Plast Reconstr Surg. 1982;70(1):1–10.

69 Jönsson K, Hunt TK, Mathes SJ. Oxygen as an isolated variable influences resistance to infection. Ann Surg. 1988;208(6):783–7.

70 Classen D, Evans RS, Pestotnik SL, et al. The timing of prophylactic administration of antibiotics and the risk of surgical-wound infection. N Engl J Med. 1992;326(5):281–6.

71 Raad II, Hohn DC, Gilbreath BJ, et al. Prevention of central venous catheter-related infections by using maximal sterile barrier precautions during insertion. Infect Control Hosp Epidemiol. 1994;15:231–8.

72 Chaiyakunapruk N, Veenstra DL, Lipsky BA, et al. Chlorhexidine compared with povidone-iodine solution for vascular catheter-site care: a meta-analysis. Ann Intern Med. 2002;136:792–801.

73 Mermel LA. Prevention of central venous catheter-related infections: what works other than impregnated or coated catheters? J Hosp Infect. 2007;65(Suppl 2):30–3.

74 Widmer AF. Intravenous-related infections. In Wenzel RP, editor. Prevention and Control of Nosocomial Infections. Baltimore, MD, Williams and Wilkins. 1997. pp. 771–806.

75 Gould CV, Umscheid CA, Agarwal RK, et al. Guidelines for prevention of catheter-associated urinary tract infections 2009. Centers for Disease Control and Prevention, Healthcare Infection Control Practices Advisory Committee. 2009. pp. 1–67.

76 Eachempati SR, Hydo LJ, Shou J, et al. Does de-escalation of antibiotic therapy for ventilator-associated pneumonia affect the likelihood of recurrent pneumonia or mortality in critically ill surgical patients? J Trauma Injury, Infection, and Critical Care. 2009;66:1343–8.

77 Hollenstein UM, Brunner M, Schmid R, et al. Soft tissue concentrations of ciprofloxacin in obese and lean subjects following weight-adjusted dosing. Int J Obes Relat Metab Disord. 2001;25:354–8.

78 Pai MP, Bordley J, Amsden GW. Plasma pharmacokinetics and tissue penetration of alatrofloxacin in morbidly obese individuals. Clin Drug Invest. 2001;21:175–81.

79 Meagher AK, Forrest A, Rayner CR, et al. Population pharmacokinetics of linezolid in patients treated in a compassionate-use program. Antimicrob Agents Chemother. 2003; 47:548–53.

80 Stein GE, Schooley SL, Peloquin, KV, et al. Pharmacokinetics and pharmacodynamics of linezolid in obese patients with cellulitis. Ann Pharmacother. 2005;39:427–32.

11 Management of Gastrointestinal Complications in the Critically Ill Obese Patient

Benjamin H. Levy III[1] and David A. Johnson[2]

[1]Department of Internal Medicine, University of Arizona, Tucson, AZ, USA
[2]Eastern Virginia Medical School, Norfolk, VA, USA

KEY POINTS

- Obese patients require special nutrition considerations in the ICU.
- Obese patients in the ICU are particularly more subject to severe erosive esophagitis and related complications of GERD.
- Obesity alone should not serve as a contraindication to liver transplantation.

INTRODUCTION

Obesity is a chronic and stigmatizing condition that has become a major health problem in most industrialized countries because of its prevalence, serious health consequences, and economic impact. Obesity has particular relevance for the gastroenterologist because of its association with a variety of gastrointestinal disorders, specific to the critical care setting, plus the need to assess and to treat postoperative complications in patients who have undergone obesity surgery.

GERD

Epidemiologic experts believe that the increased prevalence of gastroesophageal reflux disease (GERD), erosive esophagitis, Barrett's esophagus, and esophageal adenocarcinoma is directly linked to the obesity epidemic that has been mounting over the past two decades. Three studies have shown a 1.5–3.0-fold increase in reflux symptoms among obese individuals [1]. More seriously, estimates from pooled studies indicate a 2.1-fold increase in esophageal adenocarcinoma in patients with a body mass index (BMI) > 25 compared to individuals with a normal BMI [2].

Critically ill patients have the potential for gastric mucosal breakdown due to intensive care unit (ICU)-related stress, which may exacerbate an esophageal environment of chronic inflammation. Prolonged recumbency and altered esophageal acid clearance may put the obese patient in the ICU at particular risk for severe esophagitis. Treatment with proton pump inhibitors (PPIs) is routinely recommended in the management of these patients to reduce gastric pH and minimize the risk of gastric acid pneumonitis.

UPPER GASTROINTESTINAL BLEEDING AND ENDOSCOPY IN THE ICU

Upper gastrointestinal (UGI) bleeding is a common event in critically ill patients. Optimal therapeutic management requires careful determination of both the bleeding's sources and its characteristics. Complicating conditions include coagulopathy and splanchnic ischemia. Hemostatic disorders and derangements of coagulation factors present considerable problems.

In a Canadian study of over 2000 critically ill patients by Cook and colleagues, approximately 1.5–4% of patients developed clinically significant bleeding with an associated mortality rate of 6–10% [3]. Patients who bled

---

earlier in their ICU stay had a lower chance of dying than patients who bled later. The use of PPIs may decrease the chance of death for critically ill patients despite the fact that it takes approximately 3 days for PPI medication to reach clinically maximum potential [3]. Two robust independent risk factors were identified that place critically ill patients at risk for stress-induced ulcer bleeding: respiratory failure (odds ratio of 15.6) and coagulopathy (odds ratio of 4.3). Aside from the known etiologies of gastrointestinal (GI) bleeding in critically ill patients, obese patients pose additional risks due to the following factors:

1 **History of bariatric surgery** The risk of bleeding after open gastric bypass is reported at 0.6%, while the incidence of hemorrhage after laparoscopic Roux-en-Y gastric bypass (LRYGB) ranges from 1.1 to 4% [4]. This wide range may be due to technical variations, reporting accuracy, or the threshold

parameters used to differentiate bleeding from normal postoperative hemodilution. A review of the literature reveals that stomal ulceration is reported in 2–16% of patients following bariatric surgery [5]. This ulceration is typically due to ischemia at the anastomosis, nonsteroidal antiinflammatory agent (NSAID) use, or both (Figure 11.1). Additionally, these ulcerations may be associated with foreign material (e.g. staples or sutures) (Figure 11.2) at the anastomosis or erosion of mesh into the gastric wall (Figures 11.3 and 11.4). Ulcers can also occur in the native stomach/duodenum – typically due to NSAIDs or *H. pylori* (which should be excluded routinely before gastrojejunal (GJ) bypass is done) (Figure 11.5). This area is difficult if not impossible to visualize with standard endoscopy, limiting both the diagnostic and the therapeutic applications. Use of single- or double-balloon

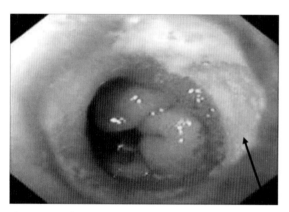

Figure 11.1 Ulcer at GJ anastomosis.

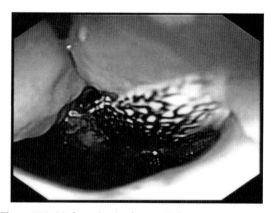

Figure 11.3 Mesh erosion in ulcer at GJ ulceration.

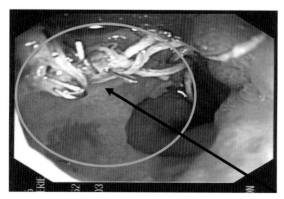

Figure 11.2 Ulcer on jejunal side of GJ anastomosis with visible sutures and staples.

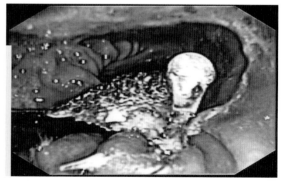

Figure 11.4 Retroflexed view from native stomach (endoscope at 9 o'clock) mesh erosion with disruption of gastric partitioning.

or spiral overtube endoscopy however has been particularly successful (in centers which have this capability) (Figure 11.6).

2 **Use of nonsteroidal anti-inflammatory agents (NSAIDs)** Obese patients may be consuming large amounts of NSAIDs for multiple reasons (e.g. osteoarthritis). The risk of GI bleeding is significantly increased when NSAIDs are combined with other antiplatelet agents (e.g. aspirin or clopidogrel for cardiovascular diseases).

Management priorities include the maintenance of hemodynamic function and the prevention of complications such as pulmonary aspiration. Strategies comprise protection of the airway during massive bleeding, restoration of circulating blood volume, and correction of precipitating conditions. Endoscopy remains the primary diagnostic and therapeutic tool for the management of

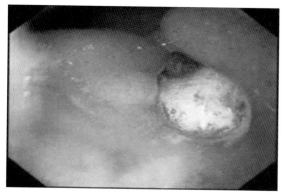

Figure 11.5 Marginal ulcer-NSAID.

GI bleeds. Endoscopy in the obese patients may present unique challenges to the endoscopist. A full understanding of the specific anatomical changes is critical (before the endoscopy is done) to ensure the optimal diagnostic and therapeutic interventions. As many surgeons may vary somewhat from the standard operative changes, it is optimal, whenever possible, to review the surgical records (and if possible speak with the surgeon) prior to any endoscopic evaluation.

Gastroenterologists have often debated whether patients should be intubated prophylacticly for airway protection during an acute UGI hemorrhage. Until recently, there has been a relative lack of medical literature to provide guidance. A study of 307 patients from the Mayo Clinic evaluated the clinical effectiveness of selectively intubating at-risk patients with acute UGI hemorrhage [6]. It concluded that cardiopulmonary complications, duration of ICU stay, and mortality were unaltered by prophylactic intubation. However, additional prospective multicenter studies examining a more diverse patient population should be performed to validate this data. In obese patients, who may be particularly prone to obstructive airway disease or sleep apnea, intubation should be considered for procedures with significant risk of aspiration (high-volume bleed), for lengthy procedures necessitating prolonged sedation, or if the patient is combative or exhibits resistance to standard sedation (e.g. patients taking chronic narcotics or anxiolytics).

The need for operative intervention of acute hemorrhage following gastric bypass depends on the clinical presentation and the timing of presentation. In the comprehensive review by Spaw et al. [7] of acute

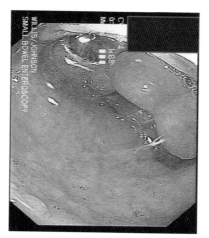

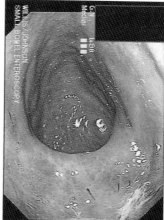

Figure 11.6 Retrograde endoscopy via Roux limb into native stomach (GJ bypass).

bleeding after LRYGB, 89 of 2895 total patients had clinically significant postoperative hemorrhage and only 20% required reoperation. The remainder of patients were successfully managed with observation, resuscitation with fluid and/or blood, and, in some cases, endoscopy. Early surgical intervention should be performed for patients with hemodynamic instability and possibly patients with early onset of hemorrhage (12 hours) after bypass surgery [8]. Some authors propose initial laparoscopy to treat complications with timely progression to laparotomy if laparoscopy fails [9]. Operative therapy is guided by the site of bleeding and may include oversewing of one or all staple lines, gastrotomy (for pouch or excluded stomach) or enterotomy with evacuation of clot, and revision of anastomotic sites.

INTRAABDOMINAL INFECTION

In obese patients, the clinical appearance of intraabdominal infections is usually nonspecific compared to normal-weight patients and radiological imaging rarely helps with diagnosis. This is attributed to the increased layers of fat, which can create imaging artifact. Intraabdominal infections should be suspected in obese ICU patients who show signs of tachycardia, tachypnea, pleural effusion, fevers, or rigors. Prompt initiation of empiric antibiotics following blood cultures can be life-saving.

C. difficile colitis

Clostridium difficile (C. difficile) has become an increasingly prevalent pathogen in ICU patients. C. difficile colitis disease is promoted by broad-spectrum antibiotics, decreased acidity in the GI tract from PPI usage, and horizontal transmission from other infected patients due to improper hand-washing and sanitization techniques. This organism is a gram-positive, spore-forming anaerobic bacillus that can cause acute infection-related colitis. C. difficile is becoming the most common cause of hospital-acquired diarrhea in developed countries [10]. Despite the common practices of isolating patients, donning gowns and gloves, and treating patients with appropriate antibiotics such as metronidazole or oral vancomycin, approximately 20% of patients relapse [4]. Some of these C. difficile relapses are now believed to be caused by an "exogenous strain rather than the original strain" [10]. PPIs are believed to be an important contributor to the C. difficile problem by reducing GI defense mechanisms such as gastric acidity and leukocyte function against ingested spores and bacteria [10].

Recently reported outbreaks in North America and Europe of C. difficile, known as BI/NAP1, are distinguishable from previously identified outbreak (J-type) strains from the late 1980s and early 1990s [11]. The BI/NAP1 strains of C. difficile produce greater amounts of toxins A (TcdA) and B (TcdB) [12] and carry an additional clostridial toxin termed a "binary toxin" [13]. These strains are notably fluoroquinolone resistant.

ELEVATED INTRAABDOMINAL PRESSURE IN OBESE PATIENTS

Intraabdominal hypertension (IAH) is an insidious complication that may necessitate ICU care. This condition occurs when intraabdominal pressures rise by > 12 mm Hg, which may potentiate severe organ dysfunction. IAH can result in decreased flow within the celiac, superior mesenteric, or renal arteries and consequent end-organ damage from hypoperfusion [14]. It can cause small-bowel mucosal tension and create an environment that potentiates bacterial translocation [14]. IAH can lead to abdominal compartment syndrome (ACS), which occurs when intraabdominal pressure exceeds 20 mm Hg. ACS may occur in both medical and surgical patients. An increase in intraperitoneal volume is the most common cause of elevated intraabdominal pressures. Bowel distension, mesenteric venous obstruction, tense ascites (as seen in cirrhotic patients), peritonitis, and intraabdominal tumor are among the other causes of intraperitoneal disorders that can cause ACS. Chronic increases in intraabdominal volume, which occur in morbidly obese patients, may lead to a "stress-relation phenomenon" where organ systems are able to compensate for changes in intraabdominal pressure. As such, acute deterioration in clinical condition may not be recognized promptly in this population [14].

ICU bedside abdominal surgery may be considered if the patient is too unstable for transport to the operating room. Abdominal decompression is the recommended approach in case of impending clinical deterioration. Continuous measurement of urinary bladder pressures (see Table 11.1) should be used for early detection of ACS in at-risk patients, including those with extrinsic compression of the abdomen, those with burn eschars, and those with tight abdominal closures [7].

CHOLELITHIASIS

Obesity is associated with an increased frequency of cholelithiasis. In the Framingham Study, patients > 20% above the median weight for height were twice as likely to develop

Table 11.1 Bladder pressure measurements and management recommendations. (Adopted from [46,47].)

Gade	Bladder pressure in mm Hg	Management recommendation
I	12–15	IAP monitoring and medical attempts to reduce IAP
II	16–20	
III	21–25	Possible surgical decompression, especially if end-organ dysfunction is suspected
IV	>25	After decompression, continue IAP monitoring and medical attempts to reduce IAP

gallstone disease compared to individuals less than 90% of their weight for height [15]. Interestingly, cholelithiasis and cholecystitis may be caused by rapid weight loss due to a related change in the lithogenicity of bile [16].

Critically ill obese patients with multiple comorbidities are predisposed to the development of acalculous cholecystitis – an illness with higher rates of mortality than regular cholecysitits. Acalculous cholecysistis is seen at a higher frequency in patients with trauma [17], severe burns, diabetes, sepsis, AIDS, or patients on mechanical ventilation [18]. The abdominal exam should be focused on palpation of the right upper quadrant to evaluate for the development of gallbladder disease. There may be variability for the presence of the classic "Murphy's sign" due to abdominal-wall fat as well as depressed mentation related to sedation or systemic illness. Abdominal ultrasound, hepatobiliary imino-diacetic acid (HIDA) scans, and computed tomography (CT) scans are commonly used modalities in establishing the diagnosis, although the sensitivity of these tests is variable. In particular, HIDA scans have a lower sensitivity for acute cholecystitis when used in patients with prolonged fasting > 24 hours. Bedside ultrasound is considered the preferred modality. A thickened gallbladder wall (> 3–4 mm) and pericholecystic fluid are considered the hallmarks of the disease. Percutaneous gallbladder drainage and parenteral antibiotics are an alternative approach for patients with suspected acute cholecystitis who are too ill for acute surgical intervention.

NONALCOHOLIC STEATOHEPATITIS

With the increased incidence of obesity worldwide, nonalcoholic fatty liver disease (NAFLD) has become a growing problem. NAFLD is a common and emergent condition now recognized as the most frequent cause of abnormal liver tests, especially in obese individuals [15,19]. It is characterized by a wide spectrum of liver damage, ranging from simple macrovesicular steatosis to nonalcoholic steatohepatitis (NASH), cirrhosis, or liver carcinoma [20,21]. An autopsy study examining hepatic histopathology in obese patients showed that the degree of liver steatosis and inflammation was proportional to the degree of obesity regardless of whether the patient had diabetes as a comorbidity [22]. NAFLD is extremely common among patients undergoing bariatric surgery, ranging from 84 to 96%. Of these patients, 25–55% have NASH, 34–47% have fibrosis, and 2–12% have bridging fibrosis or cirrhosis [22]. Obese patients with metabolic syndrome (hypertension, diabetes, and hyperlipidemia) are more likely to have NASH [23].

CIRRHOSIS AND LIVER FAILURE

Cirrhotic obese patients develop severe complications that necessitate frequent ICU care including GI bleeding, hepatorenal syndrome, bacterial peritonitis, sepsis, and hepatic encephalopathy. Obese cirrhotic patients presenting with NASH-related cirrhosis have a twofold greater risk for spontaneous bacterial peritonitis compared to cirrhotic patients with a viral etiology [24].

Ascites is the most common complication of cirrhosis. If ascites is suspected, abdominal ultrasound is helpful not only in confirming the diagnosis but also in localizing a site for paracentesis. In particular, ultrasound-assisted abdominal paracentesis yields a higher success rate in obese patients than paracentesis directed by physical examination alone. The treatment of ascites is directed at the underlying pathogenesis. Cirrhotic ascites can often be managed with diuretics and sodium restriction. The most successful diuretic regimen is a combination of spironolactone and furosemide. The goal of sodium restriction should be to limit intake to 2000 mg/day. Recent evidence suggests octreotide, administered in combination with midodrine, may improve both renal and systemic hemodynamics in patients with ascites. When performing large-volume paracentesis, an infusion of 6–8 g of albumin per liter removed prevents the development of paracentesis-induced circulatory dysfunction often associated with large fluid shifts. Obese patients presenting with GI hemorrhage, cirrhosis, and known or suspected ascites should receive parenteral antibiotics (typically with ceftriaxone) as the infection risk for spontaneous bacterial peritonitis is high in these patients. These recommendations are based upon a mortality benefit that was demonstrated in randomized controlled trials [25].

The prevalence of hepatorenal syndrome in obese cirrhotic patients is unknown. Irrespective of the underlying etiology, hepatorenal syndrome portends a poor prognosis. However, before making the diagnosis, reversible prerenal azotemia should be ruled out. Various therapeutic regimens have been described but their efficacy has never been confirmed in randomized trials. At the present, liver transplantation offers the best treatment.

Acute liver failure (ALF) is a devastating clinical syndrome associated with high mortality in obese patients. Several studies have recently demonstrated that a high BMI is associated with a preexisting liver damage. Such damage can manifest as steatosis and obviously corresponds to an increasingly poor outcome in patients with ALF [26,27]. However, these statements should be viewed with caution as these studies had significant design limitations and included small numbers of patients.

PANCREATITIS

Several clinical investigations showed that obesity increases the severity of the disease by favoring local complications within the pancreas and injuries in remote organs as well as by increasing the mortality rate [28,29]. Obesity increases the incidence of early shock, renal and pulmonary failure [30], and extends the hospital stay [31]. Yet other studies have questioned such findings [32,33].

The mechanisms by which obesity increases the severity of acute pancreatitis are unclear, but one hypothesis might be that obese patients have an increased inflammatory response within the pancreas [34]. Serum concentrations of interleukin-1α (IL-1α), IL-1 receptor antagonist (IL1-ra), IL-6, IL-8, IL-10, and IL-12p70 were significantly increased in obese patients with acute pancreatitis as compared to nonobese [34]. Increased levels of free fatty acid levels (but not leptin) correlated with higher severity of acute pancreatitis [35,36]. Another hypothesis stipulates that pancreatic microcirculation is lower in obese than in nonobese patients, which increases the risk of ischemic injury and subsequent local infections. Moreover, obese patients may be immunodeficient, a condition that predisposes to local infections [37].

The presence of metabolic syndrome with hypertension, hyperlipidemia, and diabetes complicates the management of the obese patient with pancreatitis. The initial management involves aggressive volume

Table 11.2 Atlanta Criteria of Severity.

Cardiovascular shock	SBP < 90 mm Hg
Pulmonary insufficiency	$PaO_2 < 60$
Renal failure	Serum creatinine > 2 mg/dl
GI bleeding	> 500 mL in 24 hours
Necrosis	> 3 cm or > 30%
Abscess	Any abscess
Pseudocyst	Any pseudocyst

support and monitoring for progressive complications of organ failure and pancreatic necrosis. The Atlanta Criteria of Severity (Table 11.2) may also be used to help predict which obese patients should be triaged for ICU care [38]. Furthermore, Ranson criteria of 3 or more or an APCHE II of 8 or more serve as unfavorable early predictors of severe pancreatitis. Patients should have an abdominal ultrasound scan performed within 24 hours of admission to exclude gallstones, and those with signs of biliary sepsis or obstruction (with or without sepsis) should undergo urgent endoscopic retrograde cholangiopancreatography (ERCP) and sphincterotomy. A CT abdomen with contrast is performed to differentiate interstitial from necrotizing pancreatitis and may be of greatest value 2–3 days after the start of illness. Clinical suspicion of infected necrosis should prompt urgent CT-guided fine-needle aspiration for microscopy and culture and initiation of broad-spectrum intravenous antibiotics until microbiological results are available. Infected necrosis invariably requires drainage or removal of infected tissue and numerous approaches are described, including percutaneous radiological drainage, endoscopic drainage, minimally invasive surgery, and extensive open debridement.

ABDOMINAL TRAUMA

The Hybrid III crash test dummy used by the automotive industry to test automotive safety has been used to account for the disparity in injury specifics and severity among obese patients. Two separate research studies led by Boulanger in 1992 and Choban in 1991 showed that a higher BMI was less likely to be associated with abdominal injuries in car accidents [39]. Obesity may be a protective factor that mitigates the potential for gastrointestinal injuries requiring ICU care; however, obese patients are more likely to suffer rib fractures, pulmonary contusions, and pelvic fractures [39].

ADIPOSIS DOLORSA

Obese patients may also suffer from adiposis dolorsa, a painful disorder characterized by pain upon palpation of subcutaneous fat [40]. This diagnosis is almost always missed unless a physician is educated enough to specifically seek it out. The pain can be incredibly severe and debilitating. In adiposis dolorosa, the pain usually presents as abdominal pain, flank pain, or occasionally pain radiating across the back [40]. Typically, potent analgesics do not provide adequate relief of the pain. These patients frequently receive unnecessary exploratory laparotomy or gallbladder surgery because the abdominal pain is usually suggestive of an underlying intraabdominal gastrointestinal pathology, yet the etiology is causally related to the extraneous subcutaneous fat.

Adiposis dolorosa has been shown to respond to intravenous lidocaine, but sometimes requires multiple infusions for permanent relief [40]. The physical finding of Carnett's sign may be quite helpful in discriminating abdominal-wall tenderness from intraabdominal etiology of pain. "Carnett's sign" refers to increased local tenderness during muscle tensing [41]. While supine, the patient is asked to perform a straight-leg-raising maneuver (raising both legs off the table at the same time) while the examining finger is on the painful site. Raising only the head while in the supine position can serve the same purpose. These maneuvers tighten the rectus abdominis muscles, increasing the pain from the entrapped nerve. Conversely, true visceral sources of pain are associated with less tenderness when abdominal muscles are tense. The sensitivity and specificity of the Carnett's sign have not been well established. Carnett's sign may not be interpretable in patients who cannot comply adequately with leg or head-raising maneuvers. False positive results may occur from visceral causes of pain that involve the local parietal peritoneum [40,41].

BARIATRIC SURGERY

Bariatric surgery has become an increasingly popular weight-loss option for morbidly obese patients over the past 10–15 years. Close monitoring in an intensive care setting may be warranted during the first 24 hours as anastamosis leaks or intraabdominal infections can first be detected during this period [42]. Morbidly obese patients may not exhibit the classic signs and symptoms of peritonitis. Worrisome signs include a heart rate > 120, temperature of >102 °F (39 °C), patient restlessness, and

tenesemus [42]. Barium swallow studies are helpful for detecting anastamotic leaks, but the sensitivity is variable [42]. Direct communication with the radiologist to alert them about specific concerns is crucial to making an accurate diagnosis. The use of water-soluble gastrografin initially, followed with dilute barium if no leak is evident, provides better coating of the mucosa and an enhanced sensitivity for perforation/leaks. Early identification and management of a perforation is critically important given the extremely high rate of morbidity/mortality, which is particularly related to delayed recognition/treatment of this complication.

Intraabdominal infections after bariatric surgery are usually caused by either secondary peritonitis or intracavitary abscess [43]. For patients with secondary peritonitis, surgical treatment should be focused upon eliminating the contaminant, drainage of established abscesses, intense cavity washing, and primary fascia closing [43].

Metabolic complications in the post-bariatric patient

Due to the alterations in anatomy, there are clear risks for post-bariatric surgery patients to develop both macro- and micronutrient and trace element deficiencies [44]. Physicians who care for these patients need to be familiar with the common postoperative syndromes that result from these deficiencies. Nutritional consequences of bariatric surgery can include anemia, edema, and a range of neuological, visual, and dermatological disorders. Thiamine (vitamin B1) deficiency is a major nutritional complication in these patients, particularly after a Roux-en-Y gastric bypass. Although thiamine deficiency was originally described in patients with multiorgan involvement, this deficiency can be protean in the post-bariatric surgery patient and present with cardiac, gastrointestinal, or neuropsychiatric symptoms. The test of choice is whole-blood thiamine – not a general thiamine level, which may be misleading [44]. Acute psychosis and Wernicke's encephalopathy are potential sequalae of thiamine deficiency. Thiamine should ALWAYS be given before glucose, given the possible precipitation of a Wernicke's encephalopathy [44]. As for macronutrient deficiencies, serum albumin concentrations cannot discriminate between well and malnourished patients [45]. Physicians who care for post-bariatric patients need to always consider metabolic and nutritional complications on presentation as a primary or component manifestation of any critical illness.

CONCLUSION

Morbid obesity is associated with significant gastrointestinal complications that require ICU care. The manifestations of GI complications in critically ill morbidly obese patients can be subtle and may not conform to the typical presentations seen in nonobese patients. A high index of suspicion should be maintained to ensure satisfactory outcome.

BEST PRACTICE TIPS

1 Critically ill obese patients should be kept on PPI or H_2 blocker therapy whenever possible in order to prevent stress-induced ulcer bleeding. This is particularly applicable to patients on ventilators or with coagulopathy.

2 In order to promote nitrogen equilibrium, many nutritionists recommend a low-caloric high-protein diet for obese patients in the ICU.

3 The Atlanta Criteria of Severity may also be used to help predict which obese patients with pancreatitis should be triaged for ICU care.

4 In obese patients, the clinical manifestations of intraabdominal infections are nonspecific compared to normal-weight patients. Radiological imaging may not be as sensitive or specific in this cohort. Physicians should have a low threshold for placing bariatric surgery postoperative patients in the ICU for close monitoring, especially if anastamosis leaks or intraabdominal infection are suspected.

5 Intraabdominal pressures can be approximated using a Foley catheter to measure urinary bladder pressure. Bladder pressures > 21 mm Hg should be closely monitored and surgical decompression should be considered.

REFERENCES

1 Yamada T, Alpers D, Kalloo A, Kaplowitz N, Owyang C, Powell D. Textbook of Gastroenterology. 5 edn. Chichester, UK, Blackwell Publishing. 2009. pp. 2564–6.

2 Anand G, Katz PO. Gastroesophgeal reflux disease and obesity. Gastroenterol Clin NA. 2010;39(1):39–46.

3 Ali T, Harty R. Stress-induced ulcer bleeding in critically ill patients. Gastroenterol Clin NA. 2009;38:245–365.

4 Nguyen N, Longoria M, Chalifoux S, Wilson S. Gastrointestinal hemorrhage after laparoscopic gastric bypass. Obes Surg. 2004;14(10):1308–12.

5 Schreiner MA, Fennerty MD. Endoscopy in the obese patient. Gastroenterol Clin NA. 2010;39(1):87–95.

6 Rehman A, Iscimen R, Yilmaz M, et al. Prophylactic endotracheal intubation in critically ill patients undergoing endoscopy for upper GI hemorrhage. Gastrointest Endosc. 2009;69(7):55.

7 Spaw A, Husted J. Bleeding after laparoscopic gastric bypass: case report and literature review. Surg Obes Relat Dis. 2005;1(2):99–103.

8 Nguyen N, Rivers R, Wolf B. Early gastrointestinal hemorrhage after laparoscopic gastric bypass. Obes Surg. 2003;13(1):62–5.

9 Papasavas P, Caushaj P, McCormick J, et al. Laparoscopic management of complications following laparoscopic Roux-en-Y gastric bypass for morbid obesity. Surg Endosc. 2003;17(4):610–14.

10 Aseeri M, Schroeder T, Kramer J, Zackula R, et al. Gastric acid suppression by proton pump inhibitors as a risk factor for Clostridium difficile associated diarrhea in hospitalized patients. Am J Gastroenterol. 2008;103:2308–13.

11 Samore M, Killgore G, Johnson S, et al. Multicenter typing comparison of sporadic and outbreak Clostridium difficile isolates from geographically diverse hospitals. J Infect Dis. 1997;176:1233–8.

12 Warny M, Pepin J, Fang A, et al. Toxin production by an emerging strain of Clostridium difficile associated with outbreaks of severe disease in North America and Europe. Lancet. 2005;366:1079–84.

13 McDonald LC, Killgore GE, Thompson A, et al. An epidemic, toxin gene variant strain of Clostridium difficile. N Engl J Med. 2005;353:2433–4.

14 Cleva, R, Silva F, Silberstein B, Machado D. Acute renal failure due to abdominal compartment syndrome: report on four cases and literature review. Revista do Hospital das Clinicas. 2001 Jul–Aug;56(4):123–30.

15 Festi D, Colecchia A, Sacco T, Bondi M, Roda E, Marchesini G. Hepatic steatosis in obese patients: clinical aspests and prognostic significance. Obesity Reviews. 2004;5(1):27–42.

16 Kopelman P, Stock M. Clinical Obesity. Oxford, Blackwell Sciences. 1998. p. 581.

17 Hamp T, Fridrich P, Mauritz W, Hamid L, Pelinka LE. Cholecystitis after trauma. J Trauma. 2009 Feb;66(2):400–6.

18 Theodorou P, Maurer CA, Spanholtz TA, et al. Acalculous cholecystitis in severely burned patients: incidence and predisposing factors. Burns. 2009;35(3):405–11.

19 Kowdley KV, Caldwell S. Nonalcoholic steatohepatitis: a twenty-first century epidemic? J Clin Gastroenterol. 2006;40(Suppl 1):S2–4.

20 Clark JM. The epidemiology of nonalcoholic fatty liver disease in adults. J Clin Gastroenterol. 2006;40(Suppl 1):S5–10.

21 Raman M, Allard J. Nonalcoholic fatty liver disease: a clinical approach and review. Can J Gastroenterol. 2006;20(5):345–9.

22 Kaplowitz, N. Liver and biliary diseases. Baltimore, MD, Williams and Wilkens. 1996. pp. 446–50.

23 Diehl AM. Hepatic complications of obesity. Gastrointest Clin NA. 2010;39(1):57–68.

24 Sorrentino P, Tarantino G, Conca P, Perrela A, Perrela O. Clinical presentation and prevalence of spontaneous bacterial peritonitis in patients with cryptogenic cirrhosis and

features of metabolic syndrome. Can J Gastroenterol. 2004 Jun;18(6):381–6.

25 Fernández, J, Ruiz del Arbol, L, Gómez, C, et al. Norfloxacin vs ceftriaxone in the prophylaxis of infections in patients with advanced cirrhosis and hemorrhage. Gastroenterology. 2006;131:1049–55.

26 Rutherford A, Davern T, Hay JE, Murray NG, Hassanein T, Lee WM, Chung RT. Influence of high body mass index on outcome in acute liver failure. Clin Gastroenterol Hepatol. 2006;4:1544–9.

27 Canbay A, Chen S, Gieseler RK, Malago M, Karliova M, Gerken G, Broelsch CE, Treichel U. Overweight patients are more susceptible for acute liver failure. Hepatogastroenterology. 2005;52:1516–20.

28 Gabrielli A, et al. Civetta, Taylor, & Kirby's Critical Care. 3 edn. Philadelphia, PA, Lippincott Williams and Wilkins. 1997. pp. 2326–7.

29 Blomgren KB, Sundstrom A, Steineck G, Wiholm BE. Obesity and treatment of diabetes with glyburide may both be risk factors for acute pancreatitis. Diab Care. 2002;25:298–302.

30 Lankisch PG, Schirren CA. Increased body weight as a prognostic parameter for complications in the course of acute pancreatitis. Pancreas. 1990;5:626–9.

31 Blomgren KB, Sundström A, Steineck G, Wiholm BE. Obesity and treatment of diabetes with glyburide may both be risk factors for acute pancreatitis. Diabetes Care. 2002;25:298–302.

32 Stimac D, Krznarić Zrnić I, Radic M, Zuvic-Butorac M. Outcome of the biliary acute pancreatitis is not associated with body mass index. Pancreas. 2007;34:165–6; author reply 166–7.

33 Tsai CJ. Is obesity a significant prognostic factor in acute pancreatitis? Dig Dis Sci. 1998;43:2251–4.

34 Sempere L, Martinez J, de Madaria E, Lozano B, Sanchez-Paya J, Jover R, Perez-Mateo M. Obesity and fat distribution imply a greater systemic inflammatory response and a worse prognosis in acute pancreatitis. Pancreatology. 2008;8:257–64.

35 Mentula P, Kylanpaa ML, Kemppainen E, Puolakkainen P. Obesity correlates with early hyperglycemia in patients with

acute pancreatitis who developed organ failure. Pancreas. 2008;36:1.

36 Tukiainen E, Kylanpaa ML, Ebeling P, Kemppainen E, Puolakkainen P, Repo H. Leptin and adiponectin levels in acute pancreatitis. Pancreas. 2006;32:211–14.

37 Lamas O, Marti A, Martínez JA. Obesity and immunocompetence. Eur J Clin Nutr. 2002;56(Suppl 3):S42–5.

38 Banks P, Freeman ML, Practice Parameters Committee of the American College of Gastroenterology. Practice guidelines in acute pancreatitis. American J Gastroenterol. 2006;101:2379–400.

39 Joshi M, Bochicchio K, Nehman S, Tracy JK, Scalea TM. Impact of obesity in the critically ill trauma patient: a prospective study. J Am Coll Surg. 2006:203–4:533–8.

40 Wadden T, Tunkard A. Handbook of Obesity Treatment. New York, Guilford Press. 2002. pp. 180–2.

41 Carnett, JB. Intercostal neuralgia as a cause of abdominal pain and tenderness. Surg Gynecol Obstet. 1926;42:625–30.

42 Lopez J, Sung J, Anderson W, Stone J, Gallagher S, Shapiro D, Rosemurgy A, Murr MM. Is bariatric surgery safe in academic centers? Am Surg. 2002;68:820–3.

43 Pitombo C, Jones K, Higa K, Pareja J. Obesity Surgery Principals and Practice. New York, McGraw-Hill. 2007. pp. 298–303.

44 Koch TR, Finelli FC. Postoperative metabolic and nutritional complications of bariatric surgery. Gastrointest Clin NA. 2010;39(1):109–24.

45 Mason ME, Jalagani H, Vinik A. Metabolic complications of bariatric surgery: diagnosis and management issues. Gastrointest Clin NA. 2005;34(1):25–34.

46 Zenilman M, Timoney M. How we manage abdominal compartment syndrome. Available at: http://www.contemporarysurgery.com/inside.asp?ArtID=6798 [Accessed January 11, 2011.]

47 Malbrain ML, Cheatham M, Kirkpatrick A, et al. Results from the international conference of experts on intra-abdominal hypertension and abdominal compartment syndrome. Surg Gynecol Obstet. 1990;170(1):25–31.

12 Management of Endocrine Complications in the Critically Ill Obese Patient

Joseph Varon[1] and Ilse M. Espina[2]

[1]Critical Care Services, University General Hospital; The University of Texas Health Science Center at Houston; The University of Texas Medical Branch at Galveston Houston, TX, USA

[2]Dorrington Medical Associates, Houston, TX, USA; Universidad Popular Autónoma del Estado de Puebla, Puebla, Mexico

---

KEY POINTS
- Adipose tissue is an endocrine organ that regulates metabolism.
- Glucose control should only be achieved with intravenous insulin.
- Nutrition should not be withheld in obese patients to avoid protein energy malnutrition.

INTRODUCTION

Morbid obesity is one of the major health issues worldwide leading to a decreased life expectancy [1]. Obese and morbidly obese patients have an increased risk of higher morbidity and mortality from many acute and chronic medical conditions; among the most commonly observed are hypertension, dyslipidemia, vascular disease, type 2 diabetes mellitus, respiratory problems, and some types of cancer. These medical comorbidities often complicate their clinical status during a critical illness [2,3]. Endocrine disorders are fairly common in this population. In a cohort of morbidly obese patients scheduled for bariatric surgery, the overall prevalence of endocrine diseases in morbidly obese patients was 47.4%, excluding type 2 diabetes mellitus. The prevalence of primary hypothyroidism was reported at 18.1%, while pituitary disease and Cushing's syndrome were observed in 1.9 and 0.8%, respectively. Remarkably, the prevalence of newly diagnosed endocrine disorders was 16.3% (see Figure 12.1) [4].

THE FAT TISSUE AS AN ENDOCRINE ORGAN

Historically, adipose tissue was thought to be an inert tissue that solely stores energy and protects the body from temperature and injury. Contrary to this concept, it is now evident that adipose tissue is a dynamic endocrine organ responsible for the secretion of many kinds of adipocytokines, such as adiponectin, leptin, IL-6, and TNF-α, that may affect metabolism, body-weight regulation, and glucose and lipid homeostasis [5,6]. Adipocytes also secrete acute phase proteins such as amyloid A, haptoglobin, PAI-1, and ASP. Adipokines such as leptin, resistin, vascular endothelial growth factor (VEGF), and nerve growth factor (NGF) also play a role in inflammation. The concentration of these proinflammatory cytokines increases along with the growth of fat body mass. Further, the function of macrophages and adipocytes in obese patients is altered, resulting in impaired expression of these cytokines and adipokines [7,8].

GLUCOSE CONTROL

Adipokines are an important determinant of insulin sensitivity and thus a potential link between obesity and insulin resistance [9–11]. The first data about the physiological role of leptin and its significance in the development of insulin resistance come from studies in animals lacking this hormone. However, it is not the absolute deficiency of leptin that causes obesity but rather

---

Critical Care Management of the Obese Patient, First Edition. Edited by Ali A. El Solh.
© 2012 John Wiley & Sons, Ltd. Published 2012 by John Wiley & Sons, Ltd.

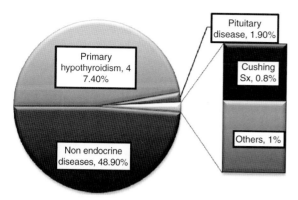

Figure 12.1 Prevalence of endocrine diseases (not including type 2 diabetes mellitus) in patients scheduled for bariatric surgery.

Table 12.1 International recommendations for glucose control in adult nondiabetic critically ill patients.

Avoid severe hyperglycemia (>10 mmol/l or 180 mg/dl) in adult ICU patients
Avoid large variations in glucose levels in ICU
The only drug recommended is intravenous insulin for glucose control
Perform glucose measurements in the laboratory
In descendent order, recommend arterial, venous, capillary samples for glucose monitoring

the lack of sensitivity to its action [12]. In fact, obese people have a higher concentration of leptin, which at the same time seems not to show the desirable anorexic effect because of leptin resistance. Disorders of transport to the brain and the presence of antileptin antibodies or leptin antagonists are considered as possible mechanisms [13], but the exact mechanism of leptin resistance is still unknown. Both leptin and insulin acting at the level of the central nervous system decrease food intake and increase energy expenditure. Insulin stimulates production of leptin by influencing glucose metabolism. Leptin, via a negative feedback, decreases the secretion of insulin and inhibits expression of its gene. Dysregulation of the adipocyte–insulin axis leads to hyperinsulinemia, which stimulates adipogenesis, causing a further increase in insulin secretion.

Adiponectin, on the other hand, improves insulin sensitivity and blood lipid levels. An inverse correlation between serum concentrations of adiponectin and insulin resistance has been found in obese and in diabetes type 2 patients [14–16]. In critically ill patients, the attenuated adrenal response reduces the secretion of adiponectin, which contributes to the state of hyperglycemia in the intensive care unit (ICU) setting [17]. Resistin is an adipocytokine that has been has been linked to obesity, type 2 diabetes, inflammation, and atherosclerosis, but the results of animal and human studies have been controversial. Resistin may represent a link between obesity and insulin resistance via proinflammatory pathways. Visfatin, also called pre-B-cell colony enhancing factor, is a newer adipocytokine that has been shown to exert insulin-mimetic effects. It has also been implicated in angiogenesis [18]. The proposed role of visfatin in obesity-related disorders still remains largely unknown, with a large potential for future research.

Additionally, increased concentration of interleukin-6 and TNF-α amplifies insulin resistance [12]. The administration of TNF-α inhibitors (etanercept, infliximab, and adalimumab) in clinical practice has led to improved control of inflammation in rheumatoid diseases. However, administration of these antibodies to obese patients with type 2 diabetes does not influence insulin resistance [19,20].

During acute illness, stress and exuberant inflammatory responses worsen hyperglycemia in critically ill obese patients. Cortisol is considered the main culprit although other stress hormones (i.e. catecholamines, glucagon, and growth hormone) play a role in the resulting hyperglycemia [21,22]. Control of glucose levels, rather than insulin administration itself, was associated with 43% reduction in intensive care mortality risk [23]. Interestingly, an analysis of a database of more than 250000 patients showed that the relationship between blood glucose and mortality was strongest after acute myocardial infarction, arrhythmia, unstable angina, or pulmonary embolism [24]. Two large-scale prospective randomized international trials could not reproduce the results of the Leuven I study advocating strict blood sugar control in the ICU [25–27]. Two subsequent metaanalyses reiterated the lack of benefit of tight glucose control by intensive insulin therapy compared to a more conservative approach [28,29]. As a consequence, the guidelines for glucose control recommend that blood glucose be kept below 180 mg/dl (10.0 mmol/l) (see Table 12.1) [27]. These recommendations are applicable to both obese and nonobese patients.

The presence of hypoglycaemia at the time of admission or during critical illness is also associated with increased mortality [30]. Analysis of a five-year database from the Australian and New Zealand Intensive Care Society including 66 184 adult admissions reported that the presence of early hypoglycemia is common and associated with lower survival rates [31]. High early blood glucose variability (that is, during the first 24 hours of

ICU stay) was also associated with higher adjusted ICU and hospital mortality.

ROUX-EN-Y GASTRIC BYPASS SURGERY AND DIABETES

The intestine, besides its digestive and absorptive capabilities, also plays a key role in the regulation of glycemic control [32]. In general, Roux-en-Y gastric bypass (RYGB) surgery produces a greater reduction in body weight compared with adjustable gastric banding (BND). After the RYGB, diabetic obese patients experience drastic improvement in their glycemic control [33], while 99–100% of those with glucose intolerance halt their progression to overt diabetes [34]. This phenomenon cannot be fully attributed to the weight loss and reduced caloric intake. These different outcomes, and the observation that insulin therapy may often be discontinued shortly after surgery, prior to significant weight loss, beg the question whether improved insulin sensitivity may be a function of the type of bariatric procedure in addition to the degree of weight loss. There are several mechanisms thought to be responsible for the antidiabetic action of the RYGB; RYGB subjects exhibit an exaggerated GLP-1 response and a suppression of gastric inhibitory polypeptide (GIP) secretion after administration of a test meal [33,35,36]. GLP-1 is an incretin that increases glucose tolerance by enhancing insulin secretion, suppressing glucagon secretion, and inhibiting gastric emptying [37,38]. After bypass, nutrients pass directly from the gastric pouch to the distal small intestine. Thus, delivery of concentrated nutrients to L-cells in the distal small intestine where GLP-1 is primarily produced may enhance GLP-1 secretion, as was described after jejunoileal bypass and total gastrectomy [39,40]. It has also been shown that postprandial levels of peptide YY (PYY), which is also produced by L-cells, are enhanced after RYGB compared with BND and body mass index (BMI)-matched controls [41]. Since GIP is synthesized primarily in the proximal small intestine, diversion of nutrients from this segment would be expected to reduce postprandial GIP levels.

THYROID FUNCTION

Morbid obesity is associated with thyroid function disturbances and a high rate of subclinical hypothyroidism. Although the range of thyroid hormone (TH) values may vary in different populations (regarding, for instance, dietary iodine intake or other factors), the usual finding is that thyroid-stimulating hormone (TSH) levels correlate with body weight [42,43]. Remarkably, thyroid autoimmunity is not the cause of high levels of TSH in morbidly obese patient [44]. The moderate increase of TSH levels is usually not associated with changes in free and total T4 in obesity. In contrast to free and total T4, the moderate increase of TSH levels is associated with moderately increased free T3 (fT3) and total T3 levels, as well as an increased thyroid volume in obesity [45,46].

Critical illness can induce many abnormalities of the hypothalamic–pituitary–thyroid axis, including diminished thyrotropin (TSH) release, reduced levels of tri-iodothyronine (T3) or thyroxine (T4), reduced thyroid-binding globulin (TBG) levels, and peripheral TH resistance. These abnormalities are referred to as the "sick euthyroid syndrome" or "nonthyroidal illness syndrome" (NTIS), an interchangeable terminology, and are characterized by low TH levels in the setting of systemic illness [47]. One hypothesis suggests that the low TH concentrations that are observed during nonthyroidal illness are a physiological response to stress and serve to decrease unnecessary energy expenditure [48]. The NTIS may also represent a maladaptive response that threatens tissue function [49]. Unfortunately, the disturbance of the hypothalamic–pituitary–thyroid axis in critically ill morbidly obese patients has not been investigated. It is worth pointing out however the following observations. In critically ill obese patients with concomitant hypothyroidism, the administration of higher doses of L-thyroxine might be necessary in order to keep TSH levels within the normal values [50]. One could argue that levothyroxine therapy in the sick euthyroid syndrome would be unlikely to have any effect because of the pronounced inhibition of conversion of T4 to T3 in the patients, which would prevent significant increases in serum T3 concentrations. Despite the poor prognosis of ICU patients with the sick euthyroid syndrome, it does not appear that treatment with either levothyroxine or LT$_3$ provides any benefit to these patients [51]. One extremely rare complication of hypothyroidism that can develop in the obese and morbidly obese critically ill patient is cardiac tamponade due to pericardial effusion. This should be suspected in subjects that present with increased TSH levels, hypotension, relative bradycardia, and an increased creatine kinase (CK) level [52]. In addition, hypothyroidism may be associated with failure to wean from mechanical ventilation and increases the complications or worsens the clinical condition overall. A close and routine monitoring for evidence of thyroid malfunction is essential with the critically ill obese patient [53].

ADRENAL INSUFFICIENCY

The mechanisms leading to dysfunction of the hypothalamic–pituitary–adrenal (HPA) axis during critical illness are poorly understood, and include decreased production of CRH, ACTH, and cortisol, as well as their receptors. TNF-α and interleukin-1 have been implicated in the reversible dysfunction of the HPA axis during critical illness [54,55]. Interleukin-1 has been demonstrated to decrease glucocorticoid receptor translocation and transcription [56]. Decreased affinity of the glucocorticoid receptor from mononuclear leukocytes of patients with sepsis has also been reported [57]. Low high-density lipoprotein (HDL) levels have shown to be an important risk factor for the development of adrenal insufficiency in ICU patients and increased morbidity and mortality [58,59]. Of interest, obese patients generally have higher lipid and lipoprotein concentrations than their leaner counterparts. These observations have led to speculation about improved survival of obese patients during critical care hospitalization [60].

The use of moderate-dose glucocorticoids in patients with septic shock, severe sepsis, and acute respiratory distress syndrome (ARDS) is controversial, and the risks and benefits of this therapy continue to be explored. Analyses of six randomized controlled trials evaluating "moderate-dose" hydrocortisone in septic shock have demonstrated greater shock reversal (at day 7); however, the benefit in terms of mortality is less clear [61–63].

If adrenal insufficiency in critical illness is identified, an immediate corticosteroid replacement therapy should be started. Dexamethasone is no longer the drug of choice due to its prolonged suppression of the HPA axis and because of its lack of significant benefit in the absence of an ACTH stimulation test. Glucocorticoid administration in patients undergoing stressful situations should be proportional to the amount of stress and the known glucocorticoid production rate associated with it [64]. Mineralocorticoid replacement is seldom necessary in the acute setting, but electrolyte and fluid status should be followed closely. Once the patient is stable and no longer in need of vasopressor therapy, steroids may be discontinued or tapered.

A recent report found that ACTH levels are significantly increased after RYGB, along with a concomitant increase of corticosterone levels [35]. One of the possible explanations for the increased ACTH levels after RYGB is the reduced leptin levels after surgery, which decrease the tonic inhibitory effect of this hormone on the HPA axis.

CONCLUSION

Critical illness due to sepsis, trauma, surgery, organ failure, or burns is associated with dramatic effects on most hormonal axes. There are also significant adverse associations of adipocytokines and inflammatory markers with multiple endocrine complications of obesity. In critical illness, uniform (predominantly hypothalamic) suppression of the (neuro)endocrine axes contributes to the low serum levels of the respective target-organ hormones. Endocrine replacement/manipulation in critical illness is controversial. Future studies will hopefully further clarify the impact of endocrine replacement on morbidity and mortality in critically ill obese patients.

> **BEST PRACTICE TIPS**
> 1 Obese and morbidly obese patients may have serious metabolic and endocrine complications.
> 2 Obesity reduction surgery may place the patient in the ICU for a variety of reasons. These procedures are associated with a variety of metabolic changes.
> 3 Glycemic control in the obese and morbidly obese patient in the ICU is no different than for nonobese patients.
> 4 Thyroid disorders are frequent in the obese patient and in some cases may have life-threatening presentations (e.g. pericardial tamponade).
> 5 Underfeeding in these patients is a common mistake that clinicians make and must be discouraged, as obese critically ill patients require aggressive nutritional support.

REFERENCES

1 Olshansky SJ, Passaro DJ, Hershow RC, Layden J, Carnes BA, Brody J, et al. A potential decline in life expectancy in the United States in the 21st century. N Engl J Med. 2005;352(11):1138–45.

2 Levin PD, Weissman C. Obesity, metabolic syndrome, and the surgical patient. Med Clin North Am. 2009; 93(5):1049–63.

3 Health implications of obesity. National Institutes of Health Consensus Development Conference Statement. Ann Intern Med. 1985;103(6 (Pt 2)):1073–7.

4 Fierabracci P, Pinchera A, Martinelli S, Scartabelli G, Salvetti G, Giannetti M, et al. Prevalence of endocrine diseases in morbidly obese patients scheduled for bariatric surgery: beyond diabetes. Obes Surg. 2011;21(1):54–60.

5 Friedman JM. Obesity in the new millennium. Nature. 2000;404(6778):632–4.

6 Libby P, Okamoto Y, Rocha VZ, Folco E. Inflammation in atherosclerosis: transition from theory to practice. Circ J. 2010;74(2):213–20.

7 Fonseca-Alaniz MH, Takada J, Alonso-Vale MI, Lima FB: Adipose tissue as an endocrine organ: from theory to practice. J Pediatr (Rio J). 2007;83(Suppl 5):S192–203.

8 Kershaw EE, Flier JS. Adipose tissue as an endocrine organ. J Clin Endocrinol Metab. 2004;89(6):2548–56.

9 Hillenbrand A, Knippschild U, Weiss M, Schrezenmeier H, Henne-Bruns D, Huber-Lang M, et al. Sepsis induced changes of adipokines and cytokines: septic patients compared to morbidly obese patients. BMC Surg. 2010;10:26.

10 Bahia L, Aguiar LG, Villela N, Bottino D, Godoy-Matos AF, Gelonese B, et al. Relationship between adipokines, inflammation, and vascular reactivity in lean controls and obese subjects with metabolic syndrome. Clinics (Sao Paulo). 2006;61(5):433–40.

11 Pittas AG, Joseph NA, Greenberg AS. Adipocytokines and insulin resistance. J Clin Endocrinol Metab. 2004;89(2): 447–52.

12 Hahn S, Tan S, Janssen O. Leptin: Neuroendokrine Wirkungen und Einflüsse auf den menstruellen Zyklus. Gynecol Endocrinol. 2006;4(1):33–8.

13 Howard JK, Cave BJ, Oksanen LJ, Tzameli I, Bjorbaek C, Flier JS: Enhanced leptin sensitivity and attenuation of diet-induced obesity in mice with haploinsufficiency of Socs3. Nat Med. 2004;10(7):734–8.

14 Pellme F, Smith U, Funahashi T, Matsuzawa Y, Brekke H, Wiklund O, et al. Circulating adiponectin levels are reduced in nonobese but insulin-resistant first-degree relatives of type 2 diabetic patients. Diabetes. 2003;52(5):1182–6.

15 Weyer C, Funahashi T, Tanaka S, Hotta K, Matsuzawa Y, Pratley RE, et al. Hypoadiponectinemia in obesity and type 2 diabetes: close association with insulin resistance and hyperinsulinemia. J Clin Endocrinol Metab. 2001;86(5): 1930–5.

16 Kern PA, Di Gregorio GB, Lu T, Rassouli N, Ranganathan G. Adiponectin expression from human adipose tissue: relation to obesity, insulin resistance, and tumor necrosis factor-alpha expression. Diabetes. 2003;52(7):1779–85.

17 Owecki M. Fat tissue and adiponectin: new players in critical care? Crit Care. 2009;13(4):174.

18 Goldstein BJ, Scalia R. Adiponectin: a novel adipokine linking adipocytes and vascular function. J Clin Endocrinol Metab. 2004;89(6):2563–8.

19 Hotamisligil GS, Arner P, Caro JF, Atkinson RL, Spiegelman BM. Increased adipose tissue expression of tumor necrosis factor-alpha in human obesity and insulin resistance. J Clin Invest. 1995;95(5):2409–15.

20 Scott DL, Kingsley GH. Tumor necrosis factor inhibitors for rheumatoid arthritis. N Engl J Med. 2006;355(7):704–12.

21 Van den Berghe G. Neuroendocrine pathobiology of chronic critical illness. Crit Care Clin. 2002;18(3):509–28.

22 Langouche L, Van den Berghe G. The dynamic neuroendocrine response to critical illness. Endocrinol Metab Clin North Am. 2006;35(4):777–91,ix.

23 Van den Berghe G. Beyond diabetes: saving lives with insulin in the ICU. Int J Obes Relat Metab Disord. 2002;26(Suppl 3):S3–8.

24 Falciglia M, Freyberg RW, Almenoff PL, D'Alessio DA, Render ML. Hyperglycemia-related mortality in critically ill patients varies with admission diagnosis. Crit Care Med. 2009;37(12):3001–9.

25 Preiser JC, Devos P, Ruiz-Santana S, Melot C, Annane D, Groeneveld J, et al. A prospective randomised multi-centre controlled trial on tight glucose control by intensive insulin therapy in adult intensive care units: the Glucontrol study. Intensive Care Med. 2009;35(10):1738–48.

26 Finfer S, Chittock DR, Su SY, Blair D, Foster D, Dhingra V, et al. Intensive versus conventional glucose control in critically ill patients. N Engl J Med. 2009;360(13):1283–97.

27 van den Berghe G, Wouters P, Weekers F, Verwaest C, Bruyninckx F, Schetz M, et al. Intensive insulin therapy in the critically ill patients. N Engl J Med. 2001;345(19):1359–67.

28 Marik PE, Preiser JC. Toward understanding tight glycemic control in the ICU: a systematic review and metaanalysis. Chest. 2010;137(3):544–51.

29 Griesdale DE, de Souza RJ, van Dam RM, Heyland DK, Cook DJ, Malhotra A, et al. Intensive insulin therapy and mortality among critically ill patients: a meta-analysis including NICE-SUGAR study data. CMAJ. 2009;180(8):821–7.

30 Lacherade JC, Jacqueminet S, Preiser JC. An overview of hypoglycemia in the critically ill. J Diabetes Sci Technol. 2009;3(6):1242–9.

31 Bagshaw SM, Bellomo R, Jacka MJ, Egi M, Hart GK, George C. The impact of early hypoglycemia and blood glucose variability on outcome in critical illness. Crit Care. 2009;13(3):R91.

32 Andreelli F, Amouyal C, Magnan C, Mithieux G. What can bariatric surgery teach us about the pathophysiology of type 2 diabetes? Diabetes Metab. 2009;35(6 Pt 2):499–507.

33 Cummings DE. Endocrine mechanisms mediating remission of diabetes after gastric bypass surgery. Int J Obes (Lond). 2009;33(Suppl 1):S33–40.

34 Meneghini LF. Impact of bariatric surgery on type 2 diabetes. Cell Biochem Biophys. 2007;48(2–3):97–102.

35 Rubino F, Gagner M, Gentileschi P, Kini S, Fukuyama S, Feng J, et al. The early effect of the Roux-en-Y gastric bypass on hormones involved in body weight regulation and glucose metabolism. Ann Surg. 2004;240(2):236–42.

36 Kashyap SR, Gatmaitan P, Brethauer S, Schauer P. Bariatric surgery for type 2 diabetes: weighing the impact for obese patients. Cleve Clin J Med. 2010;77(7):468–76.

37 Drucker DJ. The role of gut hormones in glucose homeostasis. J Clin Invest. 2007;117(1):24–32.

38 Folli F, Pontiroli AE, Schwesinger WH. Metabolic aspects of bariatric surgery. Med Clin North Am. 2007;91(3): 393–414,x.

39 Holst JJ, Sorensen TI, Andersen AN, Stadil F, Andersen B, Lauritsen KB, et al. Plasma enteroglucagon after jejunoileal bypass with 3:1 or 1:3 jejunoileal ratio. Scand J Gastroenterol. 1979;14(2):205–7.

40 Miholic J, Orskov C, Holst JJ, Kotzerke J, Meyer HJ. Emptying of the gastric substitute, glucagon-like peptide-1 (GLP-1), and reactive hypoglycemia after total gastrectomy. Dig Dis Sci. 1991;36(10):1361–70.

41 le Roux CW, Aylwin SJ, Batterham RL, Borg CM, Coyle F, Prasad V, et al. Gut hormone profiles following bariatric surgery favor an anorectic state, facilitate weight loss, and improve metabolic parameters. Ann Surg. 2006;243(1):108–14.

42 Moulin de Moraes CM, Mancini MC, de Melo ME, Figueiredo DA, Villares SM, Rascovski A, et al. Prevalence of subclinical hypothyroidism in a morbidly obese population and improvement after weight loss induced by Roux-en-Y gastric bypass. Obes Surg. 2005;15(9):1287–91.

43 Iacobellis G, Ribaudo MC, Zappaterreno A, Iannucci CV, Leonetti F. Relationship of thyroid function with body mass index, leptin, insulin sensitivity and adiponectin in euthyroid obese women. Clin Endocrinol (Oxf). 2005;62(4):487–91.

44 Rotondi M, Leporati P, La Manna A, Pirali B, Mondello T, Fonte R, et al. Raised serum TSH levels in patients with morbid obesity: is it enough to diagnose subclinical hypothyroidism? Eur J Endocrinol. 2009;160(3):403–8.

45 Szomstein S, Avital S, Brasesco O, Mehran A, Cabral JM, Rosenthal R. Laparoscopic gastric bypass in patients on thyroid replacement therapy for subnormal thyroid function: prevalence and short-term outcome. Obes Surg. 2004;14(1):95–7.

46 Raftopoulos Y, Gagne DJ, Papasavas P, Hayetian F, Maurer J, Bononi P, et al. Improvement of hypothyroidism after laparoscopic Roux-en-Y gastric bypass for morbid obesity. Obes Surg. 2004;14(4):509–13.

47 Chopra IJ. Clinical review 86: euthyroid sick syndrome – is it a misnomer? J Clin Endocrinol Metab. 1997;82(2):329–34.

48 Burman KD, Wartofsky L. Thyroid function in the intensive care unit setting. Crit Care Clin. 2001;17(1):43–57.

49 Slag MF, Morley JE, Elson MK, Crowson TW, Nuttall FQ, Shafer RB. Hypothyroxinemia in critically ill patients as a predictor of high mortality. JAMA. 1981;245(1):43–5.

50 Imberti R, Ferrari M, Albertini R, Rizzo V, Tinelli C. Increased levothyroxine requirements in critically ill patients with hypothyroidism. Minerva Anestesiol. 2010;76(7):500–3.

51 Plikat K, Langgartner J, Buettner R, Bollheimer LC, Woenckhaus U, Scholmerich J, et al. Frequency and outcome of patients with nonthyroidal illness syndrome in a medical intensive care unit. Metabolism. 2007;56(2):239–44.

52 Surani SR, Garcia RO, Modak A. Hypothyroidism induced cardiac tamponade in intensive care unit: a rare presentation. Crit Care & Shock. 2006;9:52–4.

53 Datta D, Scalise P. Hypothyroidism and failure to wean in patients receiving prolonged mechanical ventilation at a regional weaning center. Chest. 2004;126(4):1307–12.

54 Jaattela M, Ilvesmaki V, Voutilainen R, Stenman UH, Saksela E. Tumor necrosis factor as a potent inhibitor of adrenocorticotropin-induced cortisol production and steroidogenic P450 enzyme gene expression in cultured human fetal adrenal cells. Endocrinology. 1991;128(1):623–9.

55 Natarajan R, Ploszaj S, Horton R, Nadler J. Tumor necrosis factor and interleukin-1 are potent inhibitors of angiotensin-II-induced aldosterone synthesis. Endocrinology. 1989; 125(6):3084–9.

56 Pariante CM, Pearce BD, Pisell TL, Sanchez CI, Po C, Su C, et al. The proinflammatory cytokine, interleukin-1alpha, reduces glucocorticoid receptor translocation and function. Endocrinology. 1999;140(9):4359–66.

57 Krasznai A, Aranyi P, Feher T, Krajcsi P, Meszaros K, Horvath I. Alterations in the number of glucocorticoid receptors of circulating lymphocytes in sepsis. Haematologia (Budap). 1986; 19(4):293–8.

58 van der Voort PH, Gerritsen RT, Bakker AJ, Boerma EC, Kuiper MA, de Heide L. HDL-cholesterol level and cortisol response to synacthen in critically ill patients. Intensive Care Med. 2003;29(12):2199–203.

59 Chien JY, Jerng JS, Yu CJ, Yang PC. Low serum level of high-density lipoprotein cholesterol is a poor prognostic factor for severe sepsis. Crit Care Med. 2005;33(8):1688–93.

60 Marik PE. The paradoxical effect of obesity on outcome in critically ill patients. Crit Care Med. 2006;34(4):1251–3.

61 Chawla K, Kupfer Y, Goldman I, Tessler S. Hydrocortisone reverses refractory septic shock. Criti Care Med. 1999; 27(1):33A.

62 Briegel J, Forst H, Haller M, Schelling G, Kilger E, Kuprat G, et al. Stress doses of hydrocortisone reverse hyperdynamic septic shock: a prospective, randomized, double-blind, single-center study. Crit Care Med. 1999;27(4):723–32.

63 Oppert M, Schindler R, Husung C, Offermann K, Graf KJ, Boenisch O, et al. Low-dose hydrocortisone improves shock reversal and reduces cytokine levels in early hyperdynamic septic shock. Crit Care Med. 2005;33(11):2457–64.

64 Cooper MS, Stewart PM. Corticosteroid insufficiency in acutely ill patients. N Engl J Med. 2003;348(8):727–34.

13 Management of Venous Thromboembolism in the Critically Ill Obese Patient

Terence K. Trow and Richard A. Matthay

Yale University School of Medicine, Department of Internal Medicine, Section of Pulmonary and Critical Care Medicine, New Haven, CT, USA

KEY POINTS

- The prevalence of the obese critically ill patient is increasing and is likely to increase for the foreseeable future.
- Obese critically ill patients are at increased risk for venous thromboembolic events and these events are more challenging to diagnose in the obese.
- Treatment strategies for deep vein thrombosis and pulmonary embolism with unfractionated heparin is the same in the critically ill obese patient as it is in the nonobese using the actual body weight dosing nomograms. There is mounting evidence that low-molecular-weight heparin can be safely and effectively used in the obese, but the critically ill obese patient may not absorb these agents the same as the non-critically ill obese and antifactor Xa monitoring is advised if this treatment strategy is elected.

INTRODUCTION

Obesity is increasing in the USA as it is in Europe and Asia [1]. It is estimated that more than half of US adults are likely to be obese by the year 2030 [2]. While the prevalence of morbidly obese patients who become critically ill is unknown it is estimated that the incidence of obese patients requiring intensive care unit (ICU) care is at least 14 cases per 1000 per year [3]. Venous thromboembolic (VTE) disease is increased in the obese [4] and proper management of deep vein thrombosis (DVT) and pulmonary embolism (PE) in this population can be a challenge.

THE SCOPE OF THE PROBLEM: THE OBESITY EPIDEMIC

Obesity was responsible for 365 000 preventable deaths in 2000 [5,6], behind only those, attributable to tobacco smoking. A rapid rise in the prevalence of overweight and obese Americans has been observed, with the prevalence of obesity doubling from 15 to 35% between 1980 and 2006 [1,7] (see Figures 13.1 and 13.2). If these trends continue, it is estimated that 86% of adults will be overweight and 51% of adults will be obese by the year 2030 [2]. While the exact prevalence of obese patients requiring ICU care is not known [3] and is dependent on the cohort studied, some authors have suggested that as many as 25% of medical/surgical ICU patients are obese [8,9].

OBESITY AS A RISK FACTOR FOR VENOUS THROMBOEMBOLIC DISEASE

While earlier studies failed to support the role of obesity as an independent risk factor for VTE [10–13], subsequent studies have strongly confirmed it [14–19]. In fact, using data from the National Hospital Discharge Survey Study, Stein et al. found the relative risk of developing a DVT was 2.5 times greater in the obese compared with the nonobese [18]. This may be due to a variety of abnormalities in hemostasis that have been described in the obese, including increased levels of platelet activator inhibitor-1 (PAI-1) [17,20–22], increased platelet activation [23], increased levels of plasma fibrinogen

---

Critical Care Management of the Obese Patient, First Edition. Edited by Ali A. El Solh.
© 2012 John Wiley & Sons, Ltd. Published 2012 by John Wiley & Sons, Ltd.

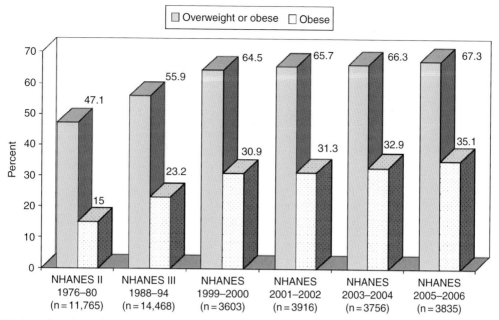

Figure 13.1 Age-adjusted prevalence rates of overweight and obesity among US adults, aged 20–74 years. (Data from National Center for Health Statistics Web site, December 2008. Available at: http://www.cdc.gov/nchs/data/hestat/obesity_adult_07_08/obesity_adult_07_08.htm. Accessed March 2011.)

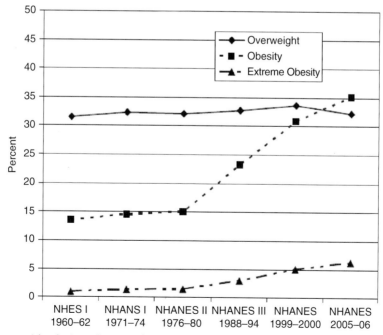

Figure 13.2 Trends in overweight, obesity, and extreme obesity among US adults, aged 20–74 years, over time. (Data from National Center for Health Statistics Web site, December 2008. Available at: http://www.cdc.gov/nchs/data/hestat/obesity_adult_07_08/obesity_adult_07_08.htm. Accessed March 2011.)

factor VII, factor VIII, and von Willebrand factor [24], as well as stasis imposed by inactivity. Thrombin generation is increased in the obese and decreases with weight loss [25]. This increased risk of thrombosis may be especially increased in women [26] on post-menopausal hormone therapy [27,28], although evidence from the ESTHER study suggests this risk may be mitigated by a transdermal delivery system as opposed to oral estrogen therapy [29].

PREVENTION OF DEEP VEIN THROMBOSIS IN THE OBESE

The optimal strategy for DVT prophylaxis in the obese is unknown. Subcutaneous (SC) unfractionated heparin (UFH) has not been well studied in the obese population. When this agent is used, standard doses of 5000 International Units (IU) SC administered every eight hours are often used [8], although higher doses have been advised by some [30], especially in the setting of bariatric surgery [30,31]. The 2008 American College of Chest Physicians (ACCP) Evidenced-Based Clinical Practice Guidelines endorse a higher than standard dose of UFH for the obese patient undergoing bariatric surgery but do not specify the appropriate dose [31]. Shepherd et al. employed individualized adjusted-dose UFH in 700 patients undergoing bariatric surgery using antifactor Xa heparin activity levels to define optimal doses. The dosing needed ranged from 3000 to 19 000 IU every 12 hours SC, with a median dose of 8000 IU [30]. Using this strategy, no patients developed DVT but 0.4% developed nonfatal PEs. Factors that affect UFH dosing requirements include weight, age, gender, and smoking status [30,31].

The use of low-molecular-weight heparin (LMWH) for the prophylaxis of DVT in the obese is controversial. Since obese patients have a lower proportion of lean body mass as a percentage of total body weight (TBW), LMWH dosing based on TBW could theoretically result in supratherapeutic anticoagulation. Obese patients have historically been excluded from the clinical studies that initially evaluated LMWH so there is little randomized, double-blind, controlled data to guide the use of these agents in this population. In a study comparing two different doses of enoxaparin prophylaxis in obese patients undergoing bariatric surgery [32], 40 mg enoxaparin SC every 12 hours was superior to a dose of 30 mg SC every 12 hours [32]. The larger dose was not associated with an increased risk of bleeding. Likewise, a multicenter retrospective study of enoxaparin therapy dosed at either 30 mg (preoperatively) or 40 mg (postoperatively) every

12 or every 24 hours after bariatric surgery resulted in very low rates of VTE [33]. Similarly, 5700 IU of nadroparin administered subcutaneously was successful in prophylaxing 60 obese patients undergoing bariatric surgery [34]. In a study of tinzaparin, anti-Xa and anti-XIa activity were consistently therapeutic over a wide range of body weights and body mass indices (BMIs), indicating that tinzaparin pharmacokinetics was not influenced by body weight or BMI [35]. In a subgroup analysis of 1118 obese patients in the PREVENT trial, dalteparin at a fixed dose of 5000 IU SC daily appeared to reduce the risk of VTE, PE, and sudden death [36]. Taken together, these studies suggest that LMWH can be safely and effectively used as prophylaxis in the obese. However, the patients in the aforementioned studies were not critically ill and the effect of LMWH may be diminished in ICU patients because of antithrombin, fluid overload, edema, vasopressor use, and other factors [37–40], making standard dosing regimens potentially inadequate in this setting. A VTE prophylaxis protocol stratifying obese patients into high- and low-risk categories has been suggested, but again this was not specifically designed for the critically ill obese patient [41].

In the event of contraindication to anticoagulant prophylaxis the 2008 ACCP Evidenced-Based Clinical Practice Guidelines endorse the use of mechanical methods of thromboprophylaxis including intermittent pneumatic compression (IPC) devices and/or graduated compression stockings [31], although their effectiveness in the obese has not been studied to our knowledge.

MAKING THE DIAGNOSIS OF VENOUS THROMBOEMBOLIC DISEASE IN THE OBESE

Establishing the diagnosis of VTE or PE in the morbidly obese can be extremely challenging. Dyspnea and arterial hypoxemia can be the result of multiple causes in critically ill obese patients, including lower-zone atelectasis and aspiration pneumonia [8]. Even when DVT or PE is suspected, diagnostic imaging may be inadequate. Compression and Doppler ultrasonographic venous imaging of the extremities is less sensitive in the obese [8,42–44]. The use of tissue harmonic imaging can improve image quality [45] but is rare in most medical centers [43]. Chest roentgenogram quality is also limited in the obese, even with adjustments in the kilovolts applied, resulting in a steady increase in habitus-limited radiology reports over the past two decades [46]. Likewise, computerized tomographic pulmonary artery angiography (CTPA) image acquisition can be problematic in the obese. The percentage of emergency rooms and hospitals with computerized tomography (CT) and magnetic resonance imaging (MRI) scanners capable of accommodating patients weighing 200 kg (450 lbs) or more has been reported at 10 and 8%, respectively [47]. While academic centers fared better at having CT scanners capable of handling patients > 200 kg (450 lbs) (28%), they fared no better for MRI capability (8%) [47]. Standard CT scanners in the past had table weight limits of 200 kg (450 lbs) with a gantry diameter of 70 cm but newer-generation scanners now exist to accommodate 300 kg (650 lbs) of weight and can offer a gantry diameter of 90 cm with a vertical diameter up to 52–53 cm [43]. Even if the critically ill obese patient can fit into the scanner, technical issues that limit image quality include inability to raise obese arms out of the field of view, inadequate beam penetration, limited field of view resulting in beam-hardening artifacts, and image cropping [43,48]. Some of these technical issues can be overcome by increasing the kilovoltage peak (kVp) to 140 and decreasing the gantry rotation speed from one rotation in 0.5 seconds to one rotation in 1.0 seconds [48,49]. These solutions, however, result in increased radiation doses for the obese patient. In addition, the proper amount of contrast agent must be increased to achieve proper vessel opacification in the obese. Given that the volume of contrast injected is the sum of the scanning delay plus the scanning duration up to a maximum volume of 125 ml [50,51], a dose of 1.2 ml of contrast per kilogram body weight injected at a rate of 4.0 ml/second is required to achieve 250 Hounsefield units of opacification for patients weighing up to 153 kg (336 lbs). Requirements for larger patients than this have not been delineated to our knowledge. All of these factors have resulted in inferior CTPA results for the detection of PE in obese adults [43,52,53].

Regarding nuclear ventilation-perfusion (V/Q) scanning, adequate image acquisition can likewise be a challenge. Unlike CTPA, no automated system exists to ensure adequate exposure in the obese, and a fixed standard dose of isotope is given. In the obese, there is no generally accepted protocol for increasing the dose. Using longer time for data acquisition may improve results [49].

While not typically used for the diagnosis of PE or DVT, MRI scanning can also prove technically challenging in the morbidly obese. Bore diameters for most MRI scanners are 60 cm, with a bore length of 149–170 cm and a table weight limit of 160 kg (350 lbs) [43]. Recently, larger-bore scanners (70 cm) with shorter bore lengths

(125 cm) have been developed to accommodate the obese patient [43]. The positioning of phase array body coils further limits the vertical diameter available for the patient, however, and while these coils provide the most optimal-quality images, they may not be able to be used with the morbidly obese [43]. Newer scanners can accommodate patients up to 250 kg (550 lbs) in weight [43,49]. Near-field artifacts and wrap-around artifacts frequently limit image quality. Caution must be taken to avoid skin burns where the skin abuts the gantry, especially in the diaphoretic, clammy, critically ill obese patient [48,49].

Finally, the use of echocardiography to assess right ventricular dysfunction has been suggested to be an important risk stratification tool in patients with PE [54]. However, the image quality of cardiac ultrasound is also adversely affected by obesity [55].

TREATING ESTABLISHED DEEP VEIN THROMBOSIS AND PULMONARY EMBOLISM IN THE CRITICALLY ILL OBESE

Unfractionated heparin

The approach to treatment of DVT and PE in the obese patient with UFH appears to be similar to that for the nonobese regarding weight-based protocols [56]. Yee and Norton found that using actual body weight (ABW) was superior in achieving initial activated partial thromboplastin time (aPTT) and target aPTT goals compared to ideal body weight (IBW) or dosing weight (defined as IBW + 0.3 × (ABW − IBW)) in 123 obese patients [57]. Similarly, a retrospective study of 20 obese and 20 non-obese patients using ABW (70 units/kg bolus followed by 1.5 units/kg/hour infusion) achieved similar initial aPTT and times to targeted aPTT goals [58]. In addition, in the ESSENCE and TIMI IIb trials, subgroup analysis revealed that the UFH when compared to LMWH dosed by ABW caused no greater major hemorrhage, death, or myocardial infarction events in the obese [59]. Likewise, in 294 out of 8845 total patients in the RIETE registry who were obese (defined as > 100 kg and not by BMI), use of UFH did not affect risk of recurrent VTE and did not result in a greater risk for major bleeding side effects [60].

Low-molecular-weight heparins

LMWH for the treatment of DVT and PE in the morbidly obese has been controversial. Theoretical concerns that the lower proportion of lean body mass as a percentage of

TBW in the obese could lead to supratherapeutic anticoagulation if LMWHs were dosed to ABW have led some to question the safety of their use in this population [61]. On the other hand, use of fixed dosing regimens or capped regimens regardless of body weight runs the risk of under dosing in the obese population [61,62]. For this reason the ACCP Evidence-Based Clinical Practice Guidelines previously recommended use of LMWH in the obese only if antifactor Xa monitoring was done 4 hours after dose administration with goals of 0.6–1.0 IU/ml for enoxaparin, 1.3 IU/ml for nadroparin, 0.85 IU/ml for tinzaparin, and 1.05 IU/ml for dalteparin [62]. However, there is accumulating evidence to suggest that weight-based LMWH dosing without a cap may be safe without increased risk of bleeding [56]. Bazinet and colleagues studied 81 obese patients treated with enoxaparin 1.5 mg/kg once daily or 1 mg/kg twice daily except those on dialysis, and found BMI did not affect antifactor-Xa levels in non-critically ill patients [63]. Sanderink et al. studied 48 normal but obese volunteers dosed with 1.5 mg/kg SC daily enoxaparin over 4 days and found no significant difference in maximum antifactor Xa levels between obese and nonobese indidviduals [63]. These investigators also found that TBW proved to be better than BMI or IBW in predicting antifactor Xa clearance [64]. In another study of 10 obese (defined as > 40% of IBW) patients with DVT or PE who were given weight-based dalteparin, there was no significant difference in antifactor Xa levels compared to patients closer to their IBW [65]. Moreover, treatment of 193 obese patients with dalteparin at a dose of 200 IU/kg of ABW over a 12-week course resulted in only two having major hemorrhage events [66]. Subgroup analysis of the ESSENCE and TIMI IIb trials also found no significant difference in major bleeding events, death, or myocardial infarctions compared with those treated with UFH [59]. Based on these data, the 2008 ACCP Evidence-Based Clinical Practice Guidelines now recommend against routine antifactor Xa monitoring in the obese but continue to recommend it for those being treated with LMWH who are pregnant or who have a creatinine clearance (CrCl) of < 30 ml/minute [67]. Because of potentially worse outcomes with LMWH in patients with significant renal impairment, weight-based UFH is recommended over LMWH for VTE treatment in these patients [67]. It is unclear if the critically ill morbidly obese patient has different absorption of LMWH [37–40] or if antifactor Xa monitoring should be done in this subset. It is advised however that antifactor Xa monitoring with subsequent dose adjustments may be wise in the extremely obese patient (> 190 kg) due to limited published experience with the morbidly obese [68]. Regarding dosing strategies, a trend toward increased recurrent VTE in 283 obese subjects receiving enoxaparin dosed once daily compared with obese patients receiving twice-daily enoxaparin (7.3 vs 3.4%, respectively) has been reported [69]. For this reason, many authors advise twice-daily dosing in the obese until further studies have been conducted [56,69,70].

One caveat, however, with all the aforementioned studies is that they were not specifically performed on critically ill obese patients, who as previously discussed may not absorb subcutaneously administered medicines the same as non-critically ill obese patients [38–40]. The critically ill obese patient may require higher dosing strategies and thus warrants further study before final recommendations can be made. It is for this reason that many intensivists prefer to use intravenously administered UFH.

PENATASACCHARIDES, DIRECT THROMBIN INHIBITORS, AND DIRECT Xa INHIBITORS

In obese patients who develop heparin-induced thrombocytopenia (HIT), alternative agents are often selected for anticoagulation. These include pentasaccarides, direct thrombin inhibitors, and direct Xa inhibitors. The role of these agents in the critically ill morbidly obese has not been sufficiently studied to make definitive recommendations at present.

Pentasaccharides

Subgroup analysis of 594 patients with a BMI > 30 from the Matisse trials suggests that once-daily fondaparinux is safe and equally as effective as UFH and LMWH in the obese [71]. The longer-acting idrabiotaparinux was recently studied in a double-blind, randomized trial of 757 patients with symptomatic DVT and compared to idraparinux at equimolar doses [72]. This study revealed that idrabiotaparinux had a similar time course to factor Xa inhibition as well as similar efficacy and safety to idraparinux, with the added safety feature of reversibility of its anticoagulation effect by avidin infusion in those experiencing major bleeding complications. Of these 757 patients, 72 in the idraparinux arm and 59 in the idrabiotaparinux arm weighed 100 kg or more. No subgroup analysis of the obese was offered and no critically ill patients were included in this trial. All of these agents are exclusively renally cleared and should not be used in those with a CrCl below 30 ml/minute [73].

Direct thrombin inhibitors

Our review of the literature has revealed no study of dabigatran in obese patients and, accordingly, no recommendation about its use in these patients can be offered [73].

Direct factor Xa inhibitors

In our review of the literature, no studies of rivaroxaban, betrixaban, or apixaban have been conducted on the obese population and therefore no recommendations about their use in this specific subpopulation can be made [73].

CONCLUSION

The obesity epidemic in the USA will result in many critically ill obese patients in ICUs across the country. These patients are at increased risk for the development of VTE and require DVT prophylaxis. The optimal strategy for prophylaxis in this population is unknown but UFH and LMWH strategies appear to be effective. Obesity often results in delayed evaluation and management of VTE [53] and practicing intensivists need to keep this high on the differential diagnosis. Diagnosing DVT or PE in the obese is challenging, with decreased sensitivity of compression ultrasonography, V/Q scanning, and CTPA. Weight and girth limitations make some patients unscannable, leaving the clinician to treat empirically in these cases. Once a diagnosis has been made, ABW-dosed UFH , twice-daily LMWH dosed on TBW, and once-daily fondiparinux are all validated options in the obese, but none have been well studied in the critically ill obese. The need to monitor antifactor Xa levels in those on LMWH remains controversial but is currently not recommended by the 2008 ACCP Evidenced-Based Clinical Practice Guidelines, except in pregnant patients or those with severely impaired renal function [31,67]. Special features of the critically ill obese patient may make extrapolation of current LMWH dosing recommendations unwise, and until further studies are done, antifactor Xa monitoring is advisable. Fondiparinux appears safe and effective in the obese [71] but has not been studied in the critically ill obese. No data exist for the use of newer pentasacchrides, direct thrombin inhibitors, or direct factor Xa inhibitors in the critically ill obese.

> **BEST PRACTICE TIPS**
>
> 1 Since obesity is an independent risk factor for venous thromboembolism, all critically ill obese patients should be prophylaxed.
> 2 To improve CT pulmonary angiography sensitivity in the obese patient, increase kVp to 140, slow the gantry rotation to once in 1 second, and increase the volume of contrast agent used.
> 3 If LMWHs are used to treat DVT or PE, twice-daily dosing may be preferable to once-daily dosing in the obese.
> 4 When using UFH to treat DVT or PE in the obese, ABW dosing is safe and appropriate.
> 5 While antifactor Xa monitoring when using LMWH is no longer advised by the ACCP Evidence-Based Clinical Practice Guidelines in the obese in general, limited data in the critically ill obese or extremely obese exist, making monitoring in this subset of patients advisable.

REFERENCES

1 Catenacci VA, Hill JO, Wyatt HR. The obesity epidemic. Clin Chest Med. 2009;30:415–44.

2 Wang Y, Beydoun MA, Liang L, et al. Will all Americans become overweight or obese? Estimating the progression and cost of the US obesity epidemic. Obesity. 2008; 16:2323–30.

3 El Solh AA. Clinical approach to the critically ill, morbidly obese patient. Am J Respir Crit Care Med. 2004;169:557–61.

4 Stein PD, Goldman J. Obesity and thromboembolic disease. Clin Chest Med. 2009;30:489–93.

5 Mokdad AH, Marks JS, Stroup DF, et al. Actual causes of death in the United States, 2000. JAMA. 2004;291:1238–45.

6 Mokdad AH, Marks JS, Stroup DF, et al. Correction: actual causes of death in the United States. JAMA. 2005;293:293.

7 Ogden CL, Yanovski SZ, Carroll MD, et al. The epidemiology of obesity. Gastroenterology. 2007;132:2087–102.

8 Honiden S, McArdle JR. Obesity in the intensive care unit. Clin Chest Med. 2009;30:581–99.

9 Joffe A, Wood K. Obesity in critical care. Anaesthesiology. 2007;20:113–18.

10 Heit JA, Silverstein MD, Mohr DN, et al. Risk factors for deep vein thrombosis and pulmonary embolism. Arch Intern Med. 2000;160:809–15.

11 Anderson FA, Wheeler HB, Goldberg RJ, et al. A population-based perspective of the hospital incidence and case-fatality rates of deep vein thrombosis and pulmonary embolism: the Worcester dvt study. Arch Intern Med. 1991;151:933–8.

12 Heit JA, Silverstein MD, Mohr DN, et al. The epidemiology of venous thromboembolism in the community. Thromb Haemost. 2001;86:452–63.

13 Coon WW, Coller FA. Some epidemiologic considerations of thromboembolism. Surg Gynecol Obstet. 1959;109:487–501.

14 Goldhaber SZ, Grodstein F, Stampfer MJ, et al. A prospective study of risk factors for pulmonary embolism in women. JAMA. 1997;277:642–5.

15 Hansson PO, Eeriksson H, Welin L, et al. Smoking and abdominal obesity: risk factors for venous thromboembolism among middle-aged men. "The study of men born in 1913". Arch Intern Med. 1999;159:1886–90.

16 Anderson FA, Wheeler HB, Goldberg RJ, et al. The prevalence of risk factors for venous thromboembolism among hospital patients. Arch Intern Med. 1992;152:1660–4.

17 Stein PD, Matta F. Epidemiology and incidence: the scope of the problem and risk factors for development of venous thromboembolism. Clin Chest Med. 2010;31:611–28.

18 Stein PD, Beemath A, Olson RE. Obesity as a risk factor in venous thromboembolism. Am J Med. 2005;118:978–80.

19 Samama MY for the Sirius Study Group. An epidemiologic study of risk factors for deep vein thrombosis in medical outpatients. The Sirius Study. Arch Inter Med. 2000;160: 3415–20.

20 Juhan-Vague I, Alessi MC, Mavri A, et al. Plasminogen activator inhibitor-1, inflammation, obesity, and insulin resistance and vascular risk. J Thromb Haemost. 2003;1:1575–9.

21 De Pergola G, Pannacciulli N. Coagulation and fibrinolysis abnormalities in obesity. J Endocrinol Invest. 2002;25:899–904.

22 Pannacciulli N, De Mitrio V, Marin R, et al. Effect of glucose tolerance status on PAI-1 plasma levels in overweight and obese subjects. Obes Res. 2002;10:717–25.

23 Basili S, Pacini G, Guagnano MT, et al. Insulin resistance as a determinant of platelet activation in obese women. J Am Coll Cardiol. 2006;48:2531–8.

24 Mertens I, Van Gaal LF. Obesity, haemostasis and the fibrinolytic system. Obes Res. 2002;3:85–101.

25 Ay L, Kopp HP, Brix JM, et al. Thrombin generation in morbid obesity: significant reduction after weight loss. J Thromb Haemost 2010;8:759–65.

26 Goldhaber SZ, Savage DD, Garrison RJ, et al. Risk factors for pulmonary embolism. The Framingham study. Am J Med. 1983;74:1023–8.

27 Coleman M, Kuller LH, Prentice R, et al. Estorgen plus progestin and risk of venous thrombosis. JAMA. 2004;292: 1573–80.

28 Nightingale AL, Lawrenson RA, Simpson EL, et al. The effects of age, body mass index, smoking and general health on the risk of venous thrombembolism in users of combined oral contraceptives. Eur J Contracept Reprod Health Care. 2000;5:265–74.

29 Canonico M, Oger E, Connard J, et al. Obesity and risk of venous thrombembolism among postmenopausal women: differential impact of hormone therapy by route of estrogen administartion. The ESTHER trial. J Thromb Haemost. 2006;4:1259–65.

30 Shepherd MF, Rosborough TK, Schwartz ML. Heparin thromboprophylaxis in gastric bypass surgery. Obes Surg. 2003;13:249–53.

31 Geerts WH, Bergqvist D, Pineo GF, et al. Prevention of thromboembolism. American College of Chest Physician Evidence-Based Guidelines (8th edition). Chest. 2008;133:S381–453.

32 Scholten DJ, Hoedema RM, Scholten SE. A comparison of two different prophylatic dose regimens of low molecular weight heparin in bariatric surgery. Obes Surg. 2002;12:19–24.

33 Hamad GG, Choban PS. Enoxaparin for thromboprophylaxis in morbidly obese patients undergoing bariatric surgery:findings of the prophylaxis against vte outcomes in bariatric sugery patients receiving enoxaparin (PROBE) study. Obes Surg. 2005;15:1368–74.

34 Kalfarentos F, Stavropoulou F, Yarmenitis S, et al. Prophylaxis of venous thromboembolism using two different low-molecular-weight heaparin (nadroparin) in bariatric sugery: a prospective randomized trial. Obes Surg. 2001;11:670–6.

35 Hainer JW, Barrett JS, Assaid CA, et al. Dosing in heavyweight/obese patients with the LMWH, tinzaparin: a pharmacodynamic study. Thromb Haemost. 2002;87:817–23.

36 Kucher N, Leizorovicz A, Vaitkus PT, et al. Efficacy and safety of fixed low-dose dalteparin in preventing venous thromboembolism among obese or elderly hospitalized patients: a subgroup analysis of the PREVENT trial. Arch Intern Med. 2005;165:341–5.

37 Dager WE. Issues in assessing and reducing the risk for venous thromboembolism. Am J Health Syst Pharm. 2010; 67:S9–16.

38 Mayr AJ, Dunser M, Jockberger S. Antifactor Xa activity in intensive care patients receiving thromboembolic prophylaxis with standard doses of enoxaparin. Thromb Res. 2002; 105:201–4.

39 Haas CE, Nelson JL, Raghavendran K, et al. Pharmacokinetics and pharmacodynamics of enoxaparin in multiple trauma patients. J Trauma. 2005;59:1336–44.

40 Prilinger U, Karth GD, Geppert A, et al. Prophylactic anticoagulation with enoxaparin: is the subcutaneous route appropriate in the critically ill? Crit Care Med. 2003;31:1405–9.

41 Frezza EE, Wachtel MS. A simple venous thormboembolism prophylaxis protocol for patients undergoing bariatric surgery. Obesity. 2006;11:1961–5.

42 Tapson VF, Carroll BA, Davidson BL, et al. The diagnostic approach to acute venous thromboembolis. Clinical practice guidelines. American Throacic Society. Am J Respir Crit Care Med. 1999;160:1043–66.

43 Uppot RN. Impact of obesity on radiology. Radiol Clin N Am. 2007;45:231–46.

44 Haage P, Krings T, Schimitz-Rode T. Nontraumatic vascular emergencies: imaging and intervention in acute venous occlusion. Eur Radiol. 2002;12:2627–43.

45 Shapiro RS, Wagreich J, Parsons RB, et al. Tissue harmonic imaging sonography: evaluation of image quality compared with conventional sonography. AJR. 1998;171:1203–6.

46 Uppot RN, Sahani DV, Hahn PF, et al. Effect of obesity on image quality: fifteen-year longitudinal study for evaluation of dictated radiology reports. Radiology. 2006;240:435–9.

47 Ginde AA, Faoinini A, Renner DM, et al. The challenge of CT and MRI imaging of obese individuals who present to the emergency department: a national survey. Obesity. 2008;16: 2549–51.

48 Uppot RN, Sahani DV, Hahn PF, et al. Impact of obesity on medical and image-guided intervention. AJR. 2007;188: 433–40.

49 Buckley O, Ward E, Ryan A, et al. European obesity and the radiology department: what can be done to help? Eur Radiol. 2009;189:298–309.

50 Bae KT, Tao C, Gurel S, et al. Effect of patient weight on scanning duration on contrast enhancement during pulmonary multidetector CT angiography. Radiology. 2007;242:582–9.

51 Bae KT, Seeck BA, Hildebolt CF, et al. Contrast enhancement in cardiovascular MDCT: effect of body weight, height, body surface area, body mass index, and obesity. AJR. 2008;190:777–84.

52 Wittmer MH, Duzak R, Lewis ER, et al. Does obesity degrade image quality of helical cTfor suspected pulmonary embolism? Abstracts of the 104th Annual Roentgen Society Meeting, Miami (FL). 2004. p. 113.

53 Smith SB. Morbid obesity is associated with delayed diagnosis and management of acute pulmonary embolism. Abstract of the Annual International Meeting of the American College of Physicians, November 3, 2010, Vancouver, Canada. 2010. p. 104.

54 Lankett M, Kostantinides S. Mortality risk assessment and the role of thrombolysis in pulmonary embolism. Clin Chest Med. 2010;312:758–69.

55 Finkelhor RS, Moallem M, Bahler RC. Characteristics and impact of obesity on the outpatient echocardiography laboratory. J Cardiol. 2006;97:1082–4.

56 Rondina MT, Pendelton RC, Wheeler M, et al. The treatment of venous thromboembolim in special populations. Thromb Res. 2007;119:391–402.

57 Yee WP, Norton LL. Optimal weight base for weight-based heparin dosing protocol. Am J Health Syst Pharm. 1998;55: 159–62.

58 Spruill WJ, Wade WE, Huckaby WG, et al. Achievment of anticoagulation by using a weight-based heparin dosing protocol for obese and nonobese patients. Am J Health Syst Pharm. 2001;58:2143–6.

59 Spinler SA, Inverso SM, Cohen M, et al. Safety and efficacy of unfractionated heparin versus enoxaparin in patients who are obese and patients with severe renal impairment: analysis from ESSENCE and TIMI IIb studies. Am Heart J. 2003;146:33–41.

60 Barba R, Marco J, Martin-Alvarez H, et al. The influence of extreme body weight on clinical outcome of patients with venous thromboembolism: findings from a prospective registry (RIETE). J Thromb Haemost. 2005;3:703–9.

61 Clark NP. Low-molecular-weight heparin use in the obese, elderly, and in renal insufficiency. Throm Res. 2008;123: S58–61.

62 Hirsh J, Raschke R. Heparin and low-molecular-weight heparin. The seventh ACCP conference on antithrombotic and thrombolytic therapy. Chest. 2004;126:S188–203.

63 Bazinet A, Almanric K, Brunet C, et al. Dosange of enoxaparin among obese and renal impairment patients. Thromb Res. 2005;116:41–50.

64 Sanderink GJ, Liboux AL, Jariwala N, et al. The pharmacokinetics and pharmacodynamics of enoxaparin in obese volunteers. Clin Pharmacol Ther. 2002;72:308–18.

65 Wilson SJ, Wilbur K, Burton E, et al. Effect of patient weight on the anticoagulant response to adjusted therapeutic dosage of low-molecular-weight heparin for the treatment of venous thromboembolism. Haemost. 2001;31:42–8.

66 Al-Yaseen E, Wells PS, Anderson J, et al. The safety and dosing of dalteparin based on actual body weight for the treatment of acute venous thromboembolism in obese patients. J Thromb Haemost. 2005;3:100–2.

67 Hirsh J, Bauer KA, Donati MB, et al. Parenteral anticoagulants. American College of Chest Physicians Evidence-Based Clinical Practice Guidelines (8th edition). Chest. 2008;133: S141–59.

68 Nutescu EA, Spinler SA, Wittkowsky A, et al. Low-molecular-weight heparins in renal impairment and obesity: available evidence and clinical practice recommendations across medical and surgical settings. Ann Pharmacother. 2009;43: 1064–83.

69 Merli G, Spiro TE, Olsson CG, et al. Subcutaneous enoxaparin once or twice daily compared with intravenous unfractionated heparin for treatment of venous thromboembolic disease. Ann Intern Med. 2001;134:191–202.

70 George-Phillips KL, Bungard TJ. Use of low-molecular-weight heparin bridge therapy in obese patients and in patients with renal dysfunction. Pharmacotherapy. 2006;26:1479–90.

71 Davidson BL, Buller HR, Decousus H, et al. Effect of obesity on outcomes after fondaparinux, enoxaparin, or heparin treatment for acute venous thromboembolism in the Matisse trial. J Thromb Haemost. 2007;5:1191–4.

72 Buller HR, Destors JM, Gallus AS, et al. Efficacy and safety of once weekly subcutaneous idrabiotaparinux in the treatment of patients with symptomatic deep venous thrombosis. J Thromb Haemost. 2010; accepted for publication; doi 10.1111/j.1538-7836.2010.04100.x.

73 Morris TA. New synthetic antithrombotic agents for veonous thromboembolism: pentasacchrides, direct thrombin inhibitors, direct Xa inhibitors. Clin Chest Med. 2010;31:707–18.

14 Nursing Care of the Critically Ill Obese Patient

Margaret E. McAtee

Baylor All Saints Medical Center, Fort Worth, TX, USA

> **KEY POINTS**
> - Caring for extremely obese critically ill patients effectively requires a planned multidisciplinary approach.
> - Critical care nurses need to understand the pathophysiological changes that occur with obesity in order to implement interventions to prevent complications.
> - Physical assessment and monitoring may require modification for the extremely obese patient.

INTRODUCTION

In the USA today, more than one third of adults are obese. These individuals have increased risk for a multitude of health disorders including diabetes, coronary artery disease, dyslipidemia, stroke, hypertension, gallbladder disease, certain cancers, osteoarthritis, sleep apnea, and other respiratory disorders [1]. As the prevalence of obesity in the population has increased there has also been an increasing trend in hospitalized patients who are obese and extremely obese. The prevalence of obese patients in critical care varies depending on the population, ranging from 5.4% in blunt trauma patients, through 17.1% in postoperative cardiac surgical patients, to almost 25% of medical/surgical intensive care unit (ICU) patients [2]. Their admission to critical care units exposes obese patients to an environment that may be unsuited to their special needs. Critically ill obese adults have unique challenges for the nurses and multidisciplinary team caring for them [3]. Critical care nurses must have additional knowledge and skills to identify health risks to obese patients and implement interventions to prevent untoward problems. Critical care nurses are also at risk of injury when taking care of obese patients [4].

Reasons for admission of obese patients to critical care include acute problems associated with gastric restrictive surgeries, problems related to medical illnesses that require intensive care monitoring and support, and traumatic injuries that require intensive care. The obese trauma patient may have injuries that are missed because of inadequate radiological assessment related to the weight restrictions of diagnostic equipment and the difficulty in obtaining high-quality images because of thick layers of soft tissue that lie over critical structures [5].

PATHOPHYSIOLOGY OF OBESITY

Adipose tissue is not just insulation around vital organs. Fat cells secrete a number of substances that help to regulate metabolic processes. These substances can also influence the patient's risk of developing other disorders, including diabetes, hypertension, and atherosclerosis. These adipokines include adiponectin, leptin, interlukin-6 (IL-6), tumor necrosis factor-alpha (TNF-α), plasminogen activator-inhibitor-1 (PAI-1), resistin, and visfatin [6]. Adiponectin plays a part in glucose metabolism by affecting insulin sensitivity. It is also recognized as a biomarker for metabolic syndrome. Adiponectin may also act as an antiinflammatory substance and protect against atherosclerosis. Low adiponectin levels are associated with an increased risk of diabetes mellitus type 2 [7]. Although leptin acts as an appetite suppressant, obesity impairs this function and can lead to a resistance to leptin. In other words, the brain does not respond to the presence of leptin by controlling the appetite and the person continues to eat. The inflammatory proteins secreted by adipose tissue, including IL-6, TNF-α, and PAI-1, interfere

Critical Care Management of the Obese Patient, First Edition. Edited by Ali A. El Solh.
© 2012 John Wiley & Sons, Ltd. Published 2012 by John Wiley & Sons, Ltd.

with the ability of insulin to remove glucose from the blood stream. They also promote the development of atherosclerosis. PAI-1, along with fibrinogen, can cause an increased risk of intravascular clotting. Resistin levels increase with increasing obesity and result in increased appetite, decrease in insulin sensitivity, and increased fat storage. Visfatin is a hormone with actions somewhat like insulin, but visfatin levels do not rise and fall in relation to food intake [6]. Adiponectin exerts an antiinflammatory effect, while resistin, leptin, and visfatin are proinflammatory [8]. Obese patients are in a chronic inflammatory state that results in diminished immune and metabolic reserves. The increased body mass index (BMI) results in increased work for the cardiovascular and pulmonary systems and increases metabolic work. All of this diminishes physiological reserve [9].

CARDIOVASCULAR

Obese patients, especially the extremely obese, often have left ventricular hypertrophy and dilatation, increases in total blood volume and resting cardiac output, and decreased ejection fraction. Fluid loading is not well tolerated and the critical care nurse must be alert for fluid volume overload and signs of heart failure or pulmonary edema [3,10–12]. Nevertheless, a higher preload may be necessary to maintain renal perfusion [13]. Because obese patients have an increased blood volume pumping against increased systemic vascular resistance, they may have compensatory tachycardia secondary to increased oxygen demands and energy needs [12].

Cardiovascular assessment of the obese patient may be difficult. Heart tones may be distant or muffled. It may help to turn off the television, close doors, and otherwise minimize extraneous noise. Placing the patient in a left lateral position or sitting them at a 45° angle so that the heart is nearer the chest wall may facilitate auscultation of heart tones. The point of maximal impulse (PMI) may be displaced laterally toward the midaxillary line because of cardiac enlargement or the horizontal position of the heart [12].

Blood pressure measurement must be done with the appropriate size of blood pressure cuff. The bladder of the cuff should be ≥80% of the patient's arm circumference, and the width of the cuff should be ≥40% of the arm circumference [12]. Noninvasive manual and automatic blood pressure readings may underestimate the arterial blood pressure. Direct intraarterial blood pressure monitoring may be preferable when patients require accurate monitoring to guide therapeutic interventions [14].

Hemodynamic measurements may include possible hypertension with increased left ventricular end-diastolic pressure (LVEDP), increased stroke volume, and increased cardiac output [3]. Increase in BMI translates into modest differences in cardiac output and stroke volume, even at the extremes of body size. Indexing hemodynamic measurements to body surface area more accurately reflects the effects of BMI. The patient's body habitus should not adversely affect the interpretation of hemodynamic measurements [14].

Peripheral pulses may need to be assessed by Doppler if the patient has extreme peripheral edema or severe peripheral vascular disease [12]. Obese critically ill patients are at increased risk of deep vein thrombosis (DVT), but this may be difficult to assess [10,12]. Excess adipose tissue and edema of extremities may mask swelling. A focused assessment of extremities, including circulation, pain, and warmth, is important. Obese patients should have prophylaxis against venous thromboembolus (VTE), with antiembolism stockings or sequential compression devices as well as a pharmacological agent, as discussed in Chapter 13. If unable to obtain equipment in the right size to fit the patient, the nurse may wrap their legs in elastic bandages [12].

Electrocardiographic (EKG) changes can occur with obesity as a result of left ventricular remodeling. The critical care nurse should be alert for changes on EKG such as prolongation of conduction intervals because of increased myocardial mass. These include PR interval, QRS complex, and QT interval. Other changes that can occur include ST depression, left-axis deviation, and low QRS voltage. Obese patients may also exhibit cardiac arrhythmias that are exacerbated by their acute or chronic conditions, especially those that lead to hypoxia, hypercapnia, and electrolyte disturbances. Obese patients have a higher incidence of atrial fibrillation related to fluid overload and atrial dilation [12]. Review of stored cardiac rhythm events in the bedside monitoring system may help to identify abnormalities [13].

PULMONARY

Pulmonary function and pulmonary assessment are compromised in extremely obese critically ill patients. The level of compromise increases with increasing BMI and weight [15]. Decreased lung volumes occur in the obese, more so in the extremely obese, because the enlarged abdomen displaces the diaphragm upward, especially when the patient is supine. This causes a decrease in functional residual capacity, perhaps to as little as one third of normal, and also causes atelectasis of basilar alveoli. Chronic underventilation of the lung bases with normal perfusion contributes to shunting and impaired oxygenation of obese patients [3]. Atelectasis or pneumonia secondary to hypoventilation because of pain can occur postoperatively, contributing to hypoxemia and poor gas exchange [11]. Fatty infiltration of the intercostals muscles and diaphragm makes it harder for the patient to breathe, leading to fatigue and increased oxygen consumption by respiratory muscles [11,15]. Obstructive sleep apnea and obesity hyperventilation syndrome commonly occur in extremely obese patients and the critical care nurse should monitor the patient closely [2,3,10].

When assessing breath sounds, the critical care nurse should listen with the diaphragm of the stethoscope by displacing skin folds over the area. Listening to the lungs over dependent areas is important because fluid may collect here and lung tissue is closer to the chest wall [15]. Guidelines for reducing ventilator-associated pneumonia (VAP) recommend head-of-bed elevation of at least 30° [16]. For the obese patient, this may result in displacement of the abdomen upward and compromise lung expansion. If the head of the bed is elevated, the hip gatch should be lowered [17]. An alternative is to place the hemodynamically stable patient in reverse Trendelenberg at 30–45° to allow the abdomen to drop down so that diaphragmatic excursion is promoted [10,15].

Avoiding mechanical ventilation if possible by use of noninvasive mechanical ventilation may be more desirable [3]. Obese patients may have longer ventilator times with higher extubation failure rates [2,3]. Intubation may be more difficult in obese patients with short, thick necks and poor neck extension [9,10]. However, mechanical ventilation may be needed for the patient in ventilatory failure. In this case, the physician may choose to rest the respiratory muscles for the first 24–48 hours of mechanical ventilation, since obese patients are prone to respiratory muscle fatigue [3]. The ideal body weight (IBW) should be used to determine lung volumes for mechanical ventilation in order to avoid high airway pressures, alveolar distention, and acute lung injury from volutrauma. Increased alveolar–arterial gradients, which occur in many obese patients, may make end-tidal CO_2 monitoring unreliable [9].

GASTROINTESTINAL

Obese patients have an enlarged abdomen, which can cause increased abdominal pressure. If the patient is also a diabetic, they may have gastroparesis. These two conditions can contribute to esophageal reflux, which, in turn, places the patient at risk for aspiration with resultant lung injury [18]. While gastrointestinal (GI) prophylaxis with either a proton pump inhibitor or histamine$_2$ blocker should be considered for all critical care patients, obese patients are at an increased risk for complications if these medications are not used. Patient positioning, as discussed below, can be used to decrease the pressure of the abdominal wall on the stomach and diaphragm to minimize reflux. Measurement of abdominal girth from a marked site can be used to evaluate abdominal distention. Asking the patient if they are passing flatus is a more accurate method of assessing bowel function, rather than listening to bowel sounds [17]. Any patient receiving narcotics should be on a bowel regimen to avoid constipation. Obese patients, who have an increased abdominal girth to begin with, should be protected from straining to have a bowel movement [4,19].

ENDOCRINE

Central obesity, as measured by a waist circumference of 40 inches or more in men and 35 inches or more in women, contributes to metabolic syndrome, a disorder of insulin resistance [20]. As discussed earlier, some of the substances secreted by adipose tissue, including resistin, IL-6, TNF-α, and PAI-1, interfere with glucose metabolism and contribute to insulin resistance [7]. As such, bariatric patients may be resistant to the standard protocols. Joseph et al. reported on a more aggressive insulin therapy protocol that demonstrated improved glycemic control without causing hypoglycemic episodes [21]. Further studies may support the adoption of more intensive glucose control protocols but improved outcomes have not been consistently shown. At any rate, critical care nurses need to be aware that obese patients require close monitoring and may need increased levels of insulin dosing to maintain glycemic control [4].

DERMATOLOGICAL

The critical care nurse faces many challenges in protecting the obese patient from skin breakdown and wound infections. Patients are difficult to turn and mobilize. Adipose tissue has decreased vascularity [10]. Comorbidities, such as diabetes, hypertension, and cardiovascular and pulmonary dysfunction, contribute to the risk for dermatological problems. Critical illnesses that result in hypoperfusion and hypoxia also increase the patient's risk. Factors in critical care such as sedation, use of paralytics, fever, incontinence, fluid overload, and mechanical trauma also contribute to skin breakdown [22]. Multiple skin folds are prone to moisture collection, which fosters growth of bacteria and yeast, making the patient more susceptible to skin breakdown and infections [12]. Patients with a BMI of 30–39.9 are at 1.5 times greater risk for pressure ulcer development than patients with a normal BMI. The risk increases to 3 times as much for patients with a BMI ≥ 40 [22].

Obese patients have a higher incidence of surgical-wound complications including incision dehiscence, seroma, and hematoma formation. Dehiscence may be caused by tension on incision, infections, or inadequate nutrition. Use of a support such as an appropriately sized abdominal binder, systemic antibiotics for infection, and nutritional support to improve wound healing should be implemented. Seromas and hematomas may be prevented with aspiration of fluids or wound drains [22].

The critical care nurse should assess the patient's skin upon admission using a standard such as the Braden scale to stratify the patient's risk for skin breakdown and repeat the assessment according to the facility policy, but at least every 48 hours [10,22]. Consultation with an enterostomal therapist should be strongly considered to assist with evidence-based interventions for patients at risk. Care should be taken to examine all skin folds daily, including under the breasts in both males and females, under the abdomen, in the perineal and gluteal folds, in the lumbar and midback areas, and behind the neck. The nurse should also carefully inspect the position of equipment such as IV tubings, urinary catheters, endotracheal and tracheostomy tube holders and ties, and other items that may be left under patients inadvertently. These patients are also at greater risk of developing postoperative necrosis of gluteal muscles, leading to renal failure and death [22]. Guidelines exist to prevent pressure ulcers, but they may be difficult to implement in the critically ill obese patient population; see Table 14.1 for guidelines specific to obese patients. Use of appropriately sized equipment, such as bariatric beds, pressure-reducing surfaces, and turn and lift equipment, in conjunction with interdisciplinary protocols, can help the critical care team to improve morbidity for these patients [22].

Table 14.1 General treatment guidelines for preventing skin breakdown. (Reproduced from [22].)

Use a validated pressure ulcer risk assessment tool such as the Braden scale to assess patient risk for pressure ulcer development. Assess on admission to ICU and with any changes in patient condition.

Prevention and treatment plans should be evidence-based and tailored to an individual's needs, taking into account patient preference and cost-effectiveness.

Treat any underlying conditions that may contribute to hypoperfusion, hypoxia, hypotension, or hyperglycemia.

Assess nutrition and feed early to prevent catabolism and malnutrition.

Perform perineal care with each episode of incontinence.

Apply barrier creams to all moist areas (products with ingredients: zinc oxide, dimethicone, or petrolatum).

Patients at risk for pressure ulcer development should be placed on pressure-reduction surfaces appropriate for their size.

Enhance early mobility using appropriately sized equipment and adequate staffing.

Encourage independent bed mobility using assistive devices such as overhead trapeze and bedrails.

Decease friction and shear using lift equipment and antishear sheets.

Carefully inspect all skin folds daily.

Develop interdisciplinary protocols to care for obese patients across the care continuum.

Work with supply-chain managers to order appropriately sized beds, linens, and patient-care equipment.

Work with clinical engineering to obtain correct diagnostic equipment (long and/or wide blood pressure cuffs, extra long instruments and needles, wide tracheotomy ties).

Begin discharge planning on admission to prevent unnecessary delays in discharge and to facilitate transition to rehabilitation.

MUSCULOSKELETAL

Obesity places excessive strain on the musculoskeletal system. Disuse of muscles leads to deconditioning and muscle atrophy. Obese patients who are able should be encouraged to do active range of motion (ROM) exercises and to get out of bed with appropriate assistance. Those who are unable to move on their own should receive passive ROM at least once per shift to promote circulation and joint mobility. Obese patients may need a physical therapy or occupational therapy consult [11].

Rhabdomyolysis can occur in any patient as a result of muscle compression and ischemia. Obese critically ill patients, especially if unconscious, have additional risks for rhabdomyolysis related to the difficulty in turning and positioning these patients. They may have had difficulty with mobility before being admitted to the hospital. Obese patients who undergo surgical procedures have an increased risk of developing rhabdomyolysis because of immobility and positioning during the operative procedure. Good assessment skills are critical in identifying this condition early so that interventions can be implemented to treat the patient and minimize complications. The critical care nurse should be suspicious of numbness or muscle pain in dependent parts. Brown urine may indicate the presence of myoglobin in the urine. Aggressive fluid replacement may be used to maintain intravascular volume [10]. These patients may also receive mannitol to mobilize fluid from the interstitial spaces and increase blood flow through the kidneys [9].

URINARY

Obese patients may experience incontinence for a number of reasons. They may have difficulty using a standard size bedpan or bedside commode. If ambulatory, the standard hospital toilet in critical care may not be appropriate for them. If they need assistance in toileting, extra time is usually needed to assemble appropriate numbers of staff and transfer equipment to move the patient. The time delay may be too long and result in the patient soiling themselves and the bed. The enlarged abdomen also places pressure on the bladder, which may result in urgency and frequency. Some intervention strategies to prevent incontinence are to offer frequent toileting and to provide appropriately sized equipment. A large portable toilet seat that fits over a standard toilet may be useful for patients who can get out of bed. Good skin care is needed for patients experiencing incontinence, paying special attention to skin folds in the lower abdomen and perineal area [11].

A urinary catheter may be necessary for frequent or urgent monitoring of urinary output, inability to void due to neurogenic bladder, to prevent skin breakdown, or to protect a wound in the perineal or sacral area [4]. When placing a urinary catheter, three staff members may be needed for insertion. For female patients, two staff members should position the legs and retract the labial folds while a third person preps the perineal area and inserts the catheter. When inserting a catheter in a male patient, two staff members may be needed to lift the abdominal folds so that the penis can be exposed for the third member to prep and insert the catheter [18].

PHARMACOLOGICAL

Pharmacokinetics of frequently used ICU medications are altered in the setting of obesity, especially distribution and excretion [23]. Consultation with a pharmacist is warranted because of the complexity of determining appropriate dosing of medications for critically ill obese patients [5,10]. With some medications, weight-based dosing is not indicated. In others, IBW may be the appropriate measure. Still others may require an adjusted weight based on IBW and a percentage of excess body weight over and above IBW. This may be termed the dosing weight (DW) [23,24]. Intravenous medication use avoids the issue of distribution but not renal clearance. Use of other forms of medication administration, including topical, intramuscular, and subcutaneous injections, results in unpredictable rates of absorption because of poor perfusion to fatty tissue [10,18].

Dosing of many of the medications used in critical care may be guided by serum levels of the drug or other assays. For some of these medications, the initial dose may be calculated using IBW or DW. After results of serum levels are available, dosing can be adjusted for the individual. Critical care nurses often initiate vasoactive drips. Little information exists on weight-based dosing of these medications. Whether to use an IBW or actual body weight (ABW) depends on the indication and urgency of the patient situation. A conservative approach may be best. In this case, the nurse may choose to use IBW and then titrate the medication based on the patient's response [4,24,25].

POSITIONING

Obese patients have a decrease in movement of the diaphragm because of excess abdominal adipose tissue [12]. Cardiac filling pressures, already elevated in the obese patient, increase even more when supine, and predispose the critically ill obese patient to pulmonary edema. When possible, the supine position should be avoided [12]. Raising the head of bed is standard in critical care to prevent aspiration, atelectasis, pulmonary edema, and gastric reflux. Obese patients who are hemodynamically stable may benefit from reverse Trendelenberg at a 45° angle rather than simple head-of-bed elevation at 45° in order to maximize movement of the diaphragm and decrease the risk of complications [2,9,12]. Use of bariatric beds to turn and position more comfortably also prevents the patient from being squeezed between bedrails and allows for full turns, thus offloading pressure areas [12]. Resource lists and algorithms for safe movement of extremely obese patients are available from the United States Department of Veterans Affairs [26].

PSYCHOSOCIAL

Obesity is a condition caused by many factors. The attitude of many in US society is that obesity is caused by a lack of willpower or laziness, without recognizing the complexity and chronicity of the condition. Critical care nurses must examine their own biases when caring for these patients. The patients themselves know that they are difficult to care for and may have feelings of low self-esteem, shame, and embarrassment. Lack of appropriate-sized equipment, including lift equipment, patient gowns, and beds, adds to their embarrassment and frustration and makes them fearful that they will not be safe in the critical care environment. Caring for the extremely obese patient population effectively requires a planned multidisciplinary approach with appropriate equipment and staffing levels. All patients must be treated with dignity and respect [10,11, 13,19,23].

CONCLUSION

Increasing numbers of obese patients are admitted to critical care units. Critical care nurses need to understand what makes these patients different from people of normal size and those who are merely overweight. Obese and extremely obese patients have increased risks of problems when admitted to the critical care environment. Critically ill obese patients provide unique challenges to the critical care nurse. In addition to the routine care that critically ill patients need, the nurse must understand the underlying physiological changes related to obesity and the risk factors unique to this patient population. Excess adipose tissue requires adjustment in normal monitoring and assessment routines. Specialized equipment and additional personnel are required to provide safe care. More research is needed to understand fully changes that should be made in critical care units so that appropriate care is delivered to optimize patient outcomes and promote safety for critically ill obese patients and critical care nurses.

> **BEST PRACTICE TIPS**
> 1 Special attention to skin assessment is required to identify patients at risk and to intervene early to prevent breakdown.
> 2 Monitoring for pulmonary problems is important because obese patients often have some level of impaired oxygenation and increased work of breathing at baseline.
> 3 Anticipate adequate numbers of staff and appropriate equipment when moving patients to protect the patient and staff from injury.
> 4 Close monitoring for glycemic control may be necessary because obese patients may exhibit insulin resistance.
> 5 Allow additional time to complete routine tasks such as assessment, bathing, and dressing changes.

REFERENCES

1 Centers for Disease Control. Obesity: halting the epidemic by making health easier. Available at: http://www.cdc.gov/NCCDPHP/publications/AAG/obesity.htm [Accessed December 25, 2010].

2 Joffe A, Wood K. Obesity in critical care. Current Opinion in Anaesthesiology. 2007;20:113–18.

3 Charlebois D, Wilmoth D. Critical care of patients with obesity. Critical Care Nurse. 2004;24(4):19–27 [Accessed from ccn.journals.org December 6, 2010].

4 McAtee M, Personett R. Obesity-related risks and prevention strategies for critically ill adults. Critical Care Nursing Clinics of North America. 2009;21(3):391–401.

5 Hurst S, Blanco K, Boyle D, et al. Bariatric implications of critical care nursing. Dimensions of Critical Care Nursing. 2004;23(2):76–83.

6 Etienne MO, Pavlovich-Danis SJ. Body fat shapes patients' health. Available at: https://lms.nurse.com/PrintTopics.aspx?topicid=1034 [Accessed December 30, 2010].

7 Ley S, Harris S, Connelly P, et al. Adipokines and incident type 2 diabetes in a Canadian aborigine population: the sandy lake health and diabetes project. Diabetes Care. 2008 Jul;31(7):1410–15.

8 Cave M, Hurt R, Frazier T, et al. Obesity, inflammation, and the potential application of pharmaconutrition. Nutrition in Clinical Practice. 2008 Feb;23(1):16–34.

9 Pieracci FM, Barie PS, Pomp A. Critical care of the bariatric patient. Crit Care Med. 2006;34(6):1796–804.

10 Barth M, Jenson C. Postoperative nursing care of gastric bypass patients. American Journal of Critical Care. 2006 Jul;15(4):378–88.

11 Harris H. Nursing care of the morbidly obese patient. Nursing Made Incredibly Easy. 2008 May;6(3):34.

12 Peavy W. Cardiovascular effects of obesity: implications for critical care. Critical Care Nursing Clinics of North America. 2009;21(3):293–300.

13 Schutz SL. Caring for the bariatric patient. In Carlson KK, editor. AACN Advanced Critical Care Nursing. Saunders Elsevier. 2009. pp. 1420–52.

14 Stelfox HT, Ahmed A, Ribeiro RA, et al. Hemodynamic monitoring in obese patients: the impact of body mass index on cardiac output and stroke volume. Crit Care Med. 2006;34:1243–6.

15 Siela D. Pulmonary aspects of obesity in critical care. Critical Care Nursing Clinics of North America. 2009;21(3): 301–10.

16 AACN Practice Alert: ventilator associated pneumonia. Available at: http://www.aacn.org/WD/Practice/Docs/Practice Alerts/Ventilator_Associated_Pneumonia_1-2008.pdf [Accessed December 29, 2010].

17 Harrington L. Postoperative care of patients undergoing bariatric surgery. MEDSURG Nursing. 2006 Dec;15(6): 357–63.

18 Ide P, Farber E, Lautz D. Perioperative nursing care of the bariatric surgical patient. AORN Journal. 2008 Jul;88(1): 30–58.

19 Wilson J, Clark J. Obesity: impediment to wound healing. Critical Care Nursing Quarterly. 2003 Apr;26(2):119–32.

20 Despres J, Lemieux I. Abdominal obesity and metabolic syndrome. Nature. 2006;444:881–7.

21 Joseph B, Genaw J, Carlin A, et al. Perioperative tight glycemic control: the challenge of bariatric surgery patients and the fear of hypoglycemic events. The Permanente Journal. 2007 Spring;11(2). Available from: http://xnet.kp.org/permanentejournal/spring07/perioperative.html [Accessed December 26, 2010].

22 Lowe J. Skin integrity in critically ill obese patients. Critical Care Nursing Clinics of North America. 2009;21(3):311–22.

23 Davidson J, Kruse M, Cox D, Duncan R. Critical care of the morbidly obese. Critical Care Nursing Quarterly. 2003 Apr;26(2):105–18.

24 Erstad BL. Dosing of medications in morbidly obese patients in the intensive care unit setting. Intensive Care Medicine. 2004 Jan;30(1):18–32.

25 Harrington L. Ask the experts. Critical Care Nurse. 2006 Oct;26(5):68–71.

26 United States Department of Veterans Affairs. Safe bariatric patient handling toolkit. Available from: www.visn8.va.gov/patientsafetycenter/safePtHandling/toolkitBariatrics.asp [Accessed December 26, 2010].

Part IV

Hemodynamic Monitoring and Radiological Investigations

15 Hemodynamic Monitoring of the Critically Ill Obese Patient

Wim K. Lagrand, Eline R. van Slobbe-Bijlsma, and Marcus J. Schultz

Academic Medical Center, Amsterdam, The Netherlands

KEY POINTS

- Literature on hemodynamic monitoring in the critically ill obese patient mostly originates from studies and reports from perioperative care in bariatric surgery.
- Although the method of hemodynamic data assessment may be more complex in the obese, when indexed for body surface area or (predicted) lean body mass, reliable hemodynamic data are comparable between obese and nonobese patients.
- Ultrasound-guided central venous catheter placement is highly advocated in critically ill obese patients.

INTRODUCTION

The obesity epidemic is still increasing in the industrialized world [1]. In line with this, the prevalence of obesity in the intensive care unit (ICU) has increased over recent years. It has been estimated from 5.4 up to 25% and is related to substantial morbidity and mortality [1–4].

There are several reasons to initiate any form of hemodynamic monitoring in critically ill patients [5]. One is the identification of a disease state and/or its complications. Another is to understand its etiology, mostly shock-like pathology, which can be classified into: hypovolemic shock, cardiogenic shock, obstructive shock, and distributive shock, all of which have different causes and treatments. A third reason is to tailor treatment, according to the underlying disease, to improve supply and meet the metabolic demands of the tissues. The ultimate goal is to improve the patient's outcome. Notably, there is a tendency over time to develop and use more non- and/or semi-invasive devices for continuous hemodynamic monitoring.

The indications for hemodynamic monitoring in critically ill obese patients are probably quite similar to those for nonobese patients. The critical care physician, however, may be confronted with unique and challenging problems in obese patients related to changes of anatomy and fat distribution with higher body weights [6]. Literature on hemodynamic monitoring in the critically ill obese patient is scarce and sketchy. Protocols with respect to hemodynamic monitoring in the obese population differ between institutions and are frequently based on individual experiences. Most information originates from studies and reports derived from perioperative care in bariatric surgery. The reasons and goals with respect to hemodynamic monitoring in perioperative care and care in the ICU are different. Perioperative care focuses on support for a short time to overcome surgery. Care in the ICU, on the other hand, is geared toward diagnostic and therapeutic goals. It is therefore questionable to what extent results from bariatric surgery patients can directly be extrapolated to critically ill obese patients.

In this chapter we will discuss means for hemodynamic monitoring, invasive and noninvasive, with respect to the critically ill obese patient.

CARDIOVASCULAR ALTERATIONS IN OBESITY

The cardiovascular effects of obesity, as outlined in Chapter 1, comprise an increase in total blood volume, cardiac output, and stroke volume, linearly with increasing body weight. Heart rate is unaffected. The increased

---

Critical Care Management of the Obese Patient, First Edition. Edited by Ali A. El Solh.
© 2012 John Wiley & Sons, Ltd. Published 2012 by John Wiley & Sons, Ltd.

left ventricular (LV) stroke volume results in increased LV end-diastolic diameter (i.e. dilatation) [7]. Although LV ejection fraction is increased, LV systolic function is depressed in obese individuals. Right ventricular (RV) function seems to be quite unchanged [8]. As a result of the increased cardiac output, the systemic oxygen delivery is increased, serving the metabolic demands of excess fat.

Obesity should not complicate the interpretation of hemodynamic data per se [9]. Although cardiac output is increased, when indexed for body surface area (i.e. cardiac index (CI); CI = cardiac output/body surface area in m^2) the output is not different between obese and nonobese individuals. Other parameters (like extra vascular lung water measurement) may be indexed to predicted lean body mass, expressed as ml/kg. In view of the cardiovascular effects of obesity, however, precautions in data interpretation between the obese and nonobese patient must be taken into account, considering the technical and physiological principles and the algorithms of the applied hemodynamic monitoring devices.

NON- AND SEMI-INVASIVE HEMODYNAMIC MONITORING IN OBESITY

Table 15.1 summarizes non- and semi-invasive means of hemodynamic monitoring.

Physical examination

Central venous pressure estimation by physical examination in nonobese patients is known to have a high inter- and intraobserver variability. The case is no different in obese patients. Central venous pressure estimation may be obscured due to the high body weight. Jugular venous distention, hepatojugular reflex, cannon waves (as a sign of AV-dissociation), and tricuspid regurgitation may be diagnosed at the bedside. As in nonobese patients, low body (core) temperature and decreased diuresis in obese patients may indicate insufficient circulation.

Electrocardiography

Electrocardiograhy (EKG) or rhythm monitoring is one of the standard monitoring tools in the ICU. Obesity is associated with a wide variety of EKG abnormalities. Many of these are reversible after substantial weight loss [10]. EKG alterations with obesity include changes in electrical axes, conduction times (including corrected QT interval), and P-, QRS-, and T-wave voltages.

Such alterations may not be ominous. Some EKG changes, however, represent alterations in cardiac anatomy or morphology associated with obesity and/or its comorbidities. Other EKG abnormalities may serve as markers of risk for sudden cardiac death. Obesity itself may invalidate commonly used EKG diagnostic criteria. Indeed, LV hypertrophy may be obscured by isolation effects of the body fat, yielding lower QRS-complex voltages [10].

Obesity has also been identified as an arrhythmogenic factor and is associated with the occurrence of both supraventricular and ventricular arrhythmias and even sudden cardiac death [11,12]. Atrial fibrillation is the most prevalent supraventricular arrhythmia associated with obesity and it has been shown to be related to worse clinical outcome [13,14]. Case reports and small studies have demonstrated a variety of cardiac arrhythmias and conduction disturbances in morbidly obese patients and in less severely obese patients with LV hypertrophy and sleep apnea syndrome [15].

Pulse oximetry

Like EKG, pulse oximetry is one of the standard monitoring tools in routine critical care [16]. Pulse oximetry is based on spectrophotometric features of pulsatile arterial blood flow and absorption characteristics of oxyhemoglobin and deoxyhemoglobin with respect to two different wavelengths of light (660 nm (red light) and 940 nm (infrared), respectively) [17]. Pulse oximeters are probably the most valuable noninvasive method for the continuous monitoring of oxygen saturation in patients at risk for hypoxemia.

Although the use of pulse oximetry in the ICU is considered routine, there is still debate about the clinical benefit of early detection of hypoxemia by oximetry in the perioperative period [18]. The device is less reliable in low-perfusion states and hypothermia. Pulse oximeters are not able to measure oxygenation adequately in case of dyshemoglobinemia (e.g. in case of CO poisoning and methemoglobinemia). In perioperative care, pulse oximetry does not improve outcome [18,19]. In this respect, no differences seem to exist between critically ill nonobese and obese patients.

Capnography

Changes in a patient's cardiovascular and respiratory status can be assessed by capnography during mechanical ventilation. In case of effective cardiopulmonary resuscitation, increases in end-tidal CO_2 signify an increase in

Table 15.1 Non- and semi-invasive hemodynamic monitoring.

Monitoring tool	Object of measurement	General remarks or problems	Remarks or problems in obese patients
Physical examination			
Central venous pressure	Jugular venous distention Hepatojugular reflex Cannon waves Tricuspid regurgitation	High intra and interobserver variability	Clinical judgement may be invalidated by obesity
Temperature	Core temperature	None	
Diuresis	Urine output	None	
Electrocardiography	Heart rate Dysrhythmias Conduction disorders Previous myocardial infarction Myocardial ischemia	None	Changes related to obesity (see text)
Pulse oximetry	SpO_2 Heart rate	Inaccurate signals by motion artifacts, nail polish, hypotension, low cardiac output, vasoconstriction, hypothermia, hemoglobinopathy	None
Capnography	End-tidal CO_2	Related to minute ventilation and cardiac output Check for correct endotracheal ventilation Check for global circulation in case of resuscitation	Higher difference in end-tidal CO_2 and arterial CO_2 compared with nonobese
Arterial pressure by sphygmomanometry or oscillometric methods	Systolic and diastolic blood pressure Heart rate Pulsus paradoxus	Reliable, if proper technique used	Reliable, if proper technique used
Impedance technique Impedance cardiography Endotracheal CO monitoring	Cardiac output Extravascular water content	To be investigated/validated	To be investigated/validated
Carbondioxide rebreathing technique (NICO)	Cardiac output (by Fick's principle)	Only possible in mechanically ventilated patients	Accurate CO measurement depends on dead space ventilation and pulmonal shunts CO_2 administration in laparoscopic interventions may disturb measurements

(continued)

Table 15.1 *(cont'd)*

Monitoring tool	Object of measurement	General remarks or problems	Remarks or problems in obese patients
Echocardiography Transthoracic (TTE) Transesophageal (TEE)	Cardiac output Flow parameters Anatomical data (dimensions, congenital defects and proximal great vessels) Ventricle systolic and diastolic function Heart valve anatomy and function Detection of myocardial ischemia Pulmonary artery pressures Preload parameters Pericardial effusion Vegetation (infective endocarditis) Neoplasm	Less suitable for continuous measurements TEE is advocated in case of (suspicion of) infective endocarditis TEE is not applicable in case of esophageal/stomach diseases or severe coagulation disorders	Consider TEE in case of poor acoustic windows by TTE due to obesity
Esophageal Doppler	Cardiac output Stroke volume Preload conditions Afterload conditions Cardiac contractility Stroke volume variation	CO measurement is highly dependent on correct aortic diameter recording CO measurement is highly dependent on proper positioning of Doppler probe	Indexed hemodynamic measures are comparable for obese and nonobese
Microcirculation (NIRS, SDF, OPS, gastric tonometry, sublingual capnometry)	StO_2 PCD	To be investigated/validated	To be investigated/validated

ECOM, endotracheal cardiac output monitoring; TTE, transthoracic echocardiography; TEE, transesophageal echocardiography; NIRS, near-infrared spectroscopy; SDF, sidestream darkfield imaging; OPS, orthogonal polarization spectral imaging; PCD, perfused capillary density; StO_2, tissue O_2 saturation.

cardiac output (i.e. pulmonary capillary blood flow). On the other hand, reduction in cardiac output results in decreased end-tidal CO_2 ($EtCO_2$) values and in increased end-tidal–arterial CO_2 differences. In mechanically ventilated obese patients, capnography may be helpful in assessing (changes in) global hemodynamic status [20]. However, in spontaneously breathing, unintubated patients, sampling $EtCO_2$ through a nasal cannula is potentially problematic when expired gas mixes with ambient air. The resulting inaccurate measurements produce artificially low values compared to a closed system with minimal dead space. Intermittent mouth breathing might also contribute to underestimated $EtCO_2$ values. Since mouth breathing is common in obese patients, especially those with a history of obstructive sleep apnea (OSA), exhaled flow distribution between the mouth and nose highly affects the accuracy of capnometry. Therefore, capnography in spontaneously ventilating obese patients is not the ideal technique for adequate hemodynamic monitoring but may be used to assess the global (changes in) hemodynamic status.

Arterial blood pressure monitoring

Arterial blood pressure measurement is an essential part of hemodynamic monitoring. Importantly, noninvasive blood pressure measurements (oscillometric or auscultatory by sphygmomanometry) were shown to be inaccurate in critically ill obese patients when compared with intraarterial blood pressure readings [21]. The use of a proper-sized blood pressure cuff for accurate measurement is essential in obese patients. The length of the bladder should be at least 75–80% of the circumference of the upper arm, and the width of the bladder should be more than 50% of the length of the upper arm and approximately 40% of the circumference of the upper arm [22,23]. If a too-small cuff is used, the systolic pressure may be overestimated.

Alternatively, blood pressure and heart rate may be monitored noninvasively from the radial artery (e.g. with the Vasotrac system) [24]. Although more comfortable than oscillometric blood pressure methods, the Vasotrac measurements were found to differ considerably compared with intraarterial measurements in obese patients undergoing bariatric surgery [25].

If blood pressure readings cannot be obtained from the upper extremities, blood pressures may be measured by ankle monitoring or by Doppler technique. Ankle systolic and mean arterial pressures are significantly higher than brachial blood pressures but severe hypotension may interfere with ankle blood pressure monitoring [26,27]. Alternatively, systolic blood pressure may be assessed by Doppler technique, using an appropriate pressure cuff for the legs (calf). After reaching the systolic blood pressure, Doppler tones will be audible at the foot arteries (i.e. *arteria dorsalis pedis*, *arteria tibialis anterior*) during de-sufflation of the cuff.

Impedance techniques

Cardiac function may be noninvasively assessed by bioimpedance techniques. The theoretical basis for impedance cardiography (ICG) is founded on Ohm's law, in which the thorax is considered as a cylinder with two major components: a poorly conductive cylindrical static tissue impedance surrounding a high-conductive cylindrical blood resistance [28]. After applying a constant, low-amplitude (0.5–4.0 mA), high-frequency (50–100 kHz), alternating electrical current to the thorax, a voltage- and time-dependent induced voltage change can be measured, from which ICG-derived stroke volume can be calculated, as well as cardiac output, systemic vascular resistance (SVR), and thoracic fluid content (TFC).

The transthoracic bioimpedance technique, however, implies several assumptions, related to the characteristics of the tissues, organs, and body fluids involved. These assumptions are mostly derived from empirical geometric constructs in humans with average characteristics, including length and body weight [28]. In the obese patient, the pathophysiological assumptions may not hold true, thereby invalidating stroke volume measurements (e.g. due to differences in aortic compliance and differences in intrathoracic volume and content) [28]. Despite attempts to improve the calculation algorithms [28,29], the routine use of ICG for measurement of cardiac output in obese patients is still being questioned [28,30,31]. Alternative forms of bioimpedance techniques are being developed to improve accuracy (e.g. endotracheal cardiac output monitoring). Future studies are needed to prove the clinical application and benefit of these techniques in critical care settings, including the care of the critically ill obese patient.

CO_2 rebreathing techniques

CO_2 rebreathing techniques can be used as a noninvasive method for calculating cardiac output, using a differential Fick equation, in mechanically ventilated patients [32]. However, lack of hemodynamic stability, intrapulmonary shunting, and dead-space ventilation may alter the precision of cardiac output measurements [33,34]. Morbidly obese patients with preexisting lung disease or postoperative atelectasis also showed poor agreement when compared to the gold standard [35]. Newly developed equipment, algorithms, and software have improved the performance of these techniques [36]. Further validations are needed, however.

Esophageal Doppler

The esophageal Doppler technique measures blood flow velocity in the descending aorta by means of a Doppler transducer (4 MHz continuous-wave or 5 MHz pulsed-wave, according to manufacturers) placed at the tip of a flexible probe [33,37]. This method provides almost continuous hemodynamic information. However, esophageal doppler measurements are very sensitive to probe movement. This implies that this method can only be used in operating room settings or in well-sedated ICU patients.

The estimation of stroke volume using esophageal Doppler relies on the measurement of stroke distance in the descending aorta (= velocity–time integral), which is then converted into systemic stroke volume. The algorithms used to achieve this conversion vary slightly according to manufacturers and are highly influenced by correct aortic diameter estimation, as the conversion is determined by R^2. Esophageal Doppler has the possibility to estimate stroke volume variations, which may be indicative of fluid responsiveness and may guide fluid balance in sepsis and trauma patients [38].

Echocardiography

Echocardiography has proved to be of value in the management of patients with hemodynamic instability in the ICU as it may provide both anatomical and functional cardiovascular information [39,40]. Because of poor acoustic windows, transthoracic echocardiography (TTE) is often severely limited in obese patients [39]. Dramatic improvements in image quality have been achieved with the development of harmonic imaging [41]. This technology exploits the formation of ultrasound signals that return to the transducer at a multiple of the transmitted (fundamental) frequency, referred to as the harmonic frequency. Other enhancements include the use of contrast agents capable of producing LV cavity opacification from a venous injection to delineate the endocardial border. Several contrast agents are currently available that contain albumin microspheres filled with perfluorocarbon

gas, allowing for the passage of contrast through the lungs with the appearance of contrast in the LV [42].

Transesophageal echocardiography (TEE) can provide detailed information in most obese patients [39,40,43]. It is particularly useful in critically ill patients with unexplained hemodynamic instability to rule out LV and/or RV failure, tamponade, hypovolemia, and valvular dysfunction [44,45]. Moreover, the presence of multiple indwelling catheters, the need for parenteral nutrition, and prolonged mechanical ventilation increase the likelihood of bacteremia and subsequent endocarditis. Because the classical clinical findings suggestive of endocarditis are uncommon in this patient population, echocardiography may facilitate the noninvasive diagnosis of endocarditis as part of the diagnostic process (Duke's criteria) [46].

Microcirculation parameters

Apart from systemic hemodynamic consequences, the microcirculation may be impaired in many disease or shock states [47]. The microcirculation comprises the blood flow and perfusion of vessels smaller than 100 microns. Evaluation and modification of the microcirculation by variable means is the subject of future investigation [48]. Whether this is relevant and/or beneficial in obese critically ill patients is still to be answered.

INVASIVE HEMODYNAMIC MONITORING

Table 15.2 summarizes invasive means of hemodynamic monitoring.

Arterial catheterization

Direct intraarterial measurement of systemic blood pressure is nowadays a routine procedure in the ICU. Given the obscure anatomical landmarks and concomitant peripheral edema in critically ill obese patients, arterial cannulation facilitates repeated samplings of arterial blood gas analysis, which permits frequent assessment of oxygenation/gas exchange and ventilation, as well as acid base monitoring.

Pulse contour analysis was introduced in the early 1980s to calculate stroke volume and cardiac output by analysis of the arterial pressure pulse contour (waveform) [49]. It is based on the assumption that the contour of the arterial pressure waveform is proportional to stroke volume, which can be estimated by the integral of the change

Table 15.2 Invasive hemodynamic monitoring.

Monitoring tool	Object of measurement	General remarks or problems	Remarks or problems in obese patients

Arterial catheterization	1) Parameters:
	    a) Systolic blood pressure
	    b) Diastolic blood pressure
	    c) Mean arterial
	    d) Heart rate
	    e) Pulse pressure
	    f) Pulsus paradoxus
	2) Arterial blood gas analysis
	3) In case of arterial pressure waveform analysis:
	    a) Stroke volume
	    b) Cardiac output
	    c) Pulse pressure variation
	    d) Stroke volume variation
		Standard monitoring tool in ICU	Due to alterations in arterial compliance characteristics, cardiac output by uncalibrated arterial pressure waveform analysis is not reliable but may be used as a trend in the obese

Central venous catheterization	1) Central venous pressure, waveform, respiratory variations
	2) Central venous blood gas analysis (pH, $PcvO_2$, $ScvO_2$, $PcvCO_2$, Hb)
	3) Transpulmonal techniques (thermodilution or by indicator):
	    a) Cardiac output
	    b) Stroke volume
	    c) Stroke volume variation
	    d) Intrathoracic blood volume
	    e) Extravascular lung water
	    f) Global end-diastolic volume
	    g) DO_2
		Locations for insertion:
		internal jugular vein
		subclavian vein
		femoral vein
		Transpulmonal technique may be inaccurate in case of heart valve dysfunction (e.g. tricuspid and/or aortic valve regurgitation)
			Femoral vein less favourable because of increased infection (intertrigo) and thrombosis risk in the obese
			Ultrasound-guided central catheter placement is advocated

Pulmonary artery catheter (PAC)	1) Central venous pressure 2) Pulmonary artery pressure 3) Pulmonary capillary wedge pressure 4) Thermodilution CO 5) $SmvO_2$	CO estimation by PAC may be inaccurate in case of heart valve dysfunction (e.g. tricuspid and/or aortic valve regurgitation) PAC measurements less predictive with respect to global left ventricular function and preload conditions Option: application of external right ventricular pacemaker lead via PAC	Indexed hemodynamic measures are comparable for obese and nonobese

ICU, intensive care unit; $PcvO_2$, central venous oxygen tension (pressure) (unit: kPa or mm Hg); $ScvO_2$, central venous oxygen saturation (unit: %); $PcvCO_2$, central venous carbon dioxide tension (pressure) (unit: kPa or mm Hg); DO_2, oxygen delivery (unit: ml/minute); CO, cardiac output; PAC, pulmonary artery catheter; $SmvO_2$, mixed venous oxygen saturation (unit: %).

in pressure from end diastole to end systole over time. The estimate of stroke volume is also influenced by the impedance of the aorta. These assumptions implicate demographic variables (like age, gender, height, and weight) and vascular wall characteristics (depicted in skewness and kurtosis of the waveform, summarized in factor X), which may be quite different in obese compared with nonobese patients. Due to systematic errors by these assumptions, uncalibrated pressure pulse contour underestimates stroke volume or cardiac output in obese patients [50]. In these instances, uncalibrated cardiac output monitoring should be examined as a trend rather than a single value [51].

Central venous catheterization

Central venous pressure may be measured by single cannulation of the internal jugular, subclavian or axillary vein, or (as part of) pulmonary artery catheterization. Alternatively, peripherally inserted central catheters (PICCs) can be used in the obese to measure central venous pressure and to ensure reliable vascular access (infusion of fluids, intravenous medication, diagnostic blood draws) [52]. The utility of central venous pressure measurements in judging intravascular volume status remains controversial, in both obese and nonobese patients [53].

Pulmonary artery catheter

Since its introduction in clinical practice, the pulmonary artery catheter (PAC) has been used frequently in critically ill patients [54]. The PAC provides hemodynamic data (e.g. pulmonary artery pressure, pulmonary capillary wedge pressure, central venous pressure, and cardiac output by thermodilution) to judge cardiovascular status and to assist therapeutic decisions [55]. In case of chronotropic incompetence or hemodynamic important bradyarrhythmias, an external pacemaker can be introduced via adjusted PAC systems. Critically ill obese patients demonstrate elevated right atrial, mean pulmonary artery, and pulmonary artery wedge pressures. It should be noted that the validity of derived parameters indexed to body surface area has been questioned in morbidly obese patients. Several studies have demonstrated that these parameters indexed to body surface area are appropriate and closely approximate indexing to body mass index (BMI). In fact, the large body surface area in the obese patient does not affect these measurements [9,56].

Inappropriate use and poor interpretation of the PAC data may increase morbidity and mortality [57,58,59,60,61]. In a study involving 1994 patients, including those with BMI > 30 kg/m^2, there was no significant difference in outcome in high-risk surgical patients monitored with PAC versus central venous catheter [62]. More importantly, a higher incidence of pulmonary embolism in the PAC group was reported. Not surprisingly, use of PAC has been decreased over the years, despite critical study results in favor of the PAC in selected patients, treated by PAC-trained physicians [63].

CONCLUSION

Hemodynamic monitoring of critically ill obese patients may be technically difficult. The ICU physician may be confronted with unique, challenging problems in obese patients, related to their body weight. Most aspects of hemodynamic monitoring are quite equal between obese and nonobese patients but the clinician should be aware of the basic pathophysiological principles of the applied monitoring tools. Their theoretical assumptions and calculations may be invalidated because of the body weight. When indexed for body surface area (e.g. cardiac output) or predicted lean body weight (e.g. extravascular lung water), reliable hemodynamic data are comparable between obese and nonobese individuals. Obesity, therefore, should not complicate the interpretation of hemodynamic data.

> **BEST PRACTICE TIPS**
> 1 The use of a proper-sized cuff (with 75–80% of upper arm circumference) is necessary for adequate, noninvasive blood pressure measurement.
> 2 Cardiac output estimation by uncalibrated blood pressure pulse contour analysis may differ from the cardiac output by "gold standard" (i.e. thermodilution) but can be used for trending.
> 3 Ultrasound-guided catheter placement in central venous cannulation is advocated.
> 4 Echocardiography is recommended in critically ill obese patients with unexplained hemodynamic instability. TEE examination is preferable since "acoustic windows" are frequently inadequate in TTE.
> 5 When using pulmonary artery catheter, body habitus should not appreciably complicate the interpretation of hemodynamic measurements in critically ill obese patients.

REFERENCES

1 Joffe A, Wood K. Obesity in critical care. Curr Opin Anaesthesiol. 2007 Apr;20(2):113–18.
2 Bercault N, Boulain T, Kuteifan K, Wolf M, Runge I, Fleury JC. Obesity-related excess mortality rate in an adult intensive care unit: a risk-adjusted matched cohort study. Crit Care Med. 2004 Apr;32(4):998–1003.
3 Choban PS, Weireter LJ Jr, Maynes C. Obesity and increased mortality in blunt trauma. J Trauma. 1991 Sep;31(9):1253–7.
4 El-Solh A, Sikka P, Bozkanat E, Jaafar W, Davies J. Morbid obesity in the medical ICU. Chest. 2001 Dec;120(6):1989–97.
5 Pinsky MR. Hemodynamic evaluation and monitoring in the ICU. Chest. 2007 Dec;132(6):2020–9.
6 El Solh AA. Clinical approach to the critically ill, morbidly obese patient. Am J Respir Crit Care Med. 2004 Mar 1;169(5):557–61.

7 Lavie CJ, Messerli FH. Cardiovascular adaptation to obesity and hypertension. Chest. 1986 Aug;90(2):275–9.

8 Her C, Cerabona T, Bairamian M, McGoldrick KE. Right ventricular systolic function is not depressed in morbid obesity. Obes Surg. 2006 Oct;16(10):1287–93.

9 Stelfox HT, Ahmed SB, Ribeiro RA, Gettings EM, Pomerantsev E, Schmidt U. Hemodynamic monitoring in obese patients: the impact of body mass index on cardiac output and stroke volume. Crit Care Med. 2006 Apr;34(4):1243–6.

10 Fraley MA, Birchem JA, Senkottaiyan N, Alpert MA. Obesity and the electrocardiogram. Obes Rev. 2005 Nov;6(4):275–81.

11 Duflou J, Virmani R, Rabin I, Burke A, Farb A, Smialek J. Sudden death as a result of heart disease in morbid obesity. Am Heart J. 1995 Aug;130(2):306–13.

12 Messerli FH, Nunez BD, Ventura HO, Snyder DW. Overweight and sudden death: increased ventricular ectopy in cardiopathy of obesity. Arch Intern Med. 1987 Oct; 147(10):1725–8.

13 Dagres N, Anastasiou-Nana M. Atrial fibrillation and obesity: an association of increasing importance. J Am Coll Cardiol. 2010 May 25;55(21):2328–9.

14 Wang TJ, Parise H, Levy D et al. Obesity and the risk of new-onset atrial fibrillation. JAMA. 2004 Nov;292(20):2471–7.

15 Lattimore JD, Celermajer DS, Wilcox I. Obstructive sleep apnea and cardiovascular disease. J Am Coll Cardiol. 2003 May;41(9):1429–37.

16 Caples SM, Hubmayr RD. Respiratory monitoring tools in the intensive care unit. Curr Opin Crit Care. 2003 Jun;9(3):230–5.

17 McMorrow RC, Mythen MG. Pulse oximetry. Curr Opin Crit Care. 2006 Jun;12(3):269–71.

18 Pedersen T, Moller AM, Hovhannisyan K. Pulse oximetry for perioperative monitoring. Cochrane Database Syst Rev. 2009. CD002013.

19 Moller JT, Johannessen NW, Espersen K, et al. Randomized evaluation of pulse oximetry in 20,802 patients. II. Perioperative events and postoperative complications. Anesthesiology. 1993 Mar;78(3):445–53.

20 Cheifetz IM, Myers TR. Respiratory therapies in the critical care setting: should every mechanically ventilated patient be monitored with capnography from intubation to extubation? Respir Care. 2007 Apr;52(4):423–38.

21 Araghi A, Bander JJ, Guzman JA. Arterial blood pressure monitoring in overweight critically ill patients: invasive or noninvasive? Crit Care. 2006;10(2):R64.

22 Beevers G, Lip GY, O'Brien E. ABC of hypertension: blood pressure measurement. Part I. Sphygmomanometry: factors common to all techniques. BMJ. 2001 Apr;322(7292): 981–5.

23 Beevers G, Lip GY, O'Brien E. ABC of hypertension: blood pressure measurement. Part II. Conventional sphygmomanometry: technique of auscultatory blood pressure measurement. BMJ. 2001 Apr;322(7293):1043–7.

24 Belani K, Ozaki M, Hynson J, et al. A new noninvasive method to measure blood pressure: results of a multicenter trial. Anesthesiology. 1999 Sep;91(3):686–92.

25 Hager H, Mandadi G, Pulley D, et al. A comparison of noninvasive blood pressure measurement on the wrist with invasive arterial blood pressure monitoring in patients undergoing bariatric surgery. Obes Surg. 2009 Jun;19(6):717–24.

26 Block FE, Schulte GT. Ankle blood pressure measurement, an acceptable alternative to arm measurements. Int J Clin Monit Comput. 1996 Aug;13(3):167–71.

27 Wilkes JM, DiPalma JA. Brachial blood pressure monitoring versus ankle monitoring during colonoscopy. South Med J. 2004 Oct;97(10):939–41.

28 Bernstein DP, Lemmens HJ, Brodsky JB. Limitations of impedance cardiography. Obes Surg. 2005 May;15(5): 659–60.

29 Bernstein DP, Lemmens HJ. Stroke volume equation for impedance cardiography. Med Biol Eng Comput. 2005 Jul;43(4):443–50.

30 Brown CV, Martin MJ, Shoemaker WC, et al. The effect of obesity on bioimpedance cardiac index. Am J Surg. 2005 May;189(5):547–50.

31 El-Dawlatly A, Mansour E, Al-Shaer AA, et al. Impedance cardiography: noninvasive assessment of hemodynamics and thoracic fluid content during bariatric surgery. Obes Surg. 2005 May;15(5):655–8.

32 Gedeon A, Forslund L, Hedenstierna G, Romano E. A new method for noninvasive bedside determination of pulmonary blood flow. Med Biol Eng Comput. 1980 Jul;18(4):411–18.

33 Odenstedt H, Aneman A, Oi Y, Svensson M, Stenqvist O, Lundin S. Descending aortic blood flow and cardiac output: a clinical and experimental study of continuous oesophageal echo-Doppler flowmetry. Acta Anaesthesiol Scand. 2001 Feb;45(2):180–7.

34 Rocco M, Spadetta G, Morelli A, et al. A comparative evaluation of thermodilution and partial CO2 rebreathing techniques for cardiac output assessment in critically ill patients during assisted ventilation. Intensive Care Med. 2004 Jan;30(1):82–7.

35 Maxwell RA, Gibson JB, Slade JB, Fabian TC, Proctor KG. Noninvasive cardiac output by partial CO2 rebreathing after severe chest trauma. J Trauma. 2001 Nov;51(5):849–53.

36 Kotake Y, Yamada T, Nagata H, et al. Improved accuracy of cardiac output estimation by the partial CO2 rebreathing method. J Clin Monit Comput. 2009 Jun;23(3): 149–55.

37 Valtier B, Cholley BP, Belot JP, de la Coussaye JE, Mateo J, Payen DM. Noninvasive monitoring of cardiac output in critically ill patients using transesophageal Doppler. Am J Respir Crit Care Med. 1998 Jul;158(1):77–83.

38 Bilkovski RN, Rivers EP, Horst HM. Targeted resuscitation strategies after injury. Curr Opin Crit Care. 2004 Dec;10(6):529–38.

39 Beaulieu Y, Marik PE. Bedside ultrasonography in the ICU. Part 2. Chest. 2005 Sep;128(3):1766–81.

40 Beaulieu Y, Marik PE. Bedside ultrasonography in the ICU. Part 1. Chest. 2005 Aug;128(2):881–95.

41 Stamos TD, Soble JS. The use of echocardiography in the critical care setting. Crit Care Clin. 2001 Apr;17(2): 253–70,v.

42 Reilly JP, Tunick PA, Timmermans RJ, Stein B, Rosenzweig BP, Kronzon I. Contrast echocardiography clarifies uninterpretable wall motion in intensive care unit patients. J Am Coll Cardiol. 2000 Feb;35(2):485–90.

43 Guarracino F, Baldassarri R. Transesophageal echocardiography in the OR and ICU. Minerva Anestesiol. 2009 Sep;75(9):518–29.

44 Costachescu T, Denault A, Guimond JG, et al. The hemodynamically unstable patient in the intensive care unit: hemodynamic vs. transesophageal echocardiographic monitoring. Crit Care Med. 2002 Jun;30(6):1214–23.

45 Reichert CL, Visser CA, Koolen JJ, et al. Transesophageal echocardiography in hypotensive patients after cardiac operations. Comparison with hemodynamic parameters. J Thorac Cardiovasc Surg. 1992 Aug;104(2):321–6.

46 Slabbekoorn M, Horlings HM, van der Meer JT, Windhausen A, van der Sloot JA, Lagrand WK. Left-sided native valve Staphylococcus aureus endocarditis. Neth J Med. 2010 Nov;68(11):341–7.

47 De BD, Ortiz JA, Salgado D. Coupling microcirculation to systemic hemodynamics. Curr Opin Crit Care. 2010 Jun;16(3):250–4.

48 De BD, Ospina-Tascon G, Salgado D, Favory R, Creteur J, Vincent JL. Monitoring the microcirculation in the critically ill patient: current methods and future approaches. Intensive Care Med. 2010 Nov;36(11):1813–25.

49 Mayer J, Suttner S. Cardiac output derived from arterial pressure waveform. Curr Opin Anaesthesiol. 2009 Dec;22(6):804–8.

50 Bernstein DP. Pressure pulse contour-derived stroke volume and cardiac output in the morbidly obese patient. Obes Surg. 2008 Aug;18(8):1015–21.

51 Forfori F, Romano SM, Balderi T, Anselmino M, Giunta F. Response to Dr. Bernstein's review: pressure pulse contour-derived stroke volume and cardiac output in the morbidly obese patient. Obes Surg. 2009 Jan;19(1):128–30, author.

52 Black IH, Blosser SA, Murray WB. Central venous pressure measurements: peripherally inserted catheters versus centrally inserted catheters. Crit Care Med. 2000 Dec;28(12):3833–6.

53 Marik PE, Baram M, Vahid B. Does central venous pressure predict fluid responsiveness? A systematic review of the literature and the tale of seven mares. Chest. 2008 Jul;134(1):172–8.

54 Swan HJ, Ganz W, Forrester J, Marcus H, Diamond G, Chonette D. Catheterization of the heart in man with use of a flow-directed balloon-tipped catheter. N Engl J Med. 1970 Aug;283(9):447–51.

55 Forrester JS, Diamond GA, Swan HJ. Correlative classification of clinical and hemodynamic function after acute myocardial infarction. Am J Cardiol. 1977 Feb;39(2):137–45.

56 Beutler S, Schmidt U, Michard F. Hemodynamic monitoring in obese patients: a big issue. Crit Care Med. 2004 Sep;32(9):1981.

57 Connors AF, Jr., Speroff T, Dawson NV, et al. The effectiveness of right heart catheterization in the initial care of critically ill patients. SUPPORT Investigators. JAMA. 1996 Sep;276(11):889–97.

58 Gore JM, Goldberg RJ, Spodick DH, Alpert JS, Dalen JE. A community-wide assessment of the use of pulmonary artery catheters in patients with acute myocardial infarction. Chest. 1987 Oct;92(4):721–7.

59 Iberti TJ, Fischer EP, Leibowitz AB, Panacek EA, Silverstein JH, Albertson TE. A multicenter study of physicians' knowledge of the pulmonary artery catheter. Pulmonary Artery Catheter Study Group. JAMA. 1990 Dec;264(22):2928–32.

60 Marik PE. Pulmonary artery catheterization and esophageal doppler monitoring in the ICU. Chest. 1999 Oct;116(4): 1085–91.

61 Swan HJ, Ganz W. Complications with flow-directed balloon-tipped catheters. Ann Intern Med. 1979 Sep;91(3):494.

62 Sandham JD, Hull RD, Brant RF, et al. A randomized, controlled trial of the use of pulmonary-artery catheters in high-risk surgical patients. N Engl J Med. 2003 Jan;348(1):5–14.

63 Vincent JL, Pinsky MR, Sprung CL, et al. The pulmonary artery catheter: in medio virtus. Crit Care Med. 2008 Nov;36(11):3093–6.

16 Diagnostic Imaging of the Critically Ill Obese Patient

Venkata S. Katabathina, Neeraj Lalwani, Carlos S. Restrepo, and Srinivasa R. Prasad

Department of Radiology, University of Texas Health Science Center, San Antonio, TX, USA

KEY POINTS

- Imaging plays an important role in the diagnosis and follow-up of various conditions that affect the critically ill obese patient.
- Obtaining diagnostic-quality images and performing interventional procedures in obese sick patients presents a significant challenge.
- Selection of the appropriate imaging modality and performance of necessary technical modifications play major roles in successful imaging of the critically ill obese patient.

INTRODUCTION

The prevalence of obesity has been increasing in the USA; currently about 68% of the adult population is overweight (body mass index (BMI) ≥ 25), and approximately 32% is obese (BMI ≥ 30) [1]. The percentage of critically ill obese patients among all intensive care unit (ICU) patients ranges from 5.4% in blunt trauma and 17% in postoperative cardiac surgical patients to as high as 25% depending on the group of patients examined [2,3]. Management of the critically ill obese patient requires a multidisciplinary approach with expertise from clinicians of different subspecialties and allied health care personnel. Detailed clinical examination of these patients is difficult to perform and many of the clinical findings of the chest and the abdomen may be obscured by thick subcutaneous soft tissues. Hence radiological investigation is very important to the diagnosis of various chest and abdominal pathologies. Diagnostic imaging of these patients poses a significant challenge to radiologists due to a multitude of factors. Treating clinicians need input from the imaging personnel in the diagnosis and follow-up of several acute entities in these patients. Select thoracic conditions that may complicate the clinical course include pneumonia, acute respiratory distress syndrome (ARDS), cor pulmonale, pulmonary thromboembolism, and pulmonary edema. Some abdominal entities include acute pancreatitis, acute cholecystitis, acute renal failure, intestinal obstruction, bowel perforation, and abdominal compartment syndrome (ACS). In addition, imaging also helps in the search for possible sources of infection in the septic patient, detection of deep venous thrombosis (DVT), and assessment of complications related to bariatric surgery. The available imaging modalities include plain radiography, ultrasound, computed tomography (CT), and magnetic resonance imaging (MRI). Some common problems encountered by radiology personnel related to imaging of these patients include selection of the best imaging modality for a given indication, transportation of the obese patients to the radiology department, accommodation of those patients on the available imaging equipment, and acquisition of diagnostic-quality images with the least possible radiation dose [4]. In addition, performing diagnostic and therapeutic interventions is difficult and requires necessary modifications to suit the individual patient [4].

In this chapter, we discuss the potential challenges in the imaging of critically ill obese patients and review currently available solutions to provide optimal imaging services. We also provide useful tips and tricks for performing safe, effective interventional procedures in these patients.

Critical Care Management of the Obese Patient, First Edition. Edited by Ali A. El Solh.
© 2012 John Wiley & Sons, Ltd. Published 2012 by John Wiley & Sons, Ltd.

CHALLENGES AND SOLUTIONS IN IMAGING OF THE CRITICALLY ILL OBESE PATIENT

The common challenges while imaging the critically ill obese patient include: selection of the best imaging modality for a given indication; transportation of the obese patient to the radiology department; accommodation of such patients on the available imaging equipment; and acquisition of diagnostic-quality images.

Selection of the best imaging modality for a given indication

Selection of the appropriate imaging modality is the first step in successful imaging of the critically ill obese patient. The clinical indication, patient's weight, and body diameter are three important factors to be considered before scheduling these patients for a particular examination [5]. The commonly used imaging modalities include plain film radiography, fluoroscopy, ultrasound, CT scan, and MRI. While ultrasound and radiography may be performed at the bedside, other exams require the patient's transportation to the radiology department.

Chest radiograph is the most commonly performed examination in ICU patients and is the initial test for evaluation of chest pain and dyspnea. Pneumonia, pleural effusions, cor pulmonale, pulmonary edema, and ARDS can be diagnosed based on chest radiographs alone. In addition, chest radiographs are helpful in confirming the position of the central venous lines and the endotracheal tube. Contrast-enhanced chest CT is indicated in suspected cases of pulmonary embolism (PE). Although CT scan is necessary for confirmation, initial abdominal radiographs are helpful in the diagnosis of intestinal obstruction and perforation. Abdominal CT is also helpful in the diagnosis of acute cholecystitis, intraabdominal abscess, and acute pancreatitis. Fluoroscopy with water-soluble contrast is performed in suspected cases of anastomotic leak in bariatric surgery patients. Ultrasound is helpful in the detection of ascites and pleural effusions, diagnosis of acute cholecystitis, and identification of obstruction in acute renal failure patients. Although rarely used in critically ill obese patients, MRI has an important role in the diagnosis of acute cholecystitis, suspected biliary obstruction, and acute pancreatitis.

As table weight limits and aperture diameters vary for different modalities, it is important to know the patient's weight and body diameter before opting for a particular modality. Current maximum allowable weight limits and

Table 16.1 Weight and aperture diameter limitations per imaging modality. (Source: [5].)

Imaging modality	Weight limit	Maximum aperture diameter
Fluoroscopy	320 kg/700 lb	63 cm
Multidetector CT	310 kg /680 lb	90 cm
Cylindrical-bore MRI	250 kg /550 lb	70 cm
Vertical-field MRI	250 kg /550 lb	55 cm

aperture diameters by imaging modality are summarized in Table 16.1 [5]. It is good practice to discuss with the technologist and/or radiologist before scheduling any examination and transporting patients out of the ICU. Scanning patients who exceed the defined weight limit may potentially damage the table or its motor mechanics and the cost of the damage may not be covered under insurance [4]. Some patients who meet the weight limit may have a girth in excess of the gantry/bore diameter, limiting imaging evaluation. For CT and MRI examinations, table thickness entering the gantry/bore has to be accounted for in the vertical plane and 15–18 cm must be subtracted from the gantry diameter to allow for the table thickness [4]. Patients weighing beyond these set limits may need to be referred to special imaging suites for imaging evaluation [6].

Transportation of the obese patient to the radiology department

For fluoroscopy, CT, and MRI examinations, the patient has to be transported to the radiology department. Critically ill patients should be kept within the radiology department for the least possible time and must have uneventful transportation to and from the imaging department. To accompany these goals, larger wheelchairs, larger stretchers, and well-trained nursing and transport staff should be available before moving the patient out of the ICU [4]. Proper coordination between radiology personnel and the ICU staff is crucial in safe transportation. If possible, intrahospital transfer is best accomplished on the patient's own hospital bed [7].

Accommodation of the obese patient on the imaging equipment

In addition to limitations of table weight and aperture diameters for CT, MRI, and fluoroscopy equipment, ultrasound and radiography may also have some constraints for accommodation of obese patients. The

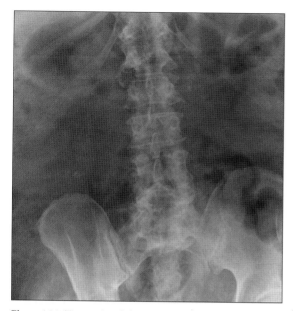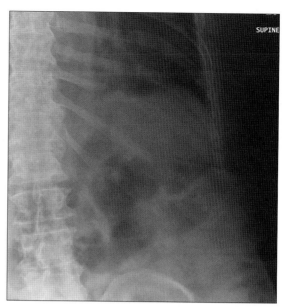

Figure 16.1 Two supine abdominal radiographs in a critically ill obese patient demonstrating the use of two 14 × 17 inch cassettes to image the entire abdomen.

maximum available size of the radiography cassette is 14 × 17 inches (approximately 35 × 43 cm) and it may be too small to cover the entire chest or abdomen in the obese patients [4]. Use of multiple cassettes to image different quadrants of the body in obese patients may help to tackle this problem (Figure 16.1). For ultrasound, appropriate position of the sick patient may be a problem for the technologists. For example, ultrasound scanning of the kidneys via a flank approach may be difficult in obese patients, and use of liver or spleen as a window may be beneficial. Proper use of pillows to support the patient's body is helpful in solving the problem of the patient's positioning [4]. While imaging the abdomen on CT and MRI, the patient's feet can be placed into the gantry/bore to avoid the girth of the upper abdomen and chest [4].

Acquisition of diagnostic-quality images

Acquisition of diagnostic-quality images is the most important and last step in optimal imaging of the critically ill obese patient. The potential challenges and possible solutions for each modality are discussed below.

Radiography and fluoroscopy

Chest and abdominal radiographs are the most commonly performed examinations in the ICU patient and are of limited diagnostic quality for obese patients. The potential causes include: 1) X-ray beam attenuation that results in decreased image contrast and increased noise; and 2) increase in exposure time resulting in motion artifacts. Use of bucky grid, and increase in kVp and mAs, helps in improving the image quality [4]. In addition, use of digital radiography allows image manipulation on the workstation and may improve proper visualization of internal structures, especially tubes and lines.

If post-bariatric surgery patient cannot fit on the fluoroscopy table, use of serial chest and/or abdominal radiographs may be beneficial in the diagnosis of anastomotic leak [4].

Sonography

Ultrasound image quality is affected by fat to a greater degree than any other imaging modality. Poor penetration of the ultrasound beam beyond the focal point and its increased attenuation as it passes through the fat are the two factors that limit the image quality [4]. The ultrasound beam is attenuated by fat at a rate of 0.63 dB/cm. However, the advantage of ultrasound for imaging of the ill obese patient is its portability. Solutions for improving image quality include use of the lowest-frequency transducer available (1.5–2 MHz), use of harmonics, and positioning of the transducer so that the organ of interest is

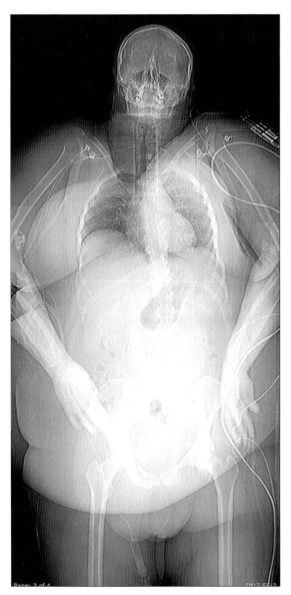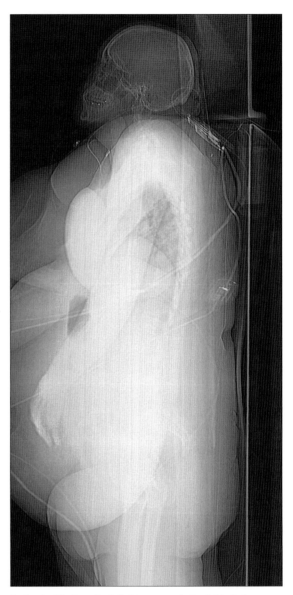

Figure 16.2 CT localizer images in a 38-year-old woman with abdominal pain. The large body habitus exceeds the field of view of the scanner on both the anteroposterior and lateral projections.

within its focal point [4]. In addition, proper positioning of the patient and application of pressure on the probe to displace the subcutaneous fat may be helpful.

CT scan

Despite limitations, CT is the most useful imaging modality for evaluation of obese patients. CT image quality is commonly diagnostic if the patient can fit within the scanner. Commonly encountered limitations while imaging the obese patient include increased image noise due to inadequate X-ray beam penetration, limited field of view, which can result in beam-hardening artifacts in the periphery of the patient's body, and image-quality limitations due to cropping (Figures 16.2 and 16.3) [4]. The graininess of a CT image is termed "image noise" and depends on the number of X-ray photos contributing to

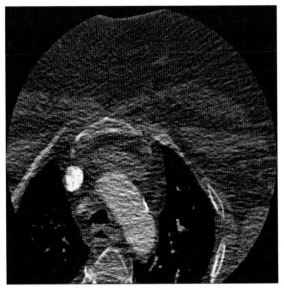 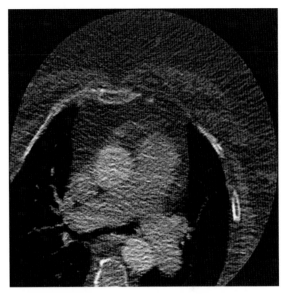

Figure 16.3 Coronary artery CT angiography in a 60-year-old morbidly obese female patient with acute chest pain. Axial images at the level of the aortic arch and pulmonary trunk. In morbidly obese patients image quality is significantly degraded, resulting in increased signal noise, producing this mottle appearance.

the image [8]. An increase in kVp and effective mAs increases the number of photons reaching the detector system, which in turn can decrease image noise [8]. Increase of kVp from 120 to 140 and switch of "fixed mAs" to "automatic mAs" are helpful in improving image quality [4,5]. In addition, a decrease in gantry speed and pitch is also useful. However, all these modifications tend to increase the radiation dose to the patient [5]. The beam-hardening artifact due to limited field of view can be avoided by adjusting the patient's position so that the area of interest doesn't exceed the field of view. It is not advisable to crop the CT image after acquisition, especially if the study is being performed to find the source of sepsis, as infection may be seen within the subcutaneous tissues.

MRI

Although MRI is rarely performed in the critically ill obese patient, certain clinical conditions (such as acute cerebrovascular accident, suspected biliary obstruction, and acute pancreatitis) may necessitate MRI evaluation. Two types are MRI machine are available: standard cylindrical-bore MRI and vertical open-field MRI. They differ in field strengths, signal-to-noise ratios (SNRs), and weight and diameter limitations. Cylindrical-bore

MRI machines have stronger gradients ($\geq 1.5\,T$) and high SNRs that result in high image quality. However, a longer bore length (about 170 cm) may be uncomfortable to the obese patient, who can become claustrophobic if the entire torso is in the bore [5]. In contradistinction, vertical-field MRIs have low SNRs and weaker gradients ($0.3–1.0\,T$) that limit the image quality; however, given the open field configuration, these MRI machines are more comfortable to obese patients. Recently released cylindrical-bore MRI machines also have larger bore diameters, shorter bore lengths, and higher table weight limits, which make them more obese-friendly [5].

Nuclear medicine

Nuclear medicine examinations such as myocardial perfusion studies and gallium and/or indium scans while searching for the source of infection are commonly performed in the critically ill obese patient. Scatter of photons within the soft tissues can decrease SNR (Figure 16.4) [4]. In addition, obese patients may exceed the maximum allowable dose and may not receive an appropriate dose for their body weight. Solutions include administration of maximum allowable radioisotope dose, use of high-field gamma cameras, and imaging for a longer time to maximize counts [5].

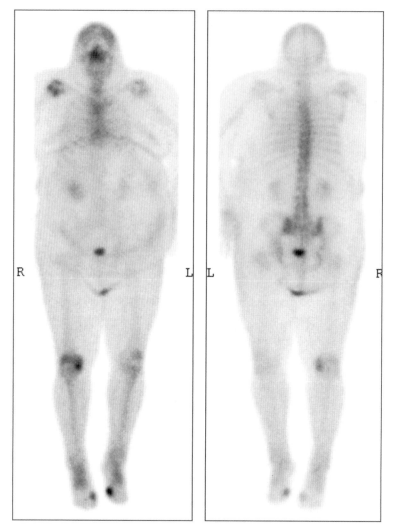

Figure 16.4 Tc-99 bone scan in a morbidly obese patient suspected for osteomyelitis, depicting significant attenuation of the radioisotopes in the bone secondary to the large amount of overlying soft tissues, making skeletal structures barely visible.

IMAGING OF COMMON THORACIC CONDITIONS

The commonly encountered thoracic conditions in critically ill obese patients that require imaging include pneumonia, pulmonary thromboembolism, ARDS, and cor pulmonale.

Pneumonia

Pneumonia is the most common cause of medical ICU admission in morbidly obese patients [9]. Obese patients are at an increased risk of pneumonia, and obesity is associated with higher risk of hospitalization with pneumonia [10,11]. In addition, the risk of gastric aspiration is increased in these patients due to a large volume of gastric fluid, increased intraabdominal pressure, and increased incidence of gastroesophageal reflux disease [12,13]. Chest radiography is the imaging test of choice for diagnosis, severity assessment, and surveillance [14,15]. On radiographs, pneumonia presents as focal or diffuse alveolar opacities with or without air bronchograms; associated pleural effusions may also be identified. Depending on the etiology, distribution of the pulmonary opacities may vary. In obese patients, the limited quality of portable radiographs may obscure distinction

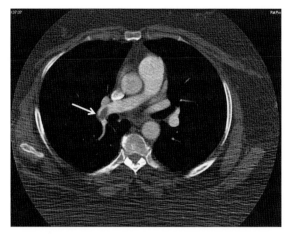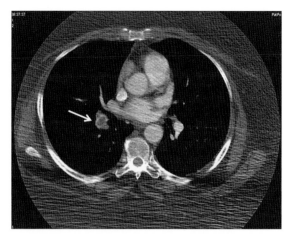

Figure 16.5 Pulmonary embolism. Contrast-enhanced CT in a morbidly obese woman presented with shortness of breath demonstrates filling defects in the right pulmonary artery (arrows).

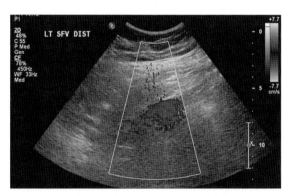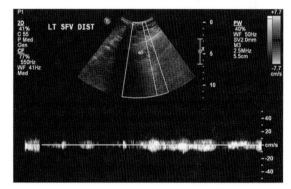

Figure 16.6 Color Doppler ultrasound of the left lower limb in an obese patient, demonstrating the use of curvilinear probe in the obese patient for definite identification of the lower-limb veins.

between pneumonic infiltrates and pulmonary edema. A confluence of shadows from overlying soft tissues can mimic pleural thickening or pleural effusions [12]. Unresolved and complicated pneumonia patients may need chest CT for further evaluation. Ultrasound is also helpful in diagnosis and aspiration of pleural effusions.

Pulmonary thromboembolism

Obesity is the single highest risk factor for PE and obese patients have a higher incidence of postoperative thromboembolic disease [16,17]. PE is the most common cause of postoperative mortality following bariatric surgery and may account for about 50% of all deaths [2]. Decreased mobility, venous stasis, and increased throm-

botic potential are possible causes for the high risk of venous thrombosis and PE. Multidetector CT scan is the imaging examination of choice and shows multiple filling defects within the pulmonary arteries, along with associated lung parenchymal changes (Figure 16.5) [18].

DVT of the lower extremity is the most common source for PE. Doppler ultrasound is the imaging modality of choice and may show acute thrombus as a hypoechoic/anechoic filling defect within the enlarged vein. In morbidly obese patients, ultrasound of the lower limbs may be limited due to subcutaneous fat and edema. Use of curvilinear ultrasound probe with 2–3 MHz frequency is recommended, instead of the routinely-used linear probe, for better demonstration of lower limb veins (Figure 16.6). Magnetic resonance venography is a potential alternative for suspected intrapelvic and proximal lower-limb thrombi [19,20]. In addition, CT venography of the lower limbs can be performed at the same time as CT pulmonary angiography without the need for additional contrast [21].

Acute respiratory distress syndrome

Acute lung injury/acute respiratory distress syndrome (ALI/ARDS) is one of the common indications for mechanical ventilation and ICU admission [9]. Although current data are inconclusive, obesity and ARDS appear to share alterations in inflammation, endothelial dysfunction, and oxidative stress. This raises the possibility that obese patients are at higher risk of developing ARDS, with poorer clinical outcome [22]. ARDS is characterized by acute onset of severe respiratory distress and unresponsive hypoxemia secondary to diffuse alveolar epithelial injury. Chest radiographs show bilateral, predominantly peripheral, asymmetrical consolidations with air bronchograms and absence of pleural effusions and septal lines. Chest radiographs help in the initial diagnosis and follow-up after resolution of the condition.

Cor pulmonale

Obese patients are at a higher risk of developing obstructive sleep apnea and obesity hypoventilation syndrome [11,13]. About one third of these patients develop pulmonary hypertension and right heart failure resulting in cor pulmonale. Cor pulmonale is one of the common causes of ICU admission in obese patients [9]. Chest radiography findings include enlargement of the central pulmonary arteries with oligemic peripheral lung parenchyma and right ventricular hypertrophy, which indicate development of pulmonary hypertension. The potential problem during interpretation of a chest radiograph in morbidly obese patients is the presence of excessive mediastinal fat, which may mimic enlarged pulmonary artery or thoracic aortic aneurysm [7].

IMAGING OF SELECT ABDOMINAL PATHOLOGIES

Imaging plays an important role in the diagnosis and management of various abdominal pathologies in the critically ill obese patient. Imaging can help in finding the source of sepsis, detecting the cause of acute abdominal pain, and diagnosing life-threatening ACS in these patients. CT is the most commonly used imaging modality in evaluating the abdominal pathologies in obese ICU patients.

Finding the source of sepsis

Sepsis is the most common cause of mortality and morbidity in noncoronary artery disease critical care units [23]. Obesity is considered as a proinflammatory state. Obese patients show an exaggerated response to external stimulus and are at increased risk of developing sepsis [24]. In addition, obese patients have greater risk of developing sepsis after surgery due to impaired wound healing related to poorly vascularized adipose tissue, and an increased incidence of diabetes mellitus and hyperglycemia [13]. The abdomen is commonly implicated as a source of sepsis in the critically ill patient, if there is no identifiable cause elsewhere in the body [25]. CT and ultrasound are common imaging modalities used; in particular, CT has been the mainstay technique for detecting intraabdominal fluid collections (Figure 16.7) [26]. In addition, CT/ultrasound also provide a roadmap and guidance for percutaneous abscess drainage in septic patients [26].

Detecting the cause of acute abdominal pain

Acute abdominal pain in the critically ill obese patient may be due to multiple inflammatory and noninflammatory causes. Common causes include acute cholecystitis, acute pancreatitis, acute appendicitis, bowel obstruction, and intestinal perforation. The incidence of cholelithiasis and acute cholecystitis is high in morbidly obese patients when compared to normal population and the risk is positively correlated with BMI [27]. Irregular gallbladder wall thickening, wall edema, pericholecystic fat stranding, and fluid collections are the common imaging findings of acute cholecystitis. In addition, complications such as gallbladder perforation, necrotizing cholecystitis, and hemorrhagic cholecystitis may be detected on imaging. Acute pancreatitis is one of the most common abdominal causes for ICU admission in obese patients [9]. Obesity is a risk factor for the development of local and systemic complications in acute pancreatitis and increases the mortality associated with this condition [28,29]. CT is the imaging modality of choice and helps in diagnosis, detection of complications, and follow-up. On CT, acute pancreatitis appears as an enlarged pancreas with peripancreatic fat stranding and fluid collections. In addition,

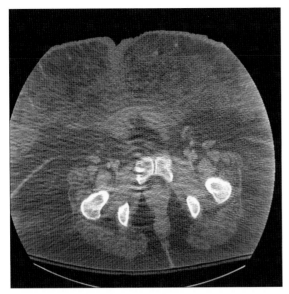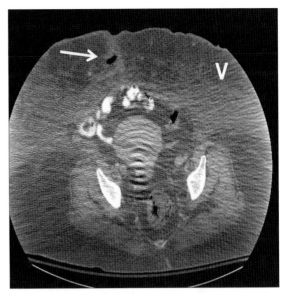

Figure 16.7 Cellulitis and soft-tissue abscess. CT of the abdomen in a morbidly obese patient demonstrates extensive stranding of the fat in the anterior abdominal wall, with a small collection of gas near the midline (arrow). Ring artifacts result from the close contact between the patient and the inner surface of the gantry (arrowhead).

identification of pseudocyst, abscess, pancreatic necrosis, and hemorrhage may be facilitated by imaging. Small bowel obstruction is common after bariatric surgery and patients present with severe abdominal pain. This topic is discussed in detail below.

Diagnosing life-threatening abdominal compartment syndrome

ACS is a potential cause of multiorgan failure in the critically ill obese patients [7]. An increase in intraabdominal pressure may be due to multiple trauma, massive hemorrhage, acute pancreatitis, or vigorous fluid resuscitation [7,12]. Although ACS is a clinical diagnosis, radiological findings such as elevated diaphragm, collapsed inferior vena cava, bowel wall thickening, bowel mucosal enhancement, hemoperitoneum, and increasing abdominal girth all suggest it [30].

Imaging of the post-bariatric surgery critically ill patient

The number of bariatric surgeries has been increasing in the USA in recent times and it is estimated that 220 000 surgeries were performed in 2008. Common bariatric surgical procedures include Roux-en-Y gastric bypass,

laparoscopic adjustable gastric banding, vertical-banded gastroplasty (VBG), jejunal bypass, and bilio-pancreatic diversion [31]. Patients undergoing bariatric surgery may require ICU admission for routine postoperative care and for management of complications. Common complications that require imaging for diagnosis include anastomotic leaks and intestinal obstruction [31]. Anastomotic leaks, occurring in up to 5% of patients, are the most dreaded complication given the high risk for sepsis [31]. Development of severe tachycardia and intractable respiratory failure during the postoperative period should arouse the suspicion of leak and immediate imaging is recommended [32]. Upper gastrointestinal contrast examination with water-soluble contrast is the investigation of choice and shows contrast extravasation about the anastomosis, extending into the peritoneal cavity [31]. If there is strong clinical suspicion for leak, exploratory laporotomy is indicated, even if imaging findings are negative [33]. Small bowel obstruction after Roux-en-Y gastric bypass surgery may occur in up to 7.5% patients, with laparoscopic procedures having higher incidence compared to open surgeries [34,35]. CT scan is the best imaging modality for confirmation of the diagnosis and detection of the etiology. Common causes of obstruction include anastomotic strictures, internal hernias, and volvulus [35].

RADIOLOGICAL INTERVENTIONS IN THE CRITICALLY ILL OBESE PATIENT

Image-guided interventions in the critically ill obese patient are technically challenging. Common difficulties include proper position for the procedure, the ability to fit the patient and the instruments into the gantry, instrument length, sedation-related issues, and greater than average risk of postprocedure complications [5]. Thoracentesis, paracentesis, placement of the cholecystostomy and gastrostomy tubes, drainage of abscesses and pancreatic pseudocysts, and biliary stenting are some of the most common procedures performed in these patients [36]. Ultrasound, CT, and fluoroscopy are the modalities available for imaging guidance. Of these, ultrasound is the preferred modality given the advantage of the easy portability of the machine, meaningtransportation of the sick patient can be avoided. Meticulous preprocedural planning with focus on tricks to tackle anticipated challenges during the procedure is key to the successful completion of the procedure. Proper review of available imaging studies helps in selection of the appropriate imaging modality, determination of the amount of subcutaneous fat, the most direct approach to the targeted tissue, and estimation of the instrument length [4]. Proper positioning of the patient during the procedure is important and appropriate use of pillows, splints, and sandbags may be helpful. For CT-guided procedures, fitting both the instruments and the patient into the gantry is a major limitation. Use of CT-fluoroscopy to guide the instrument in at a different angle, and positioning of the patient off-center into the gantry may provide the shortest distance to the target and more room on the procedure side [5,36]. The standard-length instruments may not be able to reach the intended lesion in obese patients. Preprocedural estimation of the distance and use of the appropriate instruments may overcome this problem. Use of a shorter, larger needle first and then progressively longer and thinner needles may be indicated [36]. In addition, a 1–2 cm length advantage may be gained by pushing down on and displacing the subcutaneous fat. After catheter placement in the abscess cavity, attaching the catheter to the reservoir suction and frequently irrigating the catheter may speed up the resolution. The need for redrainage can be avoided by ordering a follow-up scan to confirm the resolution before catheter removal [36]. Given the fact that critically ill patients are usually on multiple medications, sedation and pain-control issues pose a significant problem. Airway management is the most important issue to be addressed during sedation and drug dosage has to be monitored meticulously [5]. Patients with airway problems or problems with administering adequate pain medicine may need anesthesia consultation [4].

In addition, Doppler-ultrasound guidance is used by the intensivist to obtain central venous access in these patients. It has been shown that use of ultrasound guidance helps in reduction of the number of needle passes to cannulate the vein and associated complications [37]. Ultrasound guidance may also be used for the placement of arterial lines in the critically ill obese patient.

CONCLUSION

The prevalence of obese patients requiring critical care support has been increasing in the USA. Diagnostic imaging and performance of image-guided interventional procedures in the critically ill obese patient are challenging secondary to a myriad of patient-related and equipment-related issues. Radiologists and technologists should be aware of the potential problems in imaging these patients and possible solutions to tackle them, which can improve overall patient management. Selection of the appropriate imaging modality for a given indication and addition of necessary technical modifications are major factors in successful imaging of these patients.

BEST PRACTICE TIPS

1 Before scheduling the critically ill obese patient for a particular radiological examination, discussion with the radiologist regarding the clinical indication, patient's weight, and body diameter is always recommended.

2 Increase in kVp and effective mAs and decrease in gantry speed and pitch can improve CT image quality while scanning the obese patient.

3 Chest radiography is the most commonly performed radiological examination in the critically ill obese patient; CT chest is indicated in suspected cases of pulmonary thromboembolism.

4 Upper gastrointestinal contrast examination with hydro-soluble oral contrast is the investigation of choice to diagnose anastomotic leak in post-bariatric surgery patients.

5 Review of available imaging studies and meticulous preprocedural planning are important factors in the successful performance of radiological interventions in the critically ill obese patient.

REFERENCES

1 Wang Y, Beydoun MA. The obesity epidemic in the United States—gender, age, socioeconomic, racial/ethnic, and geographic characteristics: a systematic review and meta-regression analysis. Epidemiol Rev. 2007;29:6–28.

2 Joffe A, Wood K. Obesity in critical care. Curr Opin Anaesthesiol. 2007 Apr;20(2):113–18.

3 Pieracci FM, Barie PS, Pomp A. Critical care of the bariatric patient. Crit Care Med. 2006 Jun;34(6):1796–804.

4 Uppot RN, Sahani DV, Hahn PF, Gervais D, Mueller PR. Impact of obesity on medical imaging and image-guided intervention. AJR Am J Roentgenol. 2007 Feb;188(2):433–40.

5 Uppot RN. Impact of obesity on radiology. Radiol Clin North Am. 2007 Mar;45(2):231–46.

6 Ginde AA, Foianini A, Renner DM, Valley M, Camargo CA Jr. The challenge of CT and MRI imaging of obese individuals who present to the emergency department: a national survey. Obesity (Silver Spring). 2008 Nov;16(11):2549–51.

7 El Solh AA. Clinical approach to the critically ill, morbidly obese patient. Am J Respir Crit Care Med. 2004 Mar 1;169(5):557–61.

8 Goldman LW. Principles of CT: radiation dose and image quality. J Nucl Med Technol. 2007 Dec;35(4):213–25; quiz 26–8.

9 El-Solh A, Sikka P, Bozkanat E, Jaafar W, Davies J. Morbid obesity in the medical ICU. Chest. 2001 Dec;120(6):1989–97.

10 Kornum JB, Norgaard M, Dethlefsen C, Due KM, Thomsen RW, Tjonneland A, et al. Obesity and risk of subsequent hospitalisation with pneumonia. Eur Respir J. 2010 Dec;36(6):1330–6.

11 Murugan AT, Sharma G. Obesity and respiratory diseases. Chron Respir Dis. 2008;5(4):233–42.

12 Honiden S, McArdle JR. Obesity in the intensive care unit. Clin Chest Med. 2009 Sep;30(3):581–99, x.

13 Thornton K. Management of the critically ill obese patient. In Basow DS, editor. UpToDate. Waltham, MA, UpToDate. 2010.

14 Katz DS, Leung AN. Radiology of pneumonia. Clin Chest Med. 1999 Sep;20(3):549–62.

15 Sharma S, Maycher B, Eschun G. Radiological imaging in pneumonia: recent innovations. Curr Opin Pulm Med. 2007 May;13(3):159–69.

16 Goldhaber SZ, Grodstein F, Stampfer MJ, Manson JE, Colditz GA, Speizer FE, et al. A prospective study of risk factors for pulmonary embolism in women. JAMA. 1997 Feb 26;277(8):642–5.

17 Marik P, Varon J. The obese patient in the ICU. Chest. 1998 Feb;113(2):492–8.

18 MacDonald SL, Mayo JR. Computed tomography of acute pulmonary embolism. Semin Ultrasound CT MR. 2003 Aug;24(4):217–31.

19 Kanne JP, Lalani TA. Role of computed tomography and magnetic resonance imaging for deep venous thrombosis and pulmonary embolism. Circulation. 2004 Mar 30;109(12 Suppl 1): I15–21.

20 Evans AJ, Sostman HD, Knelson MH, Spritzer CE, Newman GE, Paine SS, et al. 1992 ARRS Executive Council Award. Detection of deep venous thrombosis: prospective comparison of MR imaging with contrast venography. AJR Am J Roentgenol. 1993 Jul;161(1):131–9.

21 Katz DS, Loud PA, Bruce D, Gittleman AM, Mueller R, Klippenstein DL, et al. Combined CT venography and pulmonary angiography: a comprehensive review. Radiographics. 2002 Oct;22(Spec No):S3–19; disc. S20–4.

22 McCallister JW, Adkins EJ, O'Brien JM Jr. Obesity and acute lung injury. Clin Chest Med. 2009 Sep;30(3):495–508, viii.

23 Vachharajani V, Vital S. Obesity and sepsis. J Intensive Care Med. 2006 Sep–Oct;21(5):287–95.

24 Vachharajani V. Influence of obesity on sepsis. Pathophysiology. 2008 Aug;15(2):123–34.

25 Merrell RC. The abdomen as source of sepsis in critically ill patients. Crit Care Clin. 1995 Apr;11(2):255–72.

26 Lee MJ. Non-traumatic abdominal emergencies: imaging and intervention in sepsis. Eur Radiol. 2002 Sep;12(9):2172–9.

27 Dittrick GW, Thompson JS, Campos D, Bremers D, Sudan D. Gallbladder pathology in morbid obesity. Obes Surg. 2005 Feb;15(2):238–42.

28 Abu Hilal M, Armstrong T. The impact of obesity on the course and outcome of acute pancreatitis. Obes Surg. 2008 Mar;18(3):326–8.

29 Martinez J, Johnson CD, Sanchez-Paya J, de Madaria E, Robles-Diaz G, Perez-Mateo M. Obesity is a definitive risk factor of severity and mortality in acute pancreatitis: an updated meta-analysis. Pancreatology. 2006;6(3):206–9.

30 Patel A, Lall CG, Jennings SG, Sandrasegaran K. Abdominal compartment syndrome. AJR Am J Roentgenol. 2007 Nov;189(5):1037–43.

31 Chandler RC, Srinivas G, Chintapalli KN, Schwesinger WH, Prasad SR. Imaging in bariatric surgery: a guide to post-surgical anatomy and common complications. AJR Am J Roentgenol. 2008 Jan;190(1):122–35.

32 Hamilton EC, Sims TL, Hamilton TT, Mullican MA, Jones DB, Provost DA. Clinical predictors of leak after laparoscopic Roux-en-Y gastric bypass for morbid obesity. Surg Endosc. 2003 May;17(5):679–84.

33 Jones D. Complications of bariatric surgery. In Basow DS, editor. UpToDate. Waltham, MA, UpToDate. 2010.

34 Podnos YD, Jimenez JC, Wilson SE, Stevens CM, Nguyen NT. Complications after laparoscopic gastric bypass: a review of 3464 cases. Arch Surg. 2003 Sep;138(9):957–61.

35 Sunnapwar A, Sandrasegaran K, Menias CO, Lockhart M, Chintapalli KN, Prasad SR. Taxonomy and imaging spectrum of small bowel obstruction after Roux-en-Y gastric bypass surgery. AJR Am J Roentgenol. 2010 Jan;194(1):120–8.

36 Olson M, Pohl C. Bedside and radiologic procedures in the critically ill obese patient. Crit Care Clin. 2010 Oct;26(4):665–8.

37 Gilbert TB, Seneff MG, Becker RB. Facilitation of internal jugular venous cannulation using an audio-guided Doppler ultrasound vascular access device: results from a prospective, dual-center, randomized, crossover clinical study. Crit Care Med. 1995 Jan;23(1):60–5.

Part V Postsurgical Management

17 Postoperative Care of the Obese Patient

Hui Sen Chong[1] and Robert L. Bell[2]

[1]Department of Surgery, University of Iowa Hospitals and Clinics, Iowa City, IA, USA
[2]Department of Surgery, Yale University School of Medicine, New Haven, CT, USA

KEY POINTS

- Obese patients are at a higher risk of postoperative complications from a cardiac, respiratory, and thromboembolic standpoint.
- Physicians should be wary of tachycardia and low urine output in the postoperative setting, since this might be the only sign of intraabdominal pathology in the obese patient.
- The hospital needs to be equipped with facilities to provide a safe environment for the recovering obese patient and their health care providers.

INTRODUCTION

Obesity is defined by a body mass index (BMI) $\geq 30 \, kg/m^2$. The prevalence of obesity in the US adult population has been steadily rising over the past decade [1,2]. Along with a steady rise in the number of bariatric procedures performed, surgeons in various fields are encountering an increasing volume of obese patients. This chapter serves to provide a comprehensive overview for the postoperative care of these patients.

CARDIOVASCULAR SYSTEM

Patients with obesity often have associated medical comorbidities, including hypertension, diabetes, coronary artery disease, and so on. Accordingly, these patients are at a higher risk for cardiovascular complications after surgery [3]. Multiple studies have shown a strong correlation between obesity and hypertension, cardiomyopathy, heart failure, and pulmonary hypertension [4–6]. This is especially true for obese patients with metabolic syndrome, which is defined by the presence of three of more of the following five risk factors:

1. central obesity (waist circumference > 102 cm (40 in) in men and > 88 cm (35 in) in women)
2. elevated blood pressure (> 130/85 mm Hg)
3. glucose intolerance (> 100 mg/dl)
4. elevated triglyceride level (> 150 mg/dl)
5. reduction in high-density lipoprotein cholesterol (< 40 mg/dl in men and < 50 mg/dl in women) [7,8].

Overall, obese patients have a two to threefold higher risk of cardiac adverse events when compared to those with normal weight [9]. However, BMI alone does not portend a worse prognosis. In fact, obese patients without the associated metabolic syndrome have similar perioperative cardiac adverse events to those with normal weight [3,9,10]. The American Heart Association (AHA) divides patients into low-, intermediate-, and high-risk surgical groups. This serves as a guide for physicians when it comes to preoperative workup and postoperative care. However, it is unknown if obesity, in the absence of metabolic sequelae, influences these categorizations.

There is no formal recommendation for routine postoperative telemetry in obese patients who undergo surgery. According to the AHA practice guidelines [11], continuous cardiac monitoring should be routinely placed on patients with the following conditions:

- an acute coronary event
- status post any cardiac-related surgery or intervention
- preexisting arrhythmia
- acute heart failure
- administration of an antiarrhythmic medication that has a known high risk of causing arrhythmias.

Critical Care Management of the Obese Patient, First Edition. Edited by Ali A. El Solh.
© 2012 John Wiley & Sons, Ltd. Published 2012 by John Wiley & Sons, Ltd.

Continuous cardiac monitoring may be beneficial, but is not essential, for the following conditions [11]:

- post-acute myocardial infarction
- chest pain syndromes without diagnostic electrocardiogram findings or elevated biomarkers
- status post uncomplicated, nonurgent percutaneous coronary interventions, or ablation of an arrhythmia
- syncope
- subacute heart failure.

About 1–4% of patients who undergo noncardiac surgery will sustain a perioperative myocardial infarction. Other cardiac events, such as new-onset or worsened heart failure, new-onset arrhythmias, or primary cardiac arrest, may also occur in the postoperative period [12]. Importantly, it is well established that obese patients have an increased risk of cardiac arrhythmia and sudden death, even in the absence of overt cardiac dysfunction [13,14]. Physicians must realize that perioperative ischemia or congestive heart failure often presents atypically, with patients complaining of typical chest pain only 5–28% of the time [12,15,16]. Postoperative electrocardiogram (EKG) and serial troponins should be considered for the obese patient with any of the following conditions:

- Multiple risk factors for coronary artery disease that pose a significant risk for a postoperative cardiac event.
- Intraoperative ST segment changes suggestive of ischemia. The sensitivity and specificity for predicting postoperative cardiac events in this instance ranges from 55 to 100% and 37 to 85%, respectively [12].
- Typical or atypical chest pain.

They are also indicated for obese patients with known coronary artery disease who are to undergo an intermediate- to high-risk surgical procedure [17].

Arrhythmia

Arrhythmia in the obese patient is most commonly related to hypoxia in the asleep patient in the setting of untreated obstructive sleep apnea (OSA). Nocturnal bradyarrhythmias and/or tachyarrhythmias [18] occur in approximately 80% of patients with untreated OSA. The bradycardia occurs during the initial phase of the apnea [19], and a sinus tachycardia occurs when ventilation resumes [20]. The best way to prevent these arrhythmias is to apply noninvasive positive pressure ventilation (continuous positive airway pressure, CPAP) when the patient is sleeping. Other forms of postoperative arrhythmias include atrial fibrillation, atrial flutter, and ventricular tachycardia. Postoperative atrial fibrillation occurs in about 4% of patients who undergo major noncardiotho-

racic surgery [21]. Causes of postoperative atrial fibrillation vary from left atrial enlargement, commonly encountered in obese individuals [22,23], to routine postoperative hemodynamic or electrolyte imbalance [24].

Treatment for new-onset postoperative atrial fibrillation or atrial flutter involves prompt recognition of the cause of the arrhythmia, stabilization of the patient, and electrical or pharmacological cardioversion. Electrical cardioversion should be reserved for patients who are hemodynamically unstable. More commonly, pharmacological cardioversion with drugs such as amiodarone or digoxin is extremely effective, but may result in a longer hospital stay [25]. For those patients who are asymptomatic, rate control itself may be sufficient. If the arrhythmia persists for more than 48 hours, anticoagulation should be initiated to decrease the risk of a thromboembolic event [26]. Remember that in all patients with a new-onset arrhythmia, the abnormal rhythm is merely a symptom of a homeostatic perturbation. In the postoperative setting, the arrhythmia may be the first sign of a serious surgical complication. Accordingly, the cause of the abnormal heart rhythm must be identified and treated. Never treat the rate or rhythm in isolation [21].

Hypertension

The vast majority of patients with hypertension are overweight or obese [27]. The increase in blood pressure is most pronounced when the obesity is central; that is, when there is an abdominal distribution [28]. Antihypertensives are commonly used postoperatively in patients with pre-existing hypertension, or in patients with newly diagnosed hypertension. The target blood pressure in patients with metabolic syndrome should be less than 140/90 mm Hg. However, if the hypertensive patient has associated diabetes or chronic kidney disease, the recommended goal is a blood pressure less than 130/80 mm Hg [29]. Below, we discuss some antihypertensives that are commonly used in the postoperative period.

Angiotensin converting enzyme (ACE) inhibitors/angiotensin receptor blockers (ARBs)

Fat cells produce a number of dysmetabolic hormones, including angiotensinogen. Not surprisingly, obese patients with hypertension often have a relatively elevated heart rate, high cardiac output, and hyperactivation of the renin-angiotensin-aldosterone system. Angiotensin converting enzyme (ACE) inhibitors should be considered in postoperative hypertensive patients with associated metabolic syndrome [30,31]. In addition to providing both cardio- and renoprotective benefits [30], ACE inhibitors have been proven to decrease the likelihood of developing new-onset type II diabetes, to decrease albuminuria, and to improve insulin resistance. Accordingly, ACE inhibitors are the recommended first-line agent for the obese hypertensive population [32].

Beta blockers

For patients who were on preoperative beta blockade for all indications, including the treatment of angina, symptomatic arrhythmias, hypertension, or heart failure, the medication should be continued in the postoperative period [17]. Beta blockers reduce cardiac output and inhibit rennin production [33], decreasing primary cardiac events such as cardiovascular death, myocardial infarction, and cardiac arrest in the postoperative period [34]. The goal is to achieve a targeted heart rate around 60–65 bpm [35,36]. Failure to continue preoperative beta blockade in the postoperative period could provoke a tachyarrhythmia as a result of beta blocker "withdrawal."

Calcium channel blockers

The dihydropyridine class of calcium channel blocker, such as amlodipine, is a good choice for treating hypertension in obese and/or diabetic patients [37]. Similar to the ACE inhibitors, these drugs have been shown to improve insulin resistance [30]. The nondihydropyridine class of calcium channel blocker, such as Verapamil, is more appropriately reserved for use in the setting of cardiac dysrhythmias. In these patients, Verapamil has been shown to significantly reduce the rate of incidence of ischemia and supraventricular tachycardia in the postoperative period [17].

Diuretics

The addition of spironolactone to an antihypertensive regimen that includes an ACE inhibitor or an angiotensin receptor blocker (ARB) provides additional cardio- and renoprotective benefits, especially in patients with diabetic nephropathy [30]. Thiazides, such as hydrochlorothiazide, reduce blood pressure by decreasing cardiac output via diuresis and natriuresis. They have been shown to be as effective as ACE inhibitors in lowering blood pressure [31,38].

RESPIRATORY SYSTEM

Postoperatively, obese patients are at risk for hypoxemia and hypoventilation for a variety of reasons, including: increased work of breathing, decreased functional residual

capacity, and decreased respiratory drive secondary to residual inhalational anesthetics, intravenous sedatives, or intravenous opioid analgesics [39,40]. If frequent or severe airway obstruction or hypoxemia occurs in the obese patient postoperatively, noninvasive positive airway pressure ventilation (NPPV), in the form of CPAP, should be initiated [19]. Severe and prolonged episodes of hypoxemia are especially prominent in those who are morbidly obese (BMI > 40 kg/m^2), and may occur despite the appropriate use of postoperative noninvasive positive pressure ventilation (CPAP) [39]. Therefore, the routine use of continuous pulse oximetry or telemetry is also advised.

After surgery, aggressive pulmonary toileting should be instituted as soon as the patient arrives on the surgical floor. To minimize atelectasis and prevent pneumonia, patients should be encouraged to cough, take deep breaths, and use an incentive spirometer whenever they are awake. Additionally, the head of the bed should be elevated to 30–45°, preferably in a reverse Trendelenburg position. This position reduces the abdominal pressure on the diaphragm to optimize tidal volume [41].

It is important to remember that, postoperatively, the obese patient may have difficulty maintaining an airway as a result of incomplete reversal of neuromuscular blockade and/or OSA. Patients with OSA tend to have increased oral and pharyngeal tissue, which contributes to upper airway collapse during sleep. Approximately 70% of OSA patients are obese [42]. OSA is characterized by recurrent episodes of upper airway obstruction during sleep that occur despite maintenance of neuromuscular ventilatory effort [43]. The clinical diagnosis of OSA is confirmed when the number of obstructive events is greater than fifteen episodes per hour of sleep, accompanied by episodes of choking, insomnia, or daytime sleepiness [44].

Positive airway pressure was first described by Sullivan in 1981 [45]. It is an effective method in treating OSA and can be delivered in three forms: continuous (CPAP), bilevel (BIPAP), or auto- titrating (APAP). The most common means of delivering positive pressure in patients with sleep apnea is via CPAP. For patients with documented OSA, the NPPV should be initiated during the postoperative period, starting in the recovery room. The usage should then continue once on the surgical floor or in the surgical intensive care unit (ICU), whenever the patient is asleep. CPAP should even be used in obese patients with OSA who are post gastric bypass. For post-gastric-bypass patients, there is a theoretical fear of increasing the risk of anastomotic disruption when NPPV is started in the immediate postoperative period.

In all patients who use CPAP, the incidence of gastric distension as a result of NPPV is approximately 2% [46]. Gastric distension can be minimized when the peak airway pressure is set below the resting upper esophageal sphincter pressure of 33 mm Hg ± 12 mm Hg [46]. A prospective study by Huerta et al. confirmed that there was no relationship between CPAP usage and anastomotic disruption [47]. For obese patients without documented OSA, supplemental oxygen should be administered continuously until they are able maintain their baseline oxygen saturation while breathing room air [48].

POSTOPERATIVE PARAMETERS

The patient's oxygen saturation should be kept above 90%, with supplementary oxygen per face mask or nasal canula on an as-needed basis [49]. If desaturation occurs or if the patient requires increasing supplementary oxygen, the patient's fluid status should be evaluated to ensure that they are not volume overloaded. Medications, especially narcotics and anxiolytics, should be reevaluated to ensure that they are appropriately dosed and that the patient is not overly sedated. Pulmonary processes like atelectasis, pneumonia, or pulmonary embolism (PE) should also be included in the differential diagnosis.

The presence of tachycardia is an important bedside physical finding in the postoperative period. Common causes of tachycardia must be considered, including dehydration, inadequate pain control, low oxygen saturation, myocardial ischemia, and infarction [50]. Importantly, in the obese patient with intraabdominal pathology, often a mild to moderate tachycardia and low urine output may be the only measurable clinical signs. Every physician involved in the patient's care should be wary of such physical findings. Airway assessment should always take precedence, and blood chemistry profiles (complete blood count, arterial blood gas analysis, electrolytes) will often aid in the differential diagnosis.

Postoperatively, significant third spacing of intravascular fluid may occur. Depending on the type and length of surgery, obese patients may require up to 6 liters of fluid to achieve a euvolemic state [41]. For patients with a BMI > 35 kg/m², maintenance of intravenous fluids should begin at a rate of 150 cc/hour. The rate is titrated up or down based on the patient's urine output and oral intake assessments.

In addition to frequent vital sign monitoring, accurate fluid intake and output is paramount in the obese patient. Those with dehydration and third spacing of fluids will exhibit decreased urine output (< 30 cc/hour),

but may only have relative hypotension (systolic blood pressure < 100 mm Hg) and mild tachycardia (heart rate 100–109 bpm) [51]. Assessment of blood and urine chemistry profiles (blood urea nitrogen, creatinine, fraction excretion of sodium) will also help in determining the cause of oliguria. If dehydration is the cause of a low urine output, the patient should receive a 1 liter bolus of lactated ringers and the maintenance of intravenous fluid rate should be increased. This process is repeated until the patient's urine output improves.

POSTOPERATIVE ANALGESIA

In the obese patient, a balanced, multimodal, postoperative analgesia regimen should be used to optimize the patient's pain control while minimizing opioid analgesic side effects such as respiratory depression [52]. Adequate postoperative analgesia is extremely important in that it not only improves the patient's comfort level but also decreases the risk of cardiac, pulmonary, and thromboembolic complications. A variety of options exist, but the optimal method utilizes a multimodal approach including a combination of local anesthetics in the wound, nonsteroidal antiinflammatory drugs (intravenous or oral), modest doses of opioids (intravenous or oral), and regional or epidural analgesia [52,53].

In order to minimize respiratory complications, obese patients undergoing open abdominal, open thoracic, or extremity surgery may benefit from epidural analgesia [52,54]. Epidural analgesia provides significantly better postoperative analgesia as compared to intravenous opioids [40,54–56]. The epidural solution should be opioid free in order to minimize respiratory depression [53]. Unfortunately, in some obese patients the distribution of the excess body mass can obscure anatomical landmarks, complicating epidural catheter placement [54,57,58]. Also, there is an increased risk for epidural hematoma in those who are receiving low-molecular-weight heparin (LMWH) [52]. Therefore, epidural catheters should not be placed when the postoperative use of a LMWH is anticipated.

Intramuscular injection of analgesic drugs is not recommended due to technical difficulties and unreliability in absorption [59–61]. Patient-controlled analgesia (PCA), essentially "on-demand" intravenous opioid analgesia, has been associated with greater patient satisfaction and lower pain scores as compared to other forms of parenteral opioid administration [17,62]. The patient's body weight has no significant effect on PCA dosing rate requirements [63,64]. As such, the practitioner should not adjust the PCA dose, dosing frequency, or 4-hour dose limit based on BMI alone.

THROMBOPROPHYLAXIS

Postoperative deep venous thrombosis (DVT) can be a devastating, even fatal, postoperative complication. Symptomatic venous thromboembolism occurs in 0.8–2.4% of patients [65–69]. In the surgery patient, the release of inflammatory mediators, relative immobility, and venous stasis all predisposes the postoperative patient to thromboembolic events [69,70]. Additionally, obesity is a proinflammatory state that is an independent risk factor for hypercoagulability [69,71–73].

Early and frequent ambulation is important in the postoperative period. However, studies have shown that ambulation by itself does not provide adequate thromboprophylaxis for the postoperative obese patient [74]. In addition to early ambulation, obese patients should routinely receive mechanical and pharmacological thromboprophylaxis.

Mechanical thromboprophylaxis increases venous outflow and decreases venous stasis within the leg veins. Products include graduated compression stockings, intermittent pneumatic devices, and foot pumps. As compared to no prophylaxis, graduated compression stockings or intermittent pneumatic devices reduce the risk of DVT by 57–64% in patients undergoing surgery [75,76]. Going one step further, a combination of mechanical and pharmacological thromboprophlaxis is superior to any one individually in preventing DVT and/or PE [74,77,78].

Routine postoperative pharmacologic thromboprophylaxis includes unfractionated heparin or LMWH. Both are equally effective in preventing DVT and PE in the immediate postoperative patient [79–81]. Currently, there are no studies that validate the use of one product over another in the obese patient population [74,79]. Also, the dosage regimen in this patient population remains controversial, with no established recommendations to date [68,79,82,83].In general, a review of the literature supports the following:

1. 5000 units of unfractionated heparin three times daily for patients whose BMI is $< 50\,kg/m^2$, 7500 units of unfractionated heparin three times daily for patients with a BMI $> 50\,kg/m^2$ [84].
2. For physicians who prefer using LMWH due to its once- or twice-daily administration dosing or its lower risk of heparin-induced thrombocytopenia, LMWH dosing should be based on total body weight for the treatment of obese patients [85,86]. Increasing

the prophylaxis dose of a LMWH by 30% may be appropriate in those with a BMI $\geq 40\,kg/m^2$ [82,87].
3. Once-daily dosing strategies for enoxaparin in the obese patient should be avoided [88]. Once-daily dosing for dalteparin (220 IU/kg) and tinzaparin (175 IU/kg) may be appropriate [89].
4. For patients weighing up to 190 kg, anti-Xa monitoring is not necessary [89–91]. For patients weighing more than 190 kg, LMWH dosing should be based on total body weight and adjusted based on anti-Xa levels [89].
5. The use of aspirin alone as thromboprophylaxis is not recommended [74].

When there is no contraindication, it is the standard of care to continue pharmacological thromboprophylaxis until the patient is discharged from the hospital [74]. However, delayed venous thromboembolism is known to occur after the surgical patient is discharged [92]. For high-risk surgical patients, such as those who have cancer, have experienced previous venous thromboembolic events, or are undergoing major orthopedic surgery, chemothromboprophylaxis with LMWH is recommended for at least 10 days post-discharge [74]. As for bariatric patients, this remains a controversial subject and there is no established recommendation for prolonged post-discharge administration of pharmacological thromboprophylaxis [81,83].

Inferior vena cava (IVC) filter placement is another form of prophylaxis that can be employed postoperatively. IVC filters should not be considered thromboprophylaxis as they do not inhibit clot formation. They may, however, be considered PE prophylaxis as they may prevent dislodged DVT clots from reaching the lung. Nevertheless, the placement of an IVC filter requires an invasive procedure and has both short- and long-term complications [69,93]. For the obese patient, routine postoperative use of IVC filters as the primary form of thromboprophylaxis is not recommended [74,79,93].

SKIN CARE

Obese patients are at an increased risk for skin breakdown due to the decreased vascularity of adipose tissue [51]. Additionally, the skin folds under the breast, behind the neck, and in the back, abdomen, groin, and perineum area may have underlying intertrigo as a result of chronic friction, moisture, heat, and lack of air circulation [51]. Therefore, frequent scheduled body repositioning, along with daily inspection of any involved area, is required to prevent skin breakdown in these locations. Lifting, cleansing, and drying of the skin folds should occur at least on a daily basis. The use of powders in these areas is not routinely recommended since they frequently contain abrasive particles that may lead to further skin breakdown and ulceration. Cloth or gauze is preferred, as these cause less abrasion and irritation [51].

Drainage tubes such as chest tubes, Hemovac drains, and Foley catheters should be strategically positioned so that they are not lying under the patient or hidden in between the skin folds, leading to further skin erosion and pressure ulceration. The patient's arms should be propped and padded with pillows to prevent friction against the side rail of the bed [94]. When lifts and slings are used to transfer the patient, careful attention should be paid to ensure that the skin is not pinched or sheared during the transfer process [95].

The body weight of the obese patient results in an increased pounds per square inch of pressure against the bed they are lying on, causing them to be susceptible to early formation of a decubitus ulcer [41]. Patients who are immobile should be turned in bed every 2 hours [94]. Pressure-reducing devices and mattresses with a pressure relief system should be employed to reduce shear forces on the skin when the patient is turned [61]. Linens should be kept wrinkle free to prevent pressure against the skin leading to tissue necrosis [96]. Lastly, tape removal may strip the epidermal layer, causing partial thickness skin loss. Tape should be used sparingly, and alternatives to tape such as abdominal binders, undergarments, or gauze rolls should be used whenever possible [61].

Patients with higher BMIs are also prone to surgical-site infections. Studies have shown that obese patients tend to have lower serum and tissue concentrations of prophylactic antibiotics [97], suboptimal wound tissue oxygenation due to poorly vascularized subcutaneous fat, and large potential spaces that predispose towards hematoma and seroma formation [98,99]. Practitioners should pay special attention to the surgical site for signs of infection in order to reduce the delay in diagnosis and treatment of the soft-tissue infection.

HOSPITAL CARE NEEDS

Specialized equipment such as hydraulic lift devices, transfer equipmet, and overhead trapezes should be readily available in order to decrease work-related injury in hospital personnel [100,101]. Also, nursing safety and appropriate ergonomics teaching should be incorporated into the nursing orientation and ongoing education curriculum [51]. When compared to their normal-weight counterparts, obese patients are often targets of stigmatization and discrimination in the medical setting [61,102], leading to suboptimal care in the postoperative period. Health care providers should maintain a professional attitude towards these patients and avoid judgmental or insensitive comments about their weight or food intake behavior. Sensitivity training should also be included in nursing orientation and quarterly in-service training.

Oftentimes, obese patients who are independent at home become surprisingly dependent once hospitalized. Several factors are involved, including recent surgery, unfamiliar surroundings, sedation, and altered sensorium. To promote independence and improve the health care provider's safety, the surgical floor should be well equipped for this patient population. Structurally, the rooms should be large enough to comfortably accommodate the oversized furniture. The door frames should be wide. Bathrooms should have sturdy grab bars, a walk-in shower with a handheld showerhead, and floor-mounted toilets to prevent the risk of collapse [61,102].

Early mobility during the postoperative period can be a challenge for both the obese patient and the health care provider. Physical and occupational therapists are key personnel in getting the patient mobilized with the appropriate equipment, or transitioning the patient from the nonambulatory to the ambulatory state [103]. Oversized equipment such as extra-large gowns, a bariatric bed, large bedside chairs, obesity commodes, larger bedpans, obesity wheelchairs, scales, and large and extra-large blood pressure cuffs, should be readily available for the patient's room [41,96].

Lastly, obese patients who undergo bariatric surgery should stay at a predesignated nursing care unit after surgery. This will enable them to receive consistent, skilled nursing and ancillary care. These providers will have had formal training in the dietary, activity, and medical needs of this special patient population. They will also be familiar with the standard postoperative course, as well as the common postoperative complications, unique to bariatric surgery.

CONCLUSION

With respect to the postoperative care of the obese patient, most conclusions are extrapolated from literature pertaining to patients with normal BMI, or obese patients post gastric bypass. Accordingly, high-quality data to guide a physician's care for the obese in the postoperative setting are lacking. Nevertheless, a coordinated team approach between the physician, nursing staff, and patient will allow for a smoother recovery and improve the quality of care in these patients.

BEST PRACTICE TIPS

1 ACE inhibitors or ARBs should be the first-line treatment agent for the obese patient with hypertension.

2 Obese patients with sleep apnea should be placed on NPPV (CPAP) during the postoperative period to decrease the risk of tachy- or bradyarrhythmias and respiratory complications.

3 A multimodal postoperative analgesia approach should be instituted to adequately manage obese patients' pain while minimizing respiratory depression.

4 Obesity and surgery are both risk factors for thromboembolic events. In addition to early and frequent ambulation, these patients should routinely receive both mechanical and pharmacological thromboprophylaxis in the postoperative period.

5 Obesity increases a patient's risk for skin breakdown and decubitus ulcer formation. Frequent body repositioning, careful positioning of drainage tubes, and heightened vigilance will decrease the rate of these complications.

REFERENCES

1 Flegal KM, Carroll MD, Kuczmarski RJ, Johnson CL. Overweight and obesity in the United States: prevalence and trends, 1960–1994. Int J Obes Relat Metab Disord. 1998 Jan;22(1):39–47.

2 Flegal KM, Carroll MD, Ogden CL, Johnson CL. Prevalence and trends in obesity among US adults, 1999–2000. JAMA. 2002 Oct;288(14):1723–7.

3 Mullen JT, Moorman DW, Davenport DL. The obesity paradox: body mass index and outcomes in patients undergoing nonbariatric general surgery. Ann Surg. 2009 Jul;250(1):166–72.

4 Wong CY, O'Moore-Sullivan T, Leano R, Byrne N, Beller E, Marwick TH. Alterations of left ventricular myocardial characteristics associated with obesity. Circulation. 2004 Nov;110(19):3081–7.

5 Kenchaiah S, Evans JC, Levy D, Wilson PW, Benjamin EJ, Larson MG, et al. Obesity and the risk of heart failure. N Engl J Med. 2002 Aug 1;347(5):305–13.

6 Tumuklu MM, Etikan I, Kisacik B, Kayikcioglu M. Effect of obesity on left ventricular structure and myocardial systolic function: assessment by tissue Doppler imaging and strain/strain rate imaging. Echocardiography. 2007 Sep;24(8):802–9.

7 Executive Summary of The Third Report of The National Cholesterol Education Program (NCEP) Expert Panel on Detection, Evaluation, And Treatment of High Blood Cholesterol In Adults (Adult Treatment Panel III). JAMA. 2001 May;285(19):2486–97.

8 Third Report of the National Cholesterol Education Program (NCEP) Expert Panel on Detection, Evaluation, and Treatment of High Blood Cholesterol in Adults (Adult Treatment Panel III) final report. Circulation. 2002 Dec;106 (25):3143–421.

9 Glance LG, Wissler R, Mukamel DB, Li Y, Diachun CA, Salloum R, et al. Perioperative outcomes among patients with the modified metabolic syndrome who are undergoing noncardiac surgery. Anesthesiology. 2010 Oct;113(4):859–72.

10 Klasen J, Junger A, Hartmann B, Jost A, Benson M, Virabjan T, et al. Increased body mass index and peri-operative risk in patients undergoing non-cardiac surgery. Obes Surg. 2004 Feb;14(2):275–81.

11 Drew BJ, Califf RM, Funk M, Kaufman ES, Krucoff MW, Laks MM, et al. Practice standards for electrocardiographic monitoring in hospital settings: an American Heart Association scientific statement from the Councils on Cardiovascular Nursing, Clinical Cardiology, and Cardiovascular Disease in the Young: endorsed by the International Society of Computerized Electrocardiology and the American Association of Critical-Care Nurses. Circulation. 2004 Oct 26;110(17):2721–46.

12 Wright DE, Hunt DP. Perioperative surveillance for adverse myocardial events. South Med J. 2008 Jan;101(1):52–8.

13 Messerli FH, Nunez BD, Ventura HO, Snyder DW. Overweight and sudden death. Increased ventricular ectopy in cardiopathy of obesity. Arch Intern Med. 1987 Oct;147(10):1725–8.

14 Kannel WB, Plehn JF, Cupples LA. Cardiac failure and sudden death in the Framingham Study. Am Heart J. 1988 Apr;115(4):869–75.

15 Nierman E, Zakrzewski K. Recognition and management of preoperative risk. Rheum Dis Clin North Am. 1999 Aug;25(3):585–622.

16 Devereaux PJ, Goldman L, Yusuf S, Gilbert K, Leslie K, Guyatt GH. Surveillance and prevention of major perioperative ischemic cardiac events in patients undergoing noncardiac surgery: a review. CMAJ. 2005 Sep;173(7):779–88.

17 Fleisher LA, Beckman JA, Brown KA, Calkins H, Chaikof E, Fleischmann KE, et al. ACC/AHA 2007 guidelines on perioperative cardiovascular evaluation and care for noncardiac surgery: a report of the American College of Cardiology/American Heart Association Task Force on Practice Guidelines (Writing Committee to Revise the 2002 Guidelines on Perioperative Cardiovascular Evaluation for Noncardiac Surgery): developed in collaboration with the American Society of Echocardiography, American Society of Nuclear Cardiology, Heart Rhythm Society, Society of Cardiovascular Anesthesiologists, Society for Cardiovascular Angiography and Interventions, Society for Vascular Medicine and Biology, and Society for Vascular Surgery. Circulation. 2007 Oct;116(17):E418–99.

18 Simantirakis EN, Schiza SI, Marketou ME, Chrysostomakis SI, Chlouverakis GI, Klapsinos NC, et al. Severe bradyarrhythmias in patients with sleep apnoea: the effect of

continuous positive airway pressure treatment: a long-term evaluation using an insertable loop recorder. Eur Heart J. 2004 Jun;25(12):1070–6.

19 Kryger MH, Roth T, Dement W, editors. Principles and Practice of Sleep Medicine. 2 edn. New York, NY, WB Saunders. 1994.

20 Motta J, Guilleminault C, Schroeder JS, Dement WC. Tracheostomy and hemodynamic changes in sleep-inducing apnea. Ann Intern Med. 1978 Oct;89(4):454–8.

21 Walsh SR, Tang T, Wijewardena C, Yarham SI, Boyle JR, Gaunt ME. Postoperative arrhythmias in general surgical patients. Ann R Coll Surg Engl. 2007 Mar;89(2):91–5.

22 Wang TJ, Parise H, Levy D, D'Agostino RB, Sr., Wolf PA, Vasan RS, et al. Obesity and the risk of new-onset atrial fibrillation. JAMA. 2004 Nov;292(20):2471–7.

23 Sasson Z, Rasooly Y, Gupta R, Rasooly I. Left atrial enlargement in healthy obese: prevalence and relation to left ventricular mass and diastolic function. Can J Cardiol. 1996 Mar;12(3):257–63.

24 Christians KK, Wu B, Quebbeman EJ, Brasel KJ. Postoperative atrial fibrillation in noncardiothoracic surgical patients. Am J Surg. 2001 Dec;182(6):713–15.

25 Valencia Martin J, Climent Paya VE, Marin Ortuno F, Monmeneu Menadas JV, Martinez Martinez JG, Garcia Martinez M, et al. (The efficacy of scheduled cardioversion in atrial fibrillation. Comparison of two schemes of treatment: electrical versus pharmacological cardioversion). Rev Esp Cardiol. 2002 Feb;55(2):113–20.

26 Fuster V, Ryden LE, Cannom DS, Crijns HJ, Curtis AB, Ellenbogen KA, et al. ACC/AHA/ESC 2006 Guidelines for the Management of Patients with Atrial Fibrillation: a report of the American College of Cardiology/American Heart Association Task Force on Practice Guidelines and the European Society of Cardiology Committee for Practice Guidelines (Writing Committee to Revise the 2001 Guidelines for the Management of Patients With Atrial Fibrillation): developed in collaboration with the European Heart Rhythm Association and the Heart Rhythm Society. Circulation. 2006 Aug;114(7):E257–354.

27 Stamler R, Stamler J, Riedlinger WF, Algera G, Roberts RH. Weight and blood pressure. Findings in hypertension screening of 1 million Americans. JAMA. 1978 Oct;240(15):1607–10.

28 Muller DC, Elahi D, Pratley RE, Tobin JD, Andres R. An epidemiological test of the hyperinsulinemia-hypertension hypothesis. J Clin Endocrinol Metab. 1993 Mar;76(3):544–8.

29 Chobanian AV, Bakris GL, Black HR, Cushman WC, Green LA, Izzo JL, Jr., et al. Seventh report of the Joint National Committee on Prevention, Detection, Evaluation, and Treatment of High Blood Pressure. Hypertension. 2003 Dec;42(6):1206–52.

30 Israili ZH, Lyoussi B, Hernandez-Hernandez R, Velasco M. Metabolic syndrome: treatment of hypertensive patients. Am J Ther. 2007 Jul–Aug;14(4):386–402.

31 Reisin E, Weir MR, Falkner B, Hutchinson HG, Anzalone DA, Tuck ML. Lisinopril versus hydrochlorothiazide in obese hypertensive patients: a multicenter placebo-controlled trial. Treatment in Obese Patients With Hypertension (TROPHY) Study Group. Hypertension. 1997 Jul;30(1 Pt 1):140–5.

32 Bestermann W, Houston MC, Basile J, Egan B, Ferrario CM, Lackland D, et al. Addressing the global cardiovascular risk of hypertension, dyslipidemia, diabetes mellitus, and the metabolic syndrome in the southeastern United States, part II: treatment recommendations for management of the global cardiovascular risk of hypertension, dyslipidemia, diabetes mellitus, and the metabolic syndrome. Am J Med Sci. 2005 Jun;329(6):292–305.

33 Singer GM, Setaro JF. Secondary hypertension: obesity and the metabolic syndrome. J Clin Hypertens (Greenwich). 2008 Jul;10(7):567–74.

34 Devereaux PJ, Yang H, Yusuf S, Guyatt G, Leslie K, Villar JC, et al. Effects of extended-release metoprolol succinate in patients undergoing non-cardiac surgery (POISE trial): a randomised controlled trial. Lancet. 2008 May;371 (9627):1839–47.

35 Poldermans D, Bax JJ, Schouten O, Neskovic AN, Paelinck B, Rocci G, et al. Should major vascular surgery be delayed because of preoperative cardiac testing in intermediate-risk patients receiving beta-blocker therapy with tight heart rate control? J Am Coll Cardiol. 2006 Sep;48(5):964–9.

36 Poldermans D, Boersma E, Bax JJ, Thomson IR, van de Ven LL, Blankensteijn JD, et al. The effect of bisoprolol on perioperative mortality and myocardial infarction in high-risk patients undergoing vascular surgery. Dutch Echocardiographic Cardiac Risk Evaluation Applying Stress Echocardiography Study Group. N Engl J Med. 1999 Dec;341(24):1789–94.

37 Allcock DM, Sowers JR. Best strategies for hypertension management in type 2 diabetes and obesity. Curr Diab Rep. 2010 Apr;10(2):139–44.

38 Wilson IM, Freis ED. Relationship between plasma and extracellular fluid volume depletion and the antihypertensive effect of chlorothiazide. Circulation. 1959 Dec;20: 1028–36.

39 Gallagher SF, Haines KL, Osterlund LG, Mullen M, Downs JB. Postoperative hypoxemia: common, undetected, and unsuspected after bariatric surgery. J Surg Res. 2010 Apr; 159(2):622–6.

40 Poirier P, Alpert MA, Fleisher LA, Thompson PD, Sugerman HJ, Burke LE, et al. Cardiovascular evaluation and management of severely obese patients undergoing surgery: a science advisory from the American Heart Association. Circulation. 2009 Jul;120(1):86–95.

41 Davidson JE, Kruse MW, Cox DH, Duncan R. Critical care of the morbidly obese. Crit Care Nurs Q. 2003 Apr–Jun;26(2): 105–16; quiz 17–18.

42 Miller RD, Eriksson LI, Fleisher LA, editors. Miller's Anesthesia. 7th ed. New York: Churchill Livingstone; 2009.

43 Patil SP, Schneider H, Schwartz AR, Smith PL. Adult obstructive sleep apnea: pathophysiology and diagnosis. Chest. 2007 Jul;132(1):325–37.

44 Medicine AAoS, editor. International Classification of Sleep Disorders: Diagnostic and Coding Manual. 2 edn. Westchester, IL, American Academy of Sleep Medicine. 2005.

45 Sullivan CE, Issa FG, Berthon-Jones M, Eves L. Reversal of obstructive sleep apnoea by continuous positive airway pressure applied through the nares. Lancet. 1981 Apr;1(8225):862–5.

46 Meduri GU, Turner RE, Abou-Shala N, Wunderink R, Tolley E. Noninvasive positive pressure ventilation via face mask. First-line intervention in patients with acute hypercapnic and hypoxemic respiratory failure. Chest. 1996 Jan;109(1): 179–93.

47 Ramirez A, Lalor PF, Szomstein S, Rosenthal RJ. Continuous positive airway pressure in immediate postoperative period after laparoscopic Roux-en-Y gastric bypass: is it safe? Surg Obes Relat Dis. 2009 Sep–Oct;5(5):544–6.

48 Gross JB, Bachenberg KL, Benumof JL, Caplan RA, Connis RT, Cote CJ, et al. Practice guidelines for the perioperative management of patients with obstructive sleep apnea: a report by the American Society of Anesthesiologists Task Force on Perioperative Management of patients with obstructive sleep apnea. Anesthesiology. 2006 May;104(5):1081–93; quiz 117–18.

49 Stannard D. Pulse oximetry for perioperative monitoring. AORN J. 2010 Dec;92(6):683–4.

50 Bellorin O, Abdemur A, Sucandy I, Szomstein S, Rosenthal RJ. Understanding the significance, reasons and patterns of abnormal vital signs after gastric bypass for morbid obesity. Obes Surg. 2010 Jun; 21(6):707–13.

51 Barth MM, Jenson CE. Postoperative nursing care of gastric bypass patients. Am J Crit Care. 2006 Jul;15(4):378–87; quiz 88.

52 Chand B, Gugliotti D, Schauer P, Steckner K. Perioperative management of the bariatric surgery patient: focus on cardiac and anesthesia considerations. Cleve Clin J Med. 2006 Mar;73(Suppl 1):S51–6.

53 Schumann R, Jones SB, Cooper B, Kelley SD, Bosch MV, Ortiz VE, et al. Update on best practice recommendations for anesthetic perioperative care and pain management in weight loss surgery, 2004–2007. Obesity (Silver Spring). 2009 May;17(5):889–94.

54 Ingrande J, Brodsky JB, Lemmens HJ. Regional anesthesia and obesity. Curr Opin Anaesthesiol. 2009 Oct;22(5):683–6.

55 Block BM, Liu SS, Rowlingson AJ, Cowan AR, Cowan JA, Jr., Wu CL. Efficacy of postoperative epidural analgesia: a meta-analysis. JAMA. 2003 Nov;290(18):2455–63.

56 Werawatganon T, Charuluxanun S. Patient controlled intravenous opioid analgesia versus continuous epidural analgesia for pain after intra-abdominal surgery. Cochrane Database Syst Rev. 2005(1):CD004088.

57 Mhyre JM. Anesthetic management for the morbidly obese pregnant woman. Int Anesthesiol Clin. 2007 Winter;45(1): 51–70.

58 Whitty RJ, Maxwell CV, Carvalho JC. Complications of neuraxial anesthesia in an extreme morbidly obese patient for Cesarean section. Int J Obstet Anesth. 2007 Apr;16(2): 139–44.

59 Shenkman Z, Shir Y, Brodsky JB. Perioperative management of the obese patient. Br J Anaesth. 1993 Mar;70(3):349–59.

60 Choi YK, Brolin RE, Wagner BK, Chou S, Etesham S, Pollak P. Efficacy and safety of patient-controlled analgesia for morbidly obese patients following gastric bypass surgery. Obes Surg. 2000 Apr;10(2):154–9.

61 Taggart HM, Mincer AB, Thompson AW. Caring for the orthopaedic patient who is obese. Orthop Nurs. 2004 May–Jun;23(3):204–10.

62 Hudcova J, McNicol E, Quah C, Lau J, Carr DB. Patient controlled opioid analgesia versus conventional opioid analgesia for postoperative pain. Cochrane Database Syst Rev. 2006(4): CD003348.

63 Graves DA, Batenhorst RL, Bennett RL, Wettstein JG, Griffen WO, Wright BD, et al. Morphine requirements using patient-controlled analgesia: influence of diurnal variation and morbid obesity. Clin Pharm. 1983 Jan–Feb;2(1):49–53.

64 Bennett R, Batenhorst R, Graves DA, Foster TS, Griffen WO, Wright BD. Variation in postoperative analgesic requirements in the morbidly obese following gastric bypass surgery. Pharmacotherapy. 1982 Jan–Feb;2(1):50–3.

65 Westling A, Bergqvist D, Bostrom A, Karacagil S, Gustavsson S. Incidence of deep venous thrombosis in patients undergoing obesity surgery. World J Surg. 2002 Apr;26(4):470–3.

66 Frezza EE, Chiriva-Internati M. Venous thromboembolism in morbid obesity and trauma. A review of literature. Minerva Chir. 2005 Oct;60(5):391–9.

67 Gonzalez QH, Tishler DS, Plata-Munoz JJ, Bondora A, Vickers SM, Leath T, et al. Incidence of clinically evident deep venous thrombosis after laparoscopic Roux-en-Y gastric bypass. Surg Endosc. 2004 Jul;18(7):1082–4.

68 Scholten DJ, Hoedema RM, Scholten SE. A comparison of two different prophylactic dose regimens of low molecular weight heparin in bariatric surgery. Obes Surg. 2002 Feb; 12(1):19–24.

69 Hamad GG, Bergqvist D. Venous thromboembolism in bariatric surgery patients: an update of risk and prevention. Surg Obes Relat Dis. 2007 Jan–Feb;3(1):97–102.

70 Dahl OE. Mechanisms of hypercoagulability. Thromb Haemost. 1999 Aug;82(2):902–6.

71 Anderson JA, Weitz JI. Hypercoagulable states. Clin Chest Med. 2010 Dec;31(4):659–73.

72 Samama MM. An epidemiologic study of risk factors for deep vein thrombosis in medical outpatients: the Sirius study. Arch Intern Med. 2000 Dec;160(22):3415–20.

73 Rocha AT, de Vasconcellos AG, da Luz Neto ER, Araujo DM, Alves ES, Lopes AA. Risk of venous thromboembolism and efficacy of thromboprophylaxis in hospitalized obese medical patients and in obese patients undergoing bariatric surgery. Obes Surg. 2006 Dec;16(12):1645–55.

74 Geerts WH, Bergqvist D, Pineo GF, Heit JA, Samama CM, Lassen MR, et al. Prevention of venous thromboembolism: American College of Chest Physicians Evidence-Based Clinical Practice Guidelines (8th Edition). Chest. 2008 Jun;133 (6 Suppl):S381S–453.

75 Urbankova J, Quiroz R, Kucher N, Goldhaber SZ. Intermittent pneumatic compression and deep vein thrombosis prevention. A meta-analysis in postoperative patients. Thromb Haemost. 2005 Dec;94(6):1181–5.

76 Agu O, Hamilton G, Baker D. Graduated compression stockings in the prevention of venous thromboembolism. Br J Surg. 1999 Aug;86(8):992–1004.

77 Kakkos SK, Caprini JA, Geroulakos G, Nicolaides AN, Stansby GP, Reddy DJ. Combined intermittent pneumatic leg compression and pharmacological prophylaxis for prevention of venous thromboembolism in high-risk patients. Cochrane Database Syst Rev. 2008(4):CD005258.

78 Wille-Jorgensen P, Rasmussen MS, Andersen BR, Borly L. Heparins and mechanical methods for thromboprophylaxis in colorectal surgery. Cochrane Database Syst Rev. 2003(4):CD001217.

79 King DR, Velmahos GC. Difficulties in managing the surgical patient who is morbidly obese. Crit Care Med. 2010 Sep;38(9 Suppl):S478–82.

80 Barba CA, Harrington C, Loewen M. Status of venous thromboembolism prophylaxis among bariatric surgeons: have we changed our practice during the past decade? Surg Obes Relat Dis. 2009 May–Jun;5(3):352–6.

81 Mismetti P, Laporte S, Darmon JY, Buchmuller A, Decousus H. Meta-analysis of low molecular weight heparin in the prevention of venous thromboembolism in general surgery. Br J Surg. 2001 Jul;88(7):913–30.

82 Kucher N, Leizorovicz A, Vaitkus PT, Cohen AT, Turpie AG, Olsson CG, et al. Efficacy and safety of fixed low-dose dalteparin in preventing venous thromboembolism among obese or elderly hospitalized patients: a subgroup analysis of the PREVENT trial. Arch Intern Med. 2005 Feb 14;165(3): 341–5.

83 Prophylactic measures to reduce the risk of venous thromboembolism in bariatric surgery patients. Surg Obes Relat Dis. 2007 Sep–Oct;3(5):494–5.

84 Miller MT, Rovito PF. An approach to venous thromboembolism prophylaxis in laparoscopic Roux-en-Y gastric bypass surgery. Obes Surg. 2004 Jun–Jul;14(6):731–7.

85 Spinler SA, Inverso SM, Cohen M, Goodman SG, Stringer KA, Antman EM. Safety and efficacy of unfractionated heparin versus enoxaparin in patients who are obese and patients with severe renal impairment: analysis from the ESSENCE and TIMI 11B studies. Am Heart J. 2003 Jul;146(1):33–41.

86 Yee JY, Duffull SB. The effect of body weight on dalteparin pharmacokinetics. A preliminary study. Eur J Clin Pharmacol. 2000 Jul;56(4):293–7.

87 Frederiksen SG, Hedenbro JL, Norgren L. Enoxaparin effect depends on body-weight and current doses may be inadequate in obese patients. Br J Surg. 2003 May;90(5):547–8.

88 Merli G, Spiro TE, Olsson CG, Abildgaard U, Davidson BL, Eldor A, et al. Subcutaneous enoxaparin once or twice daily compared with intravenous unfractionated heparin for treatment of venous thromboembolic disease. Ann Intern Med. 2001 Feb;134(3):191–202.

89 Nutescu EA, Spinler SA, Wittkowsky A, Dager WE. Low-molecular-weight heparins in renal impairment and obesity: available evidence and clinical practice recommendations across medical and surgical settings. Ann Pharmacother. 2009 Jun;43(6):1064–83.

90 Barrett JS, Gibiansky E, Hull RD, Planes A, Pentikis H, Hainer JW, et al. Population pharmacodynamics in patients receiving tinzaparin for the prevention and treatment of deep vein thrombosis. Int J Clin Pharmacol Ther. 2001 Oct;39(10):431–46.

91 Wilson SJ, Wilbur K, Burton E, Anderson DR. Effect of patient weight on the anticoagulant response to adjusted therapeutic dosage of low-molecular-weight heparin for the treatment of venous thromboembolism. Haemostasis. 2001 Jan–Feb;31(1):42–8.

92 Huber O, Bounameaux H, Borst F, Rohner A. Postoperative pulmonary embolism after hospital discharge. An underestimated risk. Arch Surg. 1992 Mar;127(3):310–13.

93 Ingber S, Geerts WH. Vena caval filters: current knowledge, uncertainties and practical approaches. Curr Opin Hematol. 2009 Sep;16(5):402–6.

94 Davidson JE, Callery C. Care of the obesity surgery patient requiring immediate-level care or intensive care. Obes Surg. 2001 Feb;11(1):93–7.

95 Charlebois D, Wilmoth D. Critical care of patients with obesity. Crit Care Nurse. 2004 Aug;24(4):19–27; quiz 8–9.

96 Mathison CJ. Skin and wound care challenges in the hospitalized morbidly obese patient. J Wound Ostomy Continence Nurs. 2003 Mar;30(2):78–83.

97 Edmiston CE, Krepel C, Kelly H, Larson J, Andris D, Hennen C, et al. Perioperative antibiotic prophylaxis in the gastric bypass patient: do we achieve therapeutic levels? Surgery. 2004 Oct;136(4):738–47.

98 Anaya DA, Dellinger EP. The obese surgical patient: a susceptible host for infection. Surg Infect (Larchmt). 2006 Oct;7(5):473–80.

99 Jupiter JB, Ring D, Rosen H. The complications and difficulties of management of nonunion in the severely obese. J Orthop Trauma. 1995;9(5):363–70.

100 Wilson JA, Clark JJ. Obesity: impediment to postsurgical wound healing. Adv Skin Wound Care. 2004 Oct;17(8): 426–35.

101 Rose MA, Drake DJ, Baker G, Watkins FR, Jr., Waters W, Pokorny M. Caring for morbidly obese patients: safety considerations for nurse administrators. Nurs Manage. 2008 Nov;39(11):47–50.

102 Blackwood HS. Obesity: a rapidly expanding challenge. Nurs Manage. 2004 May;35(5):27–35; quiz 6.

103 Rotkoff N. Care of the morbidly obese patient in a long-term care facility. Geriatr Nurs. 1999 Nov–Dec;20(6):309–13.

18 Management of the Obese Patient with Trauma

Hadley K. Herbert and Therèse M. Duane

Department of General Surgery, Virginia Commonwealth University, Medical College of Virginia, Richmond, VA, USA

KEY POINTS

- Obesity is an increasing epidemic in the USA and requires health care providers to adapt their practice by providing safe and appropriate care to obese patients.
- While the approach to the obese trauma patient, as outlined by the Advance Trauma Life Support (ATLS) guidelines, remains the same in terms of assessing airway, breathing, and circulation (ABC), these priorities may be adopted and modified to meet the needs of the obese patient.
- Providing safe and appropriate care for the obese trauma patient requires a multidisciplinary approach which starts in the prehospital phase and continues until the time of discharge. Strong collaboration and communication needs to occur throughout all phases of care.

INTRODUCTION

Obesity has increased dramatically throughout the USA over the last decade. Currently, more than 30% of the population has a body mass index (BMI) $\geq 30\,kg/m^2$, meeting the Centers for Disease Control (CDC) criteria for obesity. The World Health Organization (WHO) estimates that in 2005 at least 400 million adults were obese and that by 2015 this figure will reach 700 million [1]. While the health hazards of this national epidemic are well documented in terms of cardiovascular, endocrinology, and certain pulmonary diseases, less is known regarding the impact of obesity on the susceptibility to and outcome of traumatic injury.

Injury is the fifth leading cause of death in the USA and is the leading cause of death among individuals 1–24 years old. Injury results when the body is either exposed to an excessive form of energy or denied essential agents like oxygen or heat. Mechanics of injury are related to the type of injury force and subsequent tissue response. The degree of injury varies according to the presence of accompanying factors, such as severity of injury, age, gender, geography, alcohol, and obesity.

Obesity is generally defined as an abnormal increased proportion of adipose tissue or body fat in relation to muscle mass. The obese patient represents a segment of the population that is physiologically and anatomically distinct from the remaining population. Obese patients can have a higher prevalence of cardiac, respiratory, and metabolic comorbidities, which may impair their response to injury and complicate their management [2]. This chapter explores the extent to which obesity affects anatomical and physiological changes that shape the body's response to injury. In doing so, this chapter outlines an appropriate team approach to the treatment and care of an obese trauma patient during the prehospital, initial assessment, workup, operative, and hospital phases. In the last section of this chapter, we present a series of studies that illustrate that when combined with obesity, the consequences and outcome of trauma can be grave.

PREHOSPITAL PHASE

As the prevalence of obesity increases in the USA, health care providers must be able to provide appropriate care for the obese trauma patient in both the prehospital and the hospital settings. The prehospital phase includes the time from when the injury occurs to when the injured patient arrives at a health care facility and care is handed off to the hospital staff. The goal of this phase is to

---

stabilize and safely transport the patient to an appropriate level-based trauma facility.

The obese trauma patient presents unique challenges to first responders and emergency service providers during the prehospital phase, as additional equipment, such as oversized backboards, may be needed to stabilize and transport the patient. This may necessitate additional personnel, such as medics or firefighters, to help extricate the patient from the site of the injury. Cervical collars may not fit properly, and could require the prehospital team to use resources such as sandbags, blanket rolls, and tape to maintain cervical spine stabilization [3]. If an obese patient has an extremity fracture, stabilizing the fracture can be challenging. Most splints do not fit obese patients, so tape and elastic bandages will be required.

While many ambulances have added stretchers that can accommodate 340 kg (750 lbs), transport to the stretcher may require additional personnel [3]. These complications can result in increased extrication and transport times, which can delay treatment. Because time is often critical during this prehospital phase, early planning and preparation are essential. Providers must have an understanding of obese patients' anatomical and physical needs and be familiar with alterative measures to safely yet efficiently provide care.

An essential aspect of the prehospital phase is obtaining a comprehensive history of the patient. This includes a careful history of the injury and the events leading up to the injury. Additionally, it is important to obtain the patient's past medical history, including comorbidities, and past surgical history, such as bariatric surgery.

Once the patient arrives at the hospital, care is then transferred to the trauma team, often comprising surgeons, anesthesiologists, emergency medicine specialists, and various consultants, such as neurosurgeons and orthopedics. Care of the obese trauma patient thus necessitates a well-orchestrated, preplanned approach that includes a complete prehospital report, including additional equipment needed in the field (such as the number of backboards required for transport), cervical spine stabilization, extrication challenges, and the need for additional personnel for transport. The report must also include the patient's medical and surgical history to allow the trauma team to anticipate complications and provide appropriate interventions.

INITIAL ASSESSMENT

The Advance Trauma Life Support (ATLS) guidelines provide a standard approach for the care of the trauma patient, which outline the basic assessment priorities of airway, breathing, and circulation (ABC). These priorities need to be adopted with the obese patient's anatomical and physiological needs in mind.

Airway

The first step of an emergent trauma resuscitation is the assessment of airway patency. Obese patients are at risk for a compromised airway, as the presence of excess adipose tissue can increase the work of breathing, especially when the patient is in a supine position to allow for spinal immobilization. Obese patients may be predisposed to increased intraabdominal pressure or may suffer from gastroesophageal disease, such as reflux; both comorbidities increase the risk of aspiration. To reduce the risk of aspiration, critically ill patients who have undergone gastric banding should have the band deflated via the access port, usually located in the abdominal wall in the left upper quadrant or at the xiphisternum [1].

If an emergency airway is required, the obese patient may present as an intubation challenge for health care providers, given their anatomical and physiological condition [3]. Multiple factors are associated with difficult larygoscopy and intubation, such as facial hair, short neck, high arched palate, any airway deformity due to trauma, and obesity. The "LEMON" mnemonic is a quick and simple assessment to evaluate a difficult airway, as recommended by ATLS guidelines. To reinforce the role of obesity, the "O" in the mnemonic recently changed from "obstruction" to now include "obstruction and obesity" [4]. Few studies, however, have confirmed this supposition, and in fact Sifri et al.'s retrospective review showed obesity is not an independent risk factor for failed intubation in either the field or the emergency room [5].

In general, it is recommended that simple measures be made available when securing the airway of an obese patient. These measures include preparing for a range of airways adjuncts, the presence of two experienced intubators, a lengthy preoxygenation period, and supplementing cricoid pressure with adjustable-angle laryngoscopes [6]. Because hypoxia can develop quickly in obese patients, optimal preoxygenation is particularly critical in obese patients with high-risk airways [4]. If the patient requires supplemental high-oxygen delivery via face mask, the trauma team should be aware that obtaining a proper fit in the obese patient may be challenging due to excess facial tissue.

If a surgical airway is required, excess neck tissue can conceal the anatomical landmarks necessary for a tracheotomy or cricothyrotomy. Rehm et al. [7] retrospectively studied patients who had previously been endotracheally intubated and underwent an elective cricothyroidotomy for elective airway management. The primary indication to choose a cricothryoidotomy in lieu of a standard tracheotomy was the presence of technically challenging neck anatomy. In these cases, patients were morbidly obese and had other complicated anatomical challenges, such as short necks, excess adipose tissue, and malpositioning of the larynx in the thoracic inlet rather than the neck proper, resulting in intrathroacic placement of the trachestomy [7].

Breathing

Due to the presence of excess adipose tissue, assessing the obese patient's breathing status and diagnosing blunt thoracic traumatic injuries using auscultation and percussion may be challenging. Obese patients at baseline can have reduced lung volumes and compliance, resulting in ventilation/perfusion mismatch [8]. With increasing BMI, the ventilated patient will exhibit an exponential decline in functional residual capacity, lung and overall respiratory compliance, and airway resistance. The mechanical work required for ventilation can be two to four times greater than for the nonobese [6]. Obese patients also tend to have a lower oxygen saturation on high oxygen delivery.

Circulation

Obesity has a significant impact on the cardiovascular system. Obese patients have greater perfusion needs because of an increase in adipose tissue, resulting in an increased stroke volume, cardiac output, and left ventricular workload, leading to left ventricular dilation and hypertrophy [9]. A decrease in left ventricular compliance makes fluid resuscitation a challenge in the obese patient.

Obese patients have previously been found to have alterations in stroke volume and cardiac output as a result of "obesity cardiomyopathy," and a baseline decreased peripheral vascular resistance [10,11]. Obesity can decrease intrathoracic volume and simultaneously increase intrathoracic pressure from increased intraabdominal pressure. These factors can cause central venous pressure measurements to be falsely elevated [12]. If the trauma team does not take this physiological condition into account during their assessment of the obese patient, they may erroneously conclude the patient is adequately resuscitated.

Disability

Immediately following the primary ABCs, the trauma team should assess the patient's neurological status. This includes the patient's level of consciousness and papillary size and retraction. Change in mental status is an early indication of traumatic head injury. Studies have shown obese trauma patients have a lower incidence of head injuries, but the rationale as to why this occurs is not understood [13].

While the physical exam in both the primary and secondary surveys can be difficult in the obese patient, it is essential to complete a thorough physical exam in this patient population as excess adipose tissue can obscure injuries that might not otherwise be apparent. If a pelvic ring injury is present, a temporizing device may be needed to minimize potentially life-threatening consequences. While palpation of bony landmarks of the pelvis and proximal femurs is often required to allow for optimal placement of the device, in obese patients this may be nearly impossible to achieve accurately and safety [14].

Resuscitation

Trauma resuscitation requires a well-coordinated and collaborative approach. In the case of the obese trauma patient, there are many potential challenges to consider regarding the patient's anatomical and physiological conditions as well as appropriate use of equipment and diagnostic studies. Awareness and knowledge of the availability and use of such equipment, supplies, and personnel are essential. For example, pulse oximetry may not always be accurate in the obese patient, as excess adipose tissue creates a barrier for the penetration of the light sensor [15]. Alternative sites, such as the bridge of the nose, the forehead, or the earlobe, should be considered by the trauma team. Vital signs may be erroneously elevated if the blood pressure cuff is too small. To obtain an accurate measurement, the cuff should be ≥40% of the patient's arm circumference [15]. A peripheral pulse assessment can be difficult to assess in the presence of increased adipose or comorbidities such as peripheral vascular disease. The reliability of a 12-lead electrocardiogram (EKG) can be affected by inaccurate lead positioning due to indistinct landmarks and inconsistent voltages. At baseline morbid obesity can cause specific EKG changes such as low voltage, T-waves flattening or inversion, and a left shift of the P-, QRS-, and T-wave axes [6]. While large-bore intravenous access may be necessary for volume resuscitation, obtaining intravenous (IV) access in the obese patient can be challenging. Thus, alternatives such as central venous access, interosseous, or internal venous cut downs should be considered.

Radiographical studies may not be reliable in the obese population. While a portable chest X-ray is easily available, the quality of the film is often limited in the obese patient by cassette size and inadequate soft-tissue penetration. Soft-tissue artifact could be misinterpreted as a pathological finding, such as an apparent pleural thickening [6]. Thus, a computed tomography (CT) scan of the chest can be an alternative method to identify lung and chest injuries [9]. In some cases, however, CT scanners may not be advisable due to load limitations, as most scanners are limited to approximately 160 kg (350 lb) [3].

While the Focused Assessment with Sonography for Trauma (FAST) exam is often used at the bedside to diagnose internal injuries via ultrasound, the study may be of limited value in obese patients. Due to poor penetration of abdominal fat by ultrasound waves, visualization of the organs can be hampered, impairing the quality of the image and the accuracy of diagnosing an injury [6].

Operative intervention

If immediate surgical intervention is required, it is essential that the trauma team inform the operating room staff of the obese patient's needs, to ensure care is provided in a safe and timely manner. During the transport to the operating room, additional personnel may be required to assist with the transfer of the obese patient. It is important that the operating team be aware of common operating table maximum weight allowances. If an operating room table is not adequate to accommodate the patient's weight, the operating room staff and the trauma team should be familiar with alternative means by which to provide for a larger table. The additional use of arm boards or even two tables side by side may be necessary [1]. Depending on the surgical procedure, proper positioning is necessary to minimize skin breakdown and nerve damage. While safe positioning may require additional equipment, such as stirrups, arm boards, and associated fastening devices, such devices can in turn put extensive pressure on the skin, necessitating frequent skin assessments. Additionally, when positioning the patient, the surgical team should be aware that certain positions, such as Trendelenburg, prone, and lithotomy positions, can compromise chest and abdominal movement and are often tolerated poorly by obese patients.

Obese patients who require damage control laparotomy (DCL) may be at an increased risk for postoperative complications. Among patients who required a DCL, obese patients with a BMI > 30 kg/m^2 had a higher overall risk of pneumonia, sepsis, and renal failure compared to normal-weight and overweight patients. Interestingly, while BMI did not affect the rate of successful closure, the mean time to definitive closure in obese patients was on average more than 4 days longer, as compared to normal-weight patients (7.7 days vs 3.9 days; p = 0.03) [16]. Duchesne et al.'s 2009 retrospective review found that of 104 patients who underwent DCL, the severely obese with a BMI > 39 kg/m^2 were more likely to develop postoperative infections, acute renal insufficiency, and failure of primary abdominal wall facial closure. Additionally, days of ventilator support, length of stay, and mortality rates were significantly higher for severely obese patients compared to obese and nonobese patients [17].

INTRAHOSPITAL PHASE

If the critically injured obese patient is admitted to the intensive care unit (ICU), potential complications include multiorgan failure (MOF), pneumonia, sepsis, acute respiratory distress syndrome, renal failure, myocardial infarction, deep venous thrombosis (DVT), and pulmonary embolism (PE).

Mechanical ventilation may be necessary in the critically ill trauma patient to maintain appropriate ventilation and perfusion. Reiff et al.'s retrospective review of 3649 patients found that independent of age and mechanism of injury, injured patients who required mechanical ventilation were more likely to be overweight and obese [18]. Additionally, obese patients may produce large amounts of respiratory secretions, which can increase the risk of aspiration. The multidisciplinary trauma team, including nursing staff, should be aware that suctioning, oral care, and, in the absence of spinal injury, elevation of the head of bed may help to prevent aspiration and ventilator-associated pneumonia.

In patients requiring prolonged respiratory support, elective tracheostomy is the airway management of choice and is recommended 7–10 days following tracheal intubation. Percutaneous tracheostomy is now widely used for airway maintenance in critically ill patients on long-term ventilations. However, some studies suggest the decision to perform a percutaneous tracheostomy on the obese patient should be made with caution, so as not to expose the patient to adverse complications. Byhahn et al.'s 2005 prospective study found percutatenous tracheostomy in obese patients to be associated with an increased risk of perioperative complications, especially for serious adverse events [19]. Additionally, if there is a large amount of adipose tissue between the skin and trachea, the surgeon may choose to use a long-stemmed or adjustable-flange tracheostomy tube.

Obese patients are at an increased risk of DVT caused by inactivity, hypercoagulopathy, and the traumatic injury. To avoid this, the health care team must encourage early ambulation and sequential compressive devices. If sequential compression devices do not fit properly on obese patients, they should be treated with subcutaneous unfractionated or low-molecular-weight heparin (LMWH). As with the administrations of all medications, the health care team should assess the benefit of coagulation treatment against the risk. Patients with venous stasis, a $BMI > 60$, obstructive sleep apnea (OSA), truncal obesity, hypoventilation, and conditions associated with an increased risk of hypercoagulation are at an increased risk for PE [3]. If patients have a high risk of PE, the health care team may consider the insertion of an inferior vena cava filter.

Health care providers must also aggressively manage the obese patient's wound and skin care. Obese patients' excess adipose tissue may result in an increase in body temperature and perspiration; this excess of moisture can cause skin irritation and breakdown, leading to dermatitis, delayed wound healing, and ulceration. These problems can be minimized by placing gauze between skin folds and in other areas where moisture is likely to accumulate. Adipose tissue is poorly vascularized and low local oxygen tension disadvantages fibroblast and macrophage function, thus slowing healing and predisposing bacterial infection, respectively [1]. To further prevent skin breakdown and ulceration, obese patients should be repositioned every two hours.

In addition to the obese trauma patient's acute injuries, many obese patients have undiagnosed or suboptimally managed comorbidities that may affect management, such as poorly controlled diabetes, hypothyroidism, or sleep apnea. As such, early recognition of these conditions and, if necessary, involvement of appropriate physicians can be useful in optimizing care.

POSTINJURY IMPACT AND OUTCOME

During their hospitalization and rehabilitation, the obese trauma patient may require additional resources, referrals, and equipment, such as larger wheelchairs, walkers, and commodes. As part of an interdisciplinary approach, physical and occupational therapy teams can provide recommendations regarding such equipment to plan for the patient's discharge needs. Collaboration with the wound care team can prevent and treat skin breakdown. Dieticians, social services, and case managers can help establish the patient's discharge needs, keeping in mind that finding appropriate long-term facilities may pose an additional challenge. As such, discharge planning should begin as soon as possible to allow for appropriate and timely placement.

THE IMPACT OF OBESITY ON OUTCOME FOLLOWING TRAUMA

The association between obesity and mortality following trauma is inconsistent throughout the literature. Table 18.1 presents findings from 17 studies published between 1991 and 2009 illustrating the relationship between obesity and mortality or morbidity in the setting of trauma. This table includes 5 prospective and 13 retrospective studies. Of the 17 studies, 15 examined the effect of obesity on trauma mortality; 7 studies found obesity, as defined by the particular study, to be associated with a higher mortality, while 8 studies found no statistically significant difference between obese and nonobese patients. Studies also examined the role of obesity in relation to multiple organ failure, specific injuries such as distal femur and pelvic fractures, and other outcomes such as length of stay and days of mechanical ventilation. These findings again are inconsistent. For example, Neville's prospective study found critically ill obese patients sustain more complications, longer length of stay, and more days of mechanical ventilation, while Maheshwari's retrospective study of patients following motor vehicle crashes showed no significant difference in complications or length of stay [8,20].

Conclusions drawn from these study findings should be made with caution. As illustrated in Table 18.1, study populations lack homogeneity in terms of type and severity of injury, and age of the population. Additionally, definitions of obesity and study sample groupings according to BMI are inconsistent. Study sample sizes vary largely across the studies, ranging from a cohort of 19 individuals to over 12 000 enrollees. Given these limitations, it is difficult to compare and generalize the findings. The general inconsistency of the patient population and definition of obesity makes it even more challenging to draw conclusions regarding the effect of obesity on trauma mortality.

Table 18.1 Studies of obesity in trauma patients as it relates to outcome.

Author, Year	Type of study	Study population	Study sample groupings			Outcome
			Category	BMI (kg/m²)	Study size	
Smith-Choban, 1991 [21]	Retrospective	Blunt trauma patients > 15 yo	Average Overweight Severely over weight	<27 27–31 >31	140 25 19	• Severely overweight patients have a higher mortality than average and overweight patients (42.1 vs 5 and 8%, respectively)
Boulanger, 1992 [22]	Prospective	Blunt trauma patients > 15 yo who survived more than 24 hrs after injury	Nonobese Obese	<30 ≥30	5625 743	• Obese patients are more likely that nonobese patients to have rib fractures (15.7 vs 11.8; p<0.05), pulmonary contusions, pelvic fractures (13.7 vs 9.0%; p<0.01), and upper fractures (7.4 vs 9.0%; p<0.01) and lower (23.6 vs 19.4%; p<0.01) extremity fractures • Obese patients are less likely than nonobese patients to have cerebral (7.1 vs 12.6%; p<0.01) or liver (1.9 vs 3.9%; p<0.05) injuries
Mock, 2002 [23]	Retrospective	MVC patients > 15 yo	*Not stated*	<20 20–24 25–29 30–34 35–39 ≥40	2360 12278 8115 2716 837 421	• Increased BMI is associated with an increased risk of mortality (OR 1.037; 95% CI, 1.015–1.059 for each unit increase in BMI)
Arbabi, 2003 [24]	Retrospective	MCV patients > 13 yo with ≥1 AIS score > 2.	Lean Overweight Obese	≤25 25–30 >30	82 62 45	• Obese patients have a higher mortality rate than lean patients (20 vs 11.3%; p=0.04)
Neville, 2004 [8]	Prospective	Blunt trauma patients admitted to ICU	Nonobese Obese	<30 ≥30	179 63	• Obese patients have a higher mortality rate than nonobese patients (32 vs 16%; p=0.008)
Brown, 2005 [25]	Retrospective	Blunt trauma patients admitted to ICU	Nonobese Obese	<30 ≥30	870 283	• Obese patients have a higher mortality rate than nonobese patients (22 vs 17%; p=0.1) • Obese patients sustain more complications (42 vs 32%; p=0.002) and have a longer lengths of stay and more days of mechanical ventilation
Byrnes, 2005 [26]	Retrospective	Trauma patients > 18 yo	Lean Obese	<35 ≥35	1057 122	• Obese patients have a higher mortality than lean patients (10.7 vs 4.1%; p=0.003) • Obese patients are more likely to have complications during hospitalization than lean patients (27% vs 17.6%; p=0.02)

Study	Type	Population	Group	BMI	n	Findings
Alban, 2006 [27]	Retrospective	Trauma patients admitted to ICU	Nonobese Obese	≤29 ≥30	783 135	• There is no significant difference in mortality between obese and nonobese patients
Ciesla, 2006 [28]	Prospective	Trauma patients with an ISS>15, >15yo, ICU admission within 24 hrs of injury, and who survived more than 48 hrs after injury	Nonobese Obese	<30 ≥30	564 56	• Obese patients are more likely to have multiorgan failure than nonobese patients (37 vs 22%; OR 1.8; 95% CI, 1.2–2.7)
Duane, 2006 [29]	Retrospective	Blunt trauma patients	Nonobese Obese	<30 >30	338 115	• There is no significant difference in mortality between obese and nonobese patients
Porter, 2008 [14]	Prospective	Trauma patients with pelvic ring fractures	Nonobese Obese	>30 <30	186 102	• Obese patients have a higher complication rate following pelvic ring fractures than nonobese patients (39 vs 19%; p <0.001)
Tagliaferri, 2007 [30]	Retrospective	Front seat MCV patients >16yo	Nonobese Obese	<30 ≥30	4792 1127	• Obese patients have a higher mortality rate than nonobese patients (RR 1.84; 95% CI, 1.61–2.1) • Obese patients are more likely to suffer severe cerebral trauma after frontal collision (RR 1.97; 95% CI, 1.52–2.55)
Ryb, 2008 [13]	Retrospective	Blunt trauma patients >15yo in frontal and lateral crashes	Normal weight Overweight Obese	18.5–25 25–30 >30	620 561 437	• Obese and overweight patients have a higher mortality rate than normal-weight patients (20.5, 16.2, and 9.4%, respectively)
Bansal, 2009 [31]	Retrospective	Side-impact MVC patients with pelvic fractures	Normal Overweight Obese	18.5–24.9 25–29.9 ≥30	196 151 77	• Overweight and obese patients are less likely to have pelvic fractures that normal-weight patients (normal BMI adjusted OR 1.81; 95% CI, 1.17–2.86)
Diaz, 2009 [32]	Retrospective	Critically ill trauma patients	Nonobese Morbidly obese	<40 ≥40	1334 146	• There is no significant difference in mortality between obese and nonobese
Dossett, 2009 [33]	Prospective	Critically ill trauma patients	Underweight Normal Overweight Obese Severely obese	≤18.5 18.5–24.9 25–29.9 30–39.9 ≥40	23 426 403 286 81	• There is no significant difference in mortality among the groups • Obesity is not an independent risk factor for increased mortality or pulmonary complications after critical injury • Severely obese patients have longer ICU stays (4.8 days; 95% CI, 1.8–7.7 days)

(continued)

Table 18.1 (*cont'd*)

Author, Year	Type of study	Study population	Study sample groupings			Outcome
			Category	BMI (kg/m²)	Study size	
Maheshwari, 2009 [20]	Retrospective	MVC patients	Nonobese	<30	461	• Obese patients are more likely to have more severe distal femur fractures (90 vs 61%; $p < 0.01$)
			Obese	≥30	204	• There is no significant difference in length of stay, complications, or mortality
Zein, 2005 [34]	Retrospective	Trauma patients > 16yo admitted to ICU for > 48 hrs	Nonobese	*Not stated*	204	• There is no significant difference in mortality between obese and nonobese
			Obese		100	• Obese patients have longer durations of mechanical ventilation (5.3 vs 3.2 days; p=06) and ICU length of stay (9.9 vs 6.3; p=002)

yo = years old; hrs = hours

Despite conflicting evidence regarding obesity and mortality and morbidity outcomes, the problem of trauma in the obese remains significant. Trauma centers throughout the country can expect an increase in admissions of obese injured patients. Outcomes can be jeopardized during the prehospital, hospital, operative, and discharge stages, and as such the approach to the obese trauma patient must be multidisciplinary, well-coordinated, and well-communicated. Health care facilities must be adequately equipped to treat and rehabilitate these patients.

Early recognition and appropriate treatment to identify and address the particular problems outlined in this chapter can minimize poor outcomes in this potentially high-risk group. There is a need to better understand factors that predispose obese patients to trauma and how to best assess an obese trauma patient in the prehospital and resuscitation phases, as well as how to address the needs of the obese trauma patient during their hospitalization and rehabilitation. This can be achieved through effective communication and an integrated team approach.

BEST PRACTICE TIPS

1 During the prehospital phase, on-scene responders should notify emergency dispatchers if an obese patient has been injured to allow for the deployment of ambulances with appropriately equipped crews.

2 Trauma teams should establish hospital-based obese patient management guidelines, such as using load-appropriate examining tables, lifting equipment, and diagnostic imaging.

3 During the initial assessment, trauma teams should recognize the limitations of examination, investigation, and monitoring. Anticipate a difficult airway. Consider alternative sites for pulse oximetry.

4 During the obese trauma patient's hospitalization, health care providers should consider preexisting comorbidities, rather than size alone, in planning appropriate and safe management.

5 During hospitalization, health care providers much optimize DVT prophylaxis and early multidisciplinary consultation.

REFERENCES

1 Chesser TJS, Hammett RB, Norton SA. Orthopaedic trauma in the obese patient. Injury. 2010;41:247–52.

2 O'Brien JM. Obesity-related excess mortality rate in an adult intensive care unit: a risk-adjusted matched cohort study. Crit Care Med. 2004;32:1980.

3 VanHoy SN, Laidlow VT. Trauma in obese patients: implications for nursing practice. Crit Care Nurs Clin North Am. 2009;21:377–89,vi–vii.

4 Vissers RJ, Gibbs MA. The high-risk airway. Emerg Med Clin North Am. 2010;28:203–17,ix–x.

5 Sifri ZC, Kim H, Lavery R, Mohr A, Livingston DH. The impact of obesity on the outcome of emergency intubation in trauma patients. J Trauma. 2008;65:396–400.

6 Grant P, Newcombe M. Emergency management of the morbidly obese. Emerg Med Australas. 2004;16:309–17.

7 Rehm CG, Wanek SM, Gagnon EB, Pearson SK, Mullins RJ. Cricothyroidotomy for elective airway management in critically ill trauma patients with technically challenging neck anatomy. Crit Care. 2002;6:531–5.

8 Neville AL, Brown CV, Weng J, Demetriades D, Velmahos GC. Obesity is an independent risk factor of mortality in severely injured blunt trauma patients. Arch Surg. 2004;139:983–7.

9 Ziglar MK. Obesity and the trauma patient: challenges and guidelines for care. J Trauma Nurs. 2006;13:22–7.

10 Thakur V, Richards R, Reisin E. Obesity, hypertension, and the heart. Am J Med Sci. 2001;321:242–8.

11 Wong C, Marwick TH. Obesity cardiomyopathy: pathogenesis and pathophysiology. Nat Clin Pract Cardiovasc Med. 2007;4:436–43.

12 Winfield RD, Delano MJ, Lottenberg L, et al. Traditional resuscitative practices fail to resolve metabolic acidosis in morbidly obese patients after severe blunt trauma. J Trauma. 2010;68:317–30.

13 Ryb GE, Dischinger PC. Injury severity and outcome of overweight and obese patients after vehicular trauma: a crash injury research and engineering network (CIREN) study. J Trauma. 2008;64:406–11.

14 Porter SE, Graves ML, Qin Z, Russell GV. Operative experience of pelvic fractures in the obese. Obes Surg. 2008; 18:702–8.

15 Garrett K, Lauer K, Christopher BA. The effects of obesity on the cardiopulmonary system: implications for critical care nursing. Prog Cardiovasc Nurs. 2004;19:155–61.

16 Haricharan RN, Dooley AC, Weinberg JA, et al. Body mass index affects time to definitive closure after damage control surgery. J Trauma. 2009;66:1683–7.

17 Duchesne JC, Schmieg RE Jr, Simmons JD, Islam T, McGinness CL, McSwain NE Jr. Impact of obesity in damage control laparotomy patients. J Trauma. 2009;67:108–12; disc. 112–14.

18 Reiff DA, Hipp G, McGwin G Jr, Modjarrad K, MacLennan PA, Rue LW 3rd. Body mass index affects the need for and the duration of mechanical ventilation after thoracic trauma. J Trauma. 2007;62:1432–5.

19 Byhahn C, Lischke V, Meininger D, Halbig S, Westphal K. Peri-operative complications during percutaneous tracheostomy in obese patients. Anaesthesia. 2005;60:12–15.

20 Maheshwari R, Mack CD, Kaufman RP, et al. Severity of injury and outcomes among obese trauma patients with fractures of

the femur and tibia: a crash injury research and engineering network study. J Orthop Trauma. 2009;23:634–9.

21 Smith-Choban P, Weireter LJ Jr, Maynes C. Obesity and increased mortality in blunt trauma. J Trauma. 1991;31:1253–7.

22 Boulanger BR, Milzman D, Mitchell K, Rodriguez A. Body habitus as a predictor of injury pattern after blunt trauma. J Trauma. 1992;33:228–32.

23 Mock CN, Grossman DC, Kaufman RP, Mack CD, Rivara FP. The relationship between body weight and risk of death and serious injury in motor vehicle crashes. Accid Anal Prev. 2002;34:221–8.

24 Arbabi S, Wahl WL, Hemmila MR, Kohoyda-Inglis C, Taheri PA, Wang SC. The cushion effect. J Trauma. 2003;54:1090–3.

25 Brown CV, Neville AL, Rhee P, Salim A, Velmahos GC, Demetriades D. The impact of obesity on the outcomes of 1,153 critically injured blunt trauma patients. J Trauma. 2005;59:1048–51; disc. 1051.

26 Byrnes MC, McDaniel MD, Moore MB, Helmer SD, Smith RS. The effect of obesity on outcomes among injured patients. J Trauma. 2005;58:232–7.

27 Alban RF, Lyass S, Margulies DR, Shabot MM. Obesity does not affect mortality after trauma. Am Surg. 2006;72:966–9.

28 Ciesla DJ, Moore EE, Johnson JL, Burch JM, Cothren CC, Sauaia A. Obesity increases risk of organ failure after severe trauma. J Am Coll Surg. 2006;203:539–45.

29 Duane TM, Dechert T, Aboutanos MB, Malhotra AK, Ivatury RR. Obesity and outcomes after blunt trauma. J Trauma. 2006;61:1218–21.

30 Tagliaferri F, Compagnone C, Yoganandan N, Gennarelli TA. Traumatic brain injury after frontal crashes: relationship with body mass index. J Trauma. 2009;66:727–9.

31 Bansal V, Conroy C, Lee J, Schwartz A, Tominaga G, Coimbra R. Is bigger better? The effect of obesity on pelvic fractures after side impact motor vehicle crashes. J Trauma. 2009;67:709–14.

32 Diaz JJ Jr, Norris PR, Collier BR, et al. Morbid obesity is not a risk factor for mortality in critically ill trauma patients. J Trauma. 2009;66:226–31.

33 Dossett LA, Dageforde LA, Swenson BR, et al. Obesity and site-specific nosocomial infection risk in the intensive care unit. Surg Infect (Larchmt). 2009;10:137–42.

34 Zein JG, Albrecht RM, Tawk MM, Kinasewitz GT. Effect of obesity on mortality in severely injured blunt trauma patients remains unclear. Arch Surg. 2005;140:1130–1; author reply 1131.

19 Abdominal Solid Organ Transplantation in the Obese Patient

Erin C. Hall[1,2] and Dorry L. Segev[1,3]

[1]Department of Surgery, Johns Hopkins School of Medicine, Baltimore, MD, USA
[2]Department of Surgery, Georgetown University, Washington, DC, USA
[3]Department of Epidemiology, Johns Hopkins Bloomberg School of Public Health, Baltimore, MD, USA

KEY POINTS
- Carefully selected obese patients with end-stage organ disease derive survival benefit from organ transplantation.
- Obesity is independently associated with wound complications following transplantation.
- Optimization of immunosuppression regimens to decrease risk of wound complications and incident metabolic syndrome is key in post-transplant management.

INTRODUCTION

The obesity epidemic that has affected the entire USA has also affected the field of abdominal solid organ transplantation. Obesity is associated with common causes of kidney and liver failure, causing an increase in the prevalence of obesity among transplant candidates and recipients, and leading to challenges in the evaluation, waitlist management, surgical treatment, and postoperative management of obese patients undergoing kidney and liver transplants.

Obesity is associated with the top two causes of end-stage renal disease (ESRD) in the USA, diabetes and hypertension. The incidence rates of ESRD secondary to hypertension and diabetes are 99.1 per million population and 153 per million population, respectively. Unlike the stable rate of glomerulonephritis, rates of ESRD due to diabetes and hypertension are increasing [1], and the patients on the transplant waiting list reflect this increase. The percentage of kidney transplant candidates with body mass index (BMI)$\geq$35 on the waitlist has grown from 6.9% in 1999 to 11.9% in 2008 [2,3].

Obesity is also associated with the most common form of liver disease in the USA, nonalcoholic fatty liver disease (NAFLD) [4]. NAFLD cirrhosis is increasingly an indication for liver transplantation, with the percentage of liver transplants secondary to NAFLD estimated to be between 5 and 10%. A recent editorial suggests that if current trends continue, NAFLD may overtake hepatitis C as the most common primary cause of liver failure in liver transplant recipients by 2020 [5]. The patients on the waitlist for liver transplantation reflect the changing demographics of end-stage liver disease. The percentage of liver transplant candidates with BMI$\geq$35 on the waitlist has grown from 7.8% in 1999 to 11% in 2008 [6].

With increasing numbers of obese patients with end-stage organ disease, the first challenge is to determine whether or not these patients are transplant candidates. Retrospective cohort studies have shown that graft and patient survival for obese kidney recipients is decreased compared to their nonobese counterparts [7–10]. However, obese kidney recipients derive survival benefit from transplantation compared to those remaining on dialysis [11]. There is some evidence that graft and patient survival is decreased also in obese liver recipients, but this evidence is less convincing than in kidney recipients and is possibly limited to the more extreme BMIs [12–17]. Obese liver recipients also derive the same survival benefit from transplantation as their nonobese counterparts [18].

Critical Care Management of the Obese Patient, First Edition. Edited by Ali A. El Solh.
© 2012 John Wiley & Sons, Ltd. Published 2012 by John Wiley & Sons, Ltd.

Given that selected obese patients derive a survival benefit from transplantation, careful medical and surgical evaluations are important steps towards transplantation. All studies to date showing survival benefit for obese transplant recipients have been subject to selection bias. Specialized, evidence-based evaluation processes should be in place at each transplant center to identify and waitlist obese patients who are appropriate candidates for transplantation. These evaluation processes minimize risk for the patients, and help to maximize the utility gained from each transplanted organ.

Once on the waitlist, there is evidence that obese patients face disparities in time to transplantation. Obese patients are less likely to receive a transplant and more likely to be bypassed than their nonobese counterparts [3,19]. Obese transplant candidates also face different risks for death while on the waitlist than their nonobese counterparts [20]. Care must be taken to counsel obese patients about the differential risks and benefits on the waitlist.

There are also specialized considerations for post-transplant care. Obese surgical patients in general are at higher risks for cardiovascular, pulmonary, thromboembolic, and wound complications [21]. Higher rates of wound complications have been demonstrated in obese transplant recipients, but no differences have been found in perioperative rates of the other obesity-related complications listed above [22]. After transplantation, organ recipients must receive chronic immunosuppression to prevent organ rejection. In the short term, obese transplant patients on immunosuppression may be at even greater risk for wound infection and complications than their nonobese counterparts. In the long term, immunosuppression has been associated with increased incidence of the metabolic syndrome [23–25]. This risk may be amplified in obese patients, who have an increased risk for development of the metabolic syndrome at baseline [26–28]. Obese transplant patients may also be at greater risk for cardiovascular mortality than their nonobese counterparts [29]. The increased risk that obese patients face warrants aggressive monitoring and risk-factor modification post-transplantation and may require tailoring of immunosuppression regimens.

The goals of this chapter are to outline best practices and to highlight pitfalls at each step of the transplantation process for the obese patient. These steps include evaluation for candidacy, waitlist management, perioperative treatment, and long-term risk reduction. Obese transplant patients are different from the nonobese, and they face different levels of risk than their nonobese

counterparts. However, with an awareness of these differences, clinical care can be tailored to maximize the benefit derived from transplantation for obese patients with end-stage organ disease.

EVIDENCE FOR TRANSPLANTATION OF OBESE PATIENTS

Although questions remain about the efficacy and ethics of abdominal solid organ transplantation for obese patients, the preponderance of evidence suggests that benefit is derived from kidney and liver transplantation for carefully selected obese patients suffering from end-stage disease.

In kidney transplantation, most single-center studies suggest that there is no difference in graft or patient survival, although they are underpowered to detect anything but major differences [7–9]. When Meier-Kriesche et al. used national data from the USRDS (United States Renal Data System) to evaluate 51 927 first-time adult kidney transplant recipients from 1988 to 1997, extremes of BMI (BMI < 20 and > 36) were independently associated with increased rates of graft loss (aHR 1.4, 95% CI 1.3–1.6) and mortality (aHR 1.4) when compared to recipients with average BMI [10]. However, comparing obese to nonobese patients does not address the issue that is clinically relevant to the obese patient, namely choosing between the two options that are actually available to them: whether to undergo transplantation or to remain on dialysis. Interestingly, obese patients on dialysis seem to have a lower risk of death than those with lower BMI [20,30,31]. However, there is evidence to suggest that there remains a survival benefit to transplantation versus dialysis for these patients [11,32,33]. Compared to maintenance dialysis, kidney transplant recipients with a BMI ≥ 30 were shown to have a 61% lower risk for death (aHR 0.39, 95% CI 0.33–0.47) [11].

In liver transplantation, the outcomes are less controversial. There have been no independent associations found between decreased long-term graft or patient survival and recipient BMI 30–40 [12–14,16,34]. Using liver recipients in the United Network for Organ Sharing (UNOS) database between 1988 and 1996, no difference in 1- and 2-year graft survival was detected between patients in different BMI categories [14]. A BMI of ≥ 40 was independently associated with a 52% increased risk of mortality compared to those patients with a BMI ≤ 25 [14]. No other categories of BMI were found to be associated with increased risk of death post-transplant. This question was reexamined using the

National Institute of Diabetes and Digestive and Kidney Diseases Liver Transplantation Database, a prospective cohort of 1013 liver transplant recipients from 1990 to 1994 [16]. Importantly, this database included information of the amount of ascites present at transplantation and the analysis was adjusted for this variable. There was no difference in graft survival or mortality in liver recipients with BMI≥40 [16]. Using data from the Scientific Registry of Transplant Recipients (SRTR) from 2001 to 2004 on 25 647 candidates waitlisted for liver transplantation, Pelletier et al. evaluated both the risk of death associated with increasing BMI and the survival benefit to liver transplant recipients with BMI≥40 compared with remaining on the waitlist. No independent associations were found between BMI and risk of death for any BMI category [17]. Survival benefit was also demonstrated, with recipients at all BMIs deriving 83–86% (aHR 0.14–0.16, p < 0.001) decreased risk of death post-transplant compared to remaining on the waitlist [17].

EVALUATION OF THE OBESE PATIENT FOR TRANSPLANTATION

Transplantation confers survival benefit for carefully selected obese patients with end-stage kidney and liver disease. However, all of the evidence to date is subject to selection bias; in other words, only obese patients who were healthy enough to be selected by their doctors to undergo transplantation have been analysed in retrospective cohorts. It is likely that at some BMI cut point, or some combination of increased BMI and comorbidities, this survival benefit will decrease or even reverse. It has been suggested that obese patients with more than one comorbidity should not be considered candidates for liver transplantation [35], but there have been relatively few studies designed to address this question directly. Not surprisingly, there are no randomized trials to address the question of BMI-based contraindications in obese patients.

There is evidence that above a certain BMI cutoff, kidney or liver transplantation may be relatively contraindicated. Unlike those patients with a BMI between 30 and 40, Glanton et al. failed to demonstrate a survival benefit for kidney transplant recipients with BMI > 40 compared with those remaining on dialysis (aHR 0.47, 95% CI 0.17–1.25) [11]. Two national studies based on data from the UNOS have addressed BMI cutoffs in liver recipients. Using data from 1988–1996, Nair et al. demonstrated an increased risk for death of 52% (aHR 1.52,

95% CI 1.05–2.22) for those recipients with BMI > 40 compared to those with a BMI < 25 [14]. Using a UNOS cohort between 1987 and 2007, Dick et al. have found a 17% higher relative risk for death in patients with BMI >40 compared to those with BMI between 18.5 and 25. This relative risk of death was increased to 41% in the era of MELD (model for end-stage liver disease)-based liver allocation (2002–2007) [15].

Long-term post-transplant cardiovascular complications are expected to correlate with BMI. When considering transplant candidacy, proper evaluation and full cardiac risk stratification is imperative [36]. Questions remain about the interactions of particular comorbidities and obesity with respect to post-transplant risk. Identifying obese patients who are proper transplant candidates is critical to optimizing patient outcome and organ utilization.

Evaluation for kidney transplantation

All patients, including obese ones, are required to undergo standard recipient evaluation. The American Society of Transplantation's recommendation for pretransplant evaluation of cardiac risk factors includes assessment and documentation of coronary artery disease risk factors (age, cigarette smoking, diabetes, hypertension, dyslipidemia, left ventricular hypertrophy), aggressive risk-factor modification for all candidates, and a cardiac stress test for all "high-risk" candidates. High-risk candidates include those with diabetes as the primary etiology for renal disease, prior ischemia, and two or more cardiac risk factors [37].

Beyond the standard evaluation, many centers have put special procedures into place for additional evaluation of obese patients (Figure 19.1). All patients with a BMI≥30 are evaluated by a multidisciplinary team and counseled to lose weight. Given that there is emerging evidence that waist circumference is a better predictor of outcomes than BMI, weight distribution is assessed [38]. Patients with central abdominal distribution may be listed as "inactive" (still accruing time for the purposes of allocation priority, but not receiving offers) while being required to reach a certain weight-loss goal. Otherwise, eligible patients with a BMI between 30 and 40 are listed as "active" for organ offers. As BMI between 41 and 45 is a relative contraindication to kidney transplantation, patients in this category are either waitlisted as "inactive" until weight loss or "active" based on the pretransplant evaluation. Weight loss is followed every 6 months through coordinator phone calls.

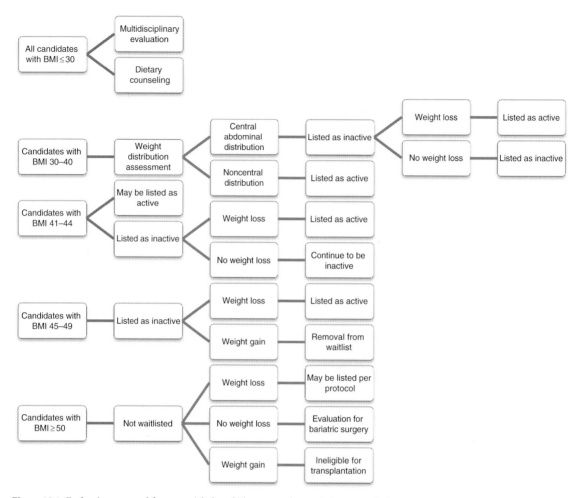

Figure 19.1 Evaluation protocol for potential obese kidney transplant recipients. Weight loss or gain is assessed at 6-month intervals.

In some centers, BMI > 45 is considered an absolute contraindication to transplantation. All patients in this BMI category are placed on the waitlist as "inactive." At the 6-month follow-up phone call, if there has been no weight loss, patients continue to be "inactive" on the waitlist. If there has been weight gain, removal from the waitlist is considered. Those patients with a BMI > 50 are not considered candidates and as such are not waitlisted. These patients undergo a medical consult with a nephrologist and multidisciplinary counseling regarding weight loss. At the 6-month follow-up call, if no weight loss, bariatric surgery is recommended to facilitate candidacy. If there has been weight gain, the patient is deemed to be ineligible for waitlisting or transplantation.

THE OBESE PATIENT ON THE WAITLIST

The obese patient on the waitlist faces a number of challenges. Obese patients on both the kidney and the liver waitlists have longer waiting times for transplantation when compared to their nonobese (BMI < 35) counterparts [3,19]. Obese patients on the kidney waitlist have a 7–44% decreased likelihood for transplantation (depending on degree of obesity) when compared to normal-weight counterparts [3]. Obese kidney transplant candidates also have a 5–22% higher likelihood of being bypassed during an organ offer. Obese liver transplant candidates have 11–29% decreased rates of transplantation, 30–38% lower odds of receiving a MELD priority exception depending on their degree of obesity, and a 10–16% higher likelihood of being turned down for an organ compared to their nonobese counterparts [19].

Controversy exists about the role of weight loss while on the waitlist. Using USRDS data on 162 284 adult kidney transplant candidates from 1990 to 2003, Schold et al. suggested that weight loss was not associated with improved transplant outcomes (either graft or patient survival) in candidates that lost weight on the waitlist [39]. One weakness of this analysis, unfortunately, was the inability to ascertain whether or not the observed weight loss was volitional. In an editorial on the subject, Schnitzler et al. contended that the majority of weight-loss episodes in the waitlisted population were related to illness and poor nutrition. It was suggested that a registry-based analysis without an intention-to-treat component was inadequate to evaluate the associations of weight loss and outcomes for obese renal transplant recipients [40]. It seems intuitive that trying to improve pretransplant cardiovascular risk factors, including obesity, through diet reeducation and focus on gradual and intentional weight loss would improve transplant outcomes, but there have been no studies to our knowledge that have addressed this topic directly.

Bariatric surgery

It has been suggested that bariatric surgery, including Roux-en-Y gastric bypass (RYGB) and laparoscopic sleeve gastrectomy, may decrease obesity-related comorbidities pretransplantation. In two small studies, obese patients with CKD have successfully undergone bariatric procedures (predominantly RYGB) with no perioperative mortality. However, not surprisingly, an increased risk of perioperative morbidity when compared to other bariatric surgery patients was shown [41,42]. Both studies reported improved obesity-related comorbidities [43,44]. Laparoscopic sleeve gastrectomy for obese liver transplant candidates has also been successful. In a case series of six cirrhotic patients undergoing laparascopic sleeve gastrectomy, no perioperative mortality was reported. Similarly to the kidney studies, obesity-associated comorbidities improved or resolved in all patients [44]. Sleeve gastrectomy is the bariatric procedure of choice in cirrhotic patients to preserve access to the gastric fundus for management of variceal bleeding [45]. For both kidney and liver transplant candidates, it remains unclear how weight reduction through bariatric surgery affects post-transplant morbidity, mortality, and graft function.

PERIOPERATIVE COMPLICATIONS IN THE OBESE TRANSPLANT RECIPIENT

Wound infection is the only perioperative complication during kidney or liver transplantation reported to be independently associated with recipient obesity [22,46,47]. A single-center retrospective study of 869 first-time kidney transplant patients from 2003 to 2008 found a BMI > 30 associated with a 2.2-fold increase in adjusted relative risk of surgical-site infections (95% CI 1.5–3.2) [22]. Possible etiologies for the increased risk of surgical-site infection in obese patients include decreased oxygen tension, immune impairment, and secondary ischemia along suture lines [21]. All potential recipients should be screened and treated for chronic skin infections (like intertriginous *Candida*) in addition to the standard perioperative skin decontamination procedures.

Perioperative wound complications, including lymphocele, seroma, dehiscence, and infection, have been associated with the use of the immunosuppression agent sirolimus. One question is how obesity and the increased risk of wound complications might affect the choice of immunosuppression in the perioperative period. A single-center study compared perioperative wound complications between immunosuppression regimens containing mycophenolatemofetil, tacrolimus, and prednisone (84 patients) with sirolimus, tacrolimus, and prednisone (74 patients). Increasing BMI was found to be an independent risk factor for wound complications in both groups, and those treated with sirolimus were found to have higher odds for any wound complication [48]. However, it does not appear that the interaction between BMI and sirolimus use was evaluated in this study. Therefore it remains unclear how increasing BMI combined with sirolimus use might (or might not) amplify the overall risk for wound complication. Given the increased risk for wound complications in recipients with increased BMI, it seems wise to avoid sirolimus immunosuppression if possible, particularly in the perioperative period.

Despite the fact that obesity has not been shown to be an independent risk factor for perioperative cardiovascular or thromboembolic events, this population warrants an increased index of suspicion for a number of perioperative complications. Obesity is associated with smaller lung volumes and decreased chest compliance. The obese transplant recipient should undergo aggressive pulmonary toilet, and be encouraged to use incentive spirometry. Continuous positive airway pressure has been advocated to prevent atelectasis and to address underlying sleep disorderedbreathinginthispopulation.Thromboembolism is the leading cause of death following bariatric surgery. Prophylaxis and a high index of suspicion with an emphasis on early ambulation are highly recommended. Obese patients who receive transplants have been highly selected and have fewer of the comorbidites associated with obese patients in general. However, as in all patients undergoing major operations, vigilance is still required.

MANAGEMENT OF LONG-TERM POSTOPERATIVE RISKS IN THE OBESE TRANSPLANT PATIENT

Once past the perioperative period, the obese transplant recipient faces a number of long-term management issues. One of the most active areas of study in obese transplant recipients is in the incidence of new-onset metabolic syndrome (abdominal obesity, hyperglycemia, dyslipidemia, and hypertension) and other previously undiagnosed cardiovascular risk factors. These markers of cardiovascular disease risk occur at higher incidence rates for obese versus nonobese transplant recipients [26–28,36,49].

Obese kidney transplant recipients have increased prevalence of metabolic syndrome post-transplant compared to their nonobese counterparts [50–52]. Each of the components of the metabolic syndrome may be associated with different degrees of increased risk for cardiovascular events, graft loss, and death among kidney transplant recipients. In a single-center study of 1666 renal transplant recipients, Kasiske et al. found a 17% (aHR 1.17, 95% CI 1.12–1.22) increased risk of death-censored graft failure and an 18% (aHR 1.18, 95% CI 1.12–1.23) increased risk of death for every 10 mm Hg increase in blood pressure [53,54]. New-onset diabetes mellitus in the post-kidney transplant patient is independently, consistently, and strongly associated with increased cardiovascular morbidity [50,52,55,56]. The Patient Outcomes in Renal Transplant (PORT) Study is an international retrospective cohort of 23 575 adult kidney transplant recipients. In it, new-onset diabetes post-transplant was associated with an 86% (aHR 1.86, 95% CI 1.43–2.43) increased risk of coronary heart disease 3 years post-transplant. The degree or magnitude of effect modification that might occur between obesity and any one of these risk factors is unclear. Post-transplant diabetes and post-transplant hypertension are both associated with increased risk of post-liver transplant mortality [45].

The metabolic syndrome should be screened for and treated aggressively in the post-transplant patient [57–59]. Goals for post-transplant diabetes management are similar to those in the general population, with a target glycosylated hemoglobin of < 7% and fasting blood sugar of 70–130 mg/dl [60]. Dietary counseling is the first line of treatment, with a low threshold for initiating an oral hypoglycemic agent. Short-acting agents with hepatic metabolism like glipizide are more appropriate for post-kidney transplant recipients, while metformin is an appropriate first-line oral hypoglycemic in post-liver transplant recipients (there is an increased risk of lactic acidosis with renal impairment and metformin) [57,61].

The current definition of hypertension is a blood pressure above 140/90 sustained over time [60]. The calcineurin inhibitors (CNIs) used for immunosuppression post-transplant can lead to hypertension through increased renal arteriolar constriction. Calcium-channel blockers are associated with improved glomerular filtration rate (GFR) post-kidney transplant and are renal protective in randomized trials of post-transplant hypertension treatment in post-liver transplant patients. Amlodipine is often used as a first-line agent [57,62]. Nifedipine is an inhibitor of intestinal cytochrome p450 and predictably increases CNI levels with potential toxicity. Angiotensin-converting enzyme (ACE) inhibitors are used in post-kidney and liver transplant patients, but they may exacerbate CNI-induced hyperkalemia [57,62].

According to guidelines, dyslipidemia is defined as triglycerides ≥ 150 mg/dl and HDL-C < 40 mg/dl for males or < 50 mg/dl for females [60]. HMG-CoA reductase inhibitors (statins) should be initiated early in the course of management for post-transplant dyslipidemias in both renal and liver transplants. Recommendations for initiation and follow-up of statin therapy include starting at low doses and frequent liver function monitoring [57,61]. Dietary modifications and control of hyperglycemia are not different between patients with a transplant and without, and include encouraging low-fat diets rich in fruits, vegetables, and fiber [63].

Care should be taken in designing an immunosuppression regimen that decreases risk for the development of the metabolic syndrome in obese post-transplant patients [64–66]. This includes steroid minimization and judicious use of CNIs when possible. Tacrolimus is associated with an increased incidence of new-onset diabetes mellitus post-liver and kidney transplant compared to cyclosporine [23–25,67]. At least one study shows evidence that steroid use may amplify the diabetogenic effects of tacrolimus [23]. Regimens that avoid steroids and minimize CNIs may be considered in obese transplant recipients, given this population's increased risk for the development of metabolic syndrome.

Another factor to take into account when prescribing immunosuppression is that obese patients may have significantly different volumes of distribution for medications compared to nonobese patients. One study of the pharmacokinetics of cyclosporine in obese kidney transplant recipients found that dosing on ideal body weight rather than actual body weight was necessary to achieve comparable drug concentrations in the early transplant period [68]. Careful monitoring of drug levels is warranted and it is recommended that drug levels are obtained even in those medications that are traditionally not monitored, such as mycophenolatemofetil, in obese patients post-transplant [69].

Post-transplant bariatric surgery is also proposed as an option for decreasing morbidity in obese transplant recipients with new-onset metabolic syndrome. Several small series of post-kidney transplant patients undergoing gastric bypass procedures report no in-hospital or 30-day mortalities [23,41,70,71]. In one series of 10 patients receiving post-renal transplant gastric bypass there was resolution of hypertension, dyslipidemias, and diabetes mellitus in over half of the recipients [41]. Post-transplant patients who undergo bariatric surgery should also have levels of immunosuppression drugs closely monitored to ensure adequate amounts are absorbed and that they stay below toxic levels, as two small-scale studies have suggested absorption and pharmacokinetics may be altered in these patients [23,72].

For liver transplant recipients, obesity is also associated with NAFLD and graft dysfunction. Increased rates of new-onset and recurrent NAFLD are associated with weight gain post-transplant [73]. A handful of small studies show that interventions, including gastric bypass surgery, aimed at weight loss in obese post-liver transplant recipients with recurrent NAFLD result in normalization of liver enzymes and glucose levels [74]. Treatment strategies include intensive diet and nutrition counseling to prevent weight gain post-transplantation, as well as monitoring and treatment for new-onset diabetes mellitus and dyslipidemias, as outlined above.

NEW FRONTIERS FOR TRANSPLANTATION IN THE OBESE PATIENT

There are new minimally invasive techniques that may prove beneficial for the obese transplant recipient. There is at least one case report of a total robotic kidney

transplant in a morbidly obese patient (BMI > 40) [75], as well as a published case series of four laparoscopic kidney transplants successfully performed [76]. Minimally invasive surgery in the obese patient is appealing because of the decreased risk for surgical-site infection and better intraoperative visualization.

CONCLUSION

The prevalence of obesity is increasing in patients with end-stage kidney and liver disease. Transplantation is the treatment of choice for obese patients who meet screening criteria. However, obese transplant patients deserve special clinical considerations at each step of the transplantation process. The survival benefit from transplantation seen in these patients is based on retrospective analyses of highly selected obese recipients. Evidence-based candidate evaluation procedures should be in place to identify appropriate obese transplantation candidates most likely to derive benefit from transplantation. On the waitlist, obese patients are less likely to receive transplantation. After transplantation, the complications associated with obese transplant recipients are not drastically different from those of any other obese surgical patient. The real difference is seen in clinical decision-making around the choices and monitoring of immunosuppression regimens. Over long-term follow-up, new-onset metabolic syndrome in the obese post-transplant patient should be treated aggressively with lifestyle changes and appropriate medical interventions. There has been some small-scale success in performing bariatric surgery on post-transplant recipients with new-onset metabolic syndrome. Currently, the obese patients considered for transplantation are otherwise healthy and have few additional comorbidities. Questions remain about "nonideal" obese patients with more than one perioperative risk factor and what the potential survival benefit and outcomes after transplantation might be for this population.

BEST PRACTICE TIPS

1 Evidence-based evaluation procedures should be instituted for candidate evaluation of obese patients.
2 Immunosuppression should be selected to minimize risk of perioperative wound complications in the obese patient.
3 Long-term immunosuppression should be tailored to minimize risk of new-onset metabolic syndrome.
4 Increased monitoring of immunosuppression levels is warranted in this population.
5 Aggressive risk-factor modification is important post-transplant for obese patients with new-onset metabolic syndrome.

REFERENCES

1 US Renal Data System, USRDS 2010: annual data report: atlas of chronic kidney disease and end-stage renal disease in the United States, National Institute of Health, National Institute of Diabetes and Digestive and Kidney Diseases. 2010.

2 United Network for Organ Sharing (UNOS) Standard Transplant Analysis and Research (STAR) Dataset, 1987–2009.

3 Segev DL, Simpkins CE, Thompson RE, Locke JE, Warren DS, Montgomery RA. Obesity impacts access to kidney transplantation. J Am Soc Nephrol. 2008 Feb;19(2):349–55.

4 Charlton M. Nonalcoholic fatty liver disease: a review of current understanding and future impact. Clin Gastroenterol Hepatol. 2004 Dec;2(12):1048–58.

5 Charlton M. Cirrhosis and liver failure in nonalcoholic fatty liver disease: molehill or mountain? Hepatology. 2008 May;47(5):1431–3.

6 2009 Annual Report of the US Organ Procurement and Transplantation Network and the Scientific Registry of Transplant Recipients: Transplant Data 1999–2008. US Department of Health and Human Services, Health Resources and Services Administration, Healthcare Systems Bureau, Division of Transplantation, Rockville, MD.

7 Yamamoto S, Hanley E, Hahn AB, Isenberg A, Singh TP, Cohen D, et al. The impact of obesity in renal transplantation: an analysis of paired cadaver kidneys. Clin Transplant. 2002 Aug;16(4):252–6.

8 Massarweh NN, Clayton JL, Mangum CA, Florman SS, Slakey DP. High body mass index and short- and long-term renal allograft survival in adults. Transplantation. 2005 Nov;80(10):1430–4.

9 Howard RJ, Thai VB, Patton PR, Hemming AW, Reed AI, Van der Werf WJ, et al. Obesity does not portend a bad outcome for kidney transplant recipients. Transplantation. 2002 Jan;73(1):53–5.

10 Meier-Kriesche HU, Arndorfer JA, Kaplan B. The impact of body mass index on renal transplant outcomes: a significant independent risk factor for graft failure and patient death. Transplantation. 2002 Jan;73(1):70–4.

11 Glanton CW, Kao TC, Cruess D, Agodoa LY, Abbott KC. Impact of renal transplantation on survival in end-stage renal disease patients with elevated body mass index. Kidney Int. 2003 Feb;63(2):647–53.

12 Nair S, Cohen DB, Cohen MP, Tan H, Maley W, Thuluvath PJ. Postoperative morbidity, mortality, costs, and long-term survival in severely obese patients undergoing orthotopic liver transplantation. Am J Gastroenterol. 2001 Mar;96(3): 842–5.

13 Sawyer RG, Pelletier SJ, Pruett TL. Increased early morbidity and mortality with acceptable long-term function in severely obese patients undergoing liver transplantation. Clin Transplant. 1999 Feb;13(1 Pt 2):126–30.

14 Nair S, Verma S, Thuluvath PJ. Obesity and its effect on survival in patients undergoing orthotopic liver transplantation in the United States. Hepatology. 2002 Jan;35(1):105–9.

15 Dick AA, Spitzer AL, Seifert CF, Deckert A, Carithers RL,Jr, Reyes JD, et al. Liver transplantation at the extremes of the body mass index. Liver Transpl. 2009 Aug;15(8):968–77.

16 Leonard J, Heimbach JK, Malinchoc M, Watt K, Charlton M. The impact of obesity on long-term outcomes in liver transplant recipients-results of the NIDDK liver transplant database. Am J Transplant. 2008 Mar;8(3):667–72.

17 Pelletier SJ, Schaubel DE, Wei G, Englesbe MJ, Punch JD, Wolfe RA, et al. Effect of body mass index on the survival benefit of liver transplantation. Liver Transpl. 2007 Dec;13(12):1678–83.

18 Pelletier SJ, Maraschio MA, Schaubel DE, Dykstra DM, Punch JD, Wolfe RA, et al. Survival benefit of kidney and liver transplantation for obese patients on the waiting list. Clin Transpl. 2003:77–88.

19 Segev DL, Thompson RE, Locke JE, Simpkins CE, Thuluvath PJ, Montgomery RA, et al. Prolonged waiting times for liver transplantation in obese patients. Ann Surg. 2008 Nov;248(5):863–70.

20 Wolfe RA, Ashby VB, Daugirdas JT, Agodoa LY, Jones CA, Port FK. Body size, dose of hemodialysis, and mortality. Am J Kidney Dis. 2000 Jan;35(1):80–8.

21 DeMaria EJ, Carmody BJ. Perioperative management of special populations: obesity. Surg Clin North Am. 2005 Dec;85(6):1283–9,xii.

22 Lynch RJ, Ranney DN, Shijie C, Lee DS, Samala N, Englesbe MJ. Obesity, surgical site infection, and outcome following renal transplantation. Ann Surg. 2009 Dec;250(6):1014–20.

23 Araki M, Flechner SM, Ismail HR, Flechner LM, Zhou L, Derweesh IH, et al. Posttransplant diabetes mellitus in kidney transplant recipients receiving calcineurin or mTOR inhibitor drugs. Transplantation. 2006 Feb 15;81(3): 335–41.

24 Burroughs TE, Lentine KL, Takemoto SK, Swindle J, Machnicki G, Hardinger K, et al. Influence of early posttransplantation prednisone and calcineurin inhibitor dosages on the incidence of new-onset diabetes. Clin J Am Soc Nephrol. 2007 May;2(3):517–23.

25 Kuo HT, Sampaio MS, Ye X, Reddy P, Martin P, Bunnapradist S. Risk factors for new-onset diabetes mellitus in adult liver transplant recipients, an analysis of the Organ Procurement and Transplant Network/United Network for Organ Sharing database. Transplantation. 2010 May 15;89(9):1134–40.

26 Goldsmith D, Pietrangeli CE. The metabolic syndrome following kidney transplantation. Kidney Int. 2010 Sep;78 Suppl 118:S8–14.

27 Hanouneh IA, Zein NN. Metabolic syndrome and liver transplantation. Minerva Gastroenterol Dietol. 2010 Sep; 56(3):297–304.

28 Pagadala M, Dasarathy S, Eghtesad B, McCullough AJ. Posttransplant metabolic syndrome: an epidemic waiting to happen. Liver Transpl. 2009 Dec;15(12):1662–70.

29 Lentine KL, Rocca-Rey LA, Bacchi G, Wasi N, Schmitz L, Salvalaggio PR, et al. Obesity and cardiac risk after kidney transplantation: experience at one center and comprehensive literature review. Transplantation. 2008 Jul;86(2):303–12.

30 Port FK, Ashby VB, Dhingra RK, Roys EC, Wolfe RA. Dialysis dose and body mass index are strongly associated with survival in hemodialysis patients. J Am Soc Nephrol. 2002 Apr;13(4):1061–6.

31 Abbott KC, Glanton CW, Trespalacios FC, Oliver DK, Ortiz MI, Agodoa LY, et al. Body mass index, dialysis modality, and survival: analysis of the United States Renal Data System Dialysis Morbidity and Mortality Wave II Study. Kidney Int. 2004 Feb;65(2):597–605.

32 Killackey M, Zhang R, Sparks K, Paramesh A, Slakey D, Florman S. Challenges of abdominal organ transplant in obesity. South Med J. 2010 Jun;103(6):532–40.

33 Marks WH, Florence LS, Chapman PH, Precht AF, Perkinson DT. Morbid obesity is not a contraindication to kidney transplantation. Am J Surg. 2004 May;187(5):635–8.

34 Schaeffer DF, Yoshida EM, Buczkowski AK, Chung SW, Steinbrecher UP, Erb SE, et al. Surgical morbidity in severely obese liver transplant recipients: a single Canadian Centre Experience. Ann Hepatol. 2009 Jan–Mar;8(1):38–40.

35 Thuluvath PJ. Morbid obesity with one or more other serious comorbidities should be a contraindication for liver transplantation. Liver Transpl. 2007 Dec;13(12):1627–9.

36 Desai S, Hong JC, Saab S. Cardiovascular risk factors following orthotopic liver transplantation: predisposing factors, incidence and management. Liver Int. 2010 Aug;30(7): 948–57.

37 Lentine KL, Hurst FP, Jindal RM, Villines TC, Kunz JS, Yuan CM, et al. Cardiovascular risk assessment among potential kidney transplant candidates: approaches and controversies. Am J Kidney Dis. 2010 Jan;55(1):152–67.

38 Kovesdy CP, Czira ME, Rudas A, Ujszaszi A, Rosivall L, Novak M, et al. Body mass index, waist circumference and mortality in kidney transplant recipients. Am J Transplant. 2010 Dec;10(12):2644–51.

39 Schold JD, Srinivas TR, Guerra G, Reed AI, Johnson RJ, Weiner ID, et al. A "weight-listing" paradox for candidates of renal transplantation? Am J Transplant. 2007 Mar;7(3): 550–9.

40 Schnitzler MA, Salvalaggio PR, Axelrod DA, Lentine KL, Takemoto SK. Lack of interventional studies in renal transplant candidates with elevated cardiovascular risk. Am J Transplant. 2007 Mar;7(3):493–4.

41 Alexander JW, Goodman H. Gastric bypass in chronic renal failure and renal transplant. Nutr Clin Pract. 2007 Feb;22(1):16–21.

42 Alexander JW, Goodman HR, Gersin K, Cardi M, Austin J, Goel S, et al. Gastric bypass in morbidly obese patients with chronic renal failure and kidney transplant. Transplantation. 2004 Aug;78(3):469–74.

43 Modanlou KA, Muthyala U, Xiao H, Schnitzler MA, Salvalaggio PR, Brennan DC, et al. Bariatric surgery among kidney transplant candidates and recipients: analysis of the United States renal data system and literature review. Transplantation. 2009 Apr 27;87(8):1167–73.

44 Takata MC, Campos GM, Ciovica R, Rabl C, Rogers SJ, Cello JP, et al. Laparoscopic bariatric surgery improves candidacy in morbidly obese patients awaiting transplantation. Surg Obes Relat Dis. 2008 Mar–Apr;4(2):159–64; disc. 164–5.

45 Charlton M. Obesity, hyperlipidemia, and metabolic syndrome. Liver Transpl. 2009 Nov;15(Suppl 2):S83–9.

46 Flechner SM, Zhou L, Derweesh I, Mastroianni B, Savas K, Goldfarb D, et al. The impact of sirolimus, mycophenolate mofetil, cyclosporine, azathioprine, and steroids on wound healing in 513 kidney-transplant recipients. Transplantation. 2003 Dec;76(12):1729–34.

47 Bennett WM, McEvoy KM, Henell KR, Pidikiti S, Douzdjian V, Batiuk T. Kidney transplantation in the morbidly obese: complicated but still better than dialysis. Clin Transplant. 2011 May;25(3):401–5.

48 Valente JF, Hricik D, Weigel K, Seaman D, Knauss T, Siegel CT, et al. Comparison of sirolimus vs. mycophenolate mofetil on surgical complications and wound healing in adult kidney transplantation. Am J Transplant. 2003 Sep;3(9):1128–34.

49 Parikh CR, Klem P, Wong C, Yalavarthy R, Chan L. Obesity as an independent predictor of posttransplant diabetes mellitus. Transplant Proc. 2003 Dec;35(8):2922–6.

50 Kasiske BL, Snyder JJ, Gilbertson D, Matas AJ. Diabetes mellitus after kidney transplantation in the United States. Am J Transplant. 2003 Feb;3(2):178–85.

51 Armstrong KA, Campbell SB, Hawley CM, Nicol DL, Johnson DW, Isbel NM. Obesity is associated with worsening cardiovascular risk factor profiles and proteinuria progression in renal transplant recipients. Am J Transplant. 2005 Nov;5(11):2710–18.

52 Cosio FG, Kudva Y, van der Velde M, Larson TS, Textor SC, Griffin MD, et al. New onset hyperglycemia and diabetes are associated with increased cardiovascular risk after kidney transplantation. Kidney Int. 2005 Jun;67(6):2415–21.

53 Kasiske BL, Cangro CB, Hariharan S, Hricik DE, Kerman RH, Roth D, et al. The evaluation of renal transplantation candidates: clinical practice guidelines. Am J Transplant. 2001; 1(Suppl 2):3–95.

54 Kasiske BL, Anjum S, Shah R, Skogen J, Kandaswamy C, Danielson B, et al. Hypertension after kidney transplantation. Am J Kidney Dis. 2004 Jun;43(6):1071–81.

55 Israni AK, Snyder JJ, Skeans MA, Peng Y, Maclean JR, Weinhandl ED, et al. Predicting coronary heart disease after kidney transplantation: Patient Outcomes in Renal Transplantation (PORT) Study. Am J Transplant. 2010 Feb;10(2):338–53.

56 Lentine KL, Brennan DC, Schnitzler MA. Incidence and predictors of myocardial infarction after kidney transplantation. J Am Soc Nephrol. 2005 Feb;16(2):496–506.

57 Watt KD, Charlton MR. Metabolic syndrome and liver transplantation: a review and guide to management. J Hepatol. 2010 Jul;53(1):199–206.

58 Reuben A. Long-term management of the liver transplant patient: diabetes, hyperlipidemia, and obesity. Liver Transpl. 2001 Nov;7(11 Suppl 1):S13–21.

59 Wilkinson A, Davidson J, Dotta F, Home PD, Keown P, Kiberd B, et al. Guidelines for the treatment and management of new-onset diabetes after transplantation. Clin Transplant. 2005 Jun;19(3):291–8.

60 Alberti KG, Eckel RH, Grundy SM, Zimmet PZ, Cleeman JI, Donato KA, et al. Harmonizing the metabolic syndrome: a joint interim statement of the International Diabetes Federation Task Force on Epidemiology and Prevention; National Heart, Lung, and Blood Institute; American Heart Association; World Heart Federation; International Atherosclerosis Society; and International Association for the Study of Obesity. Circulation. 2009 Oct 20;120(16):1640–5.

61 Markell MS, Armenti V, Danovitch G, Sumrani N. Hyperlipidemia and glucose intolerance in the post-renal transplant patient. J Am Soc Nephrol. 1994 Feb;4(8 Suppl):S37–47.

62 Mangray M, Vella JP. Hypertension after kidney transplant. Am J Kidney Dis. 2011 Feb;57(2):331–41.

63 Chan M, Patwardhan A, Ryan C, Trevillian P, Chadban S, Westgarth F, et al. Evidence-based guidelines for the nutritional management of adult kidney transplant recipients. J Ren Nutr. 2011 Jan;21(1):47–51.

64 Bodziak KA, Hricik DE. New-onset diabetes mellitus after solid organ transplantation. Transpl Int. 2009 May;22(5):519–30.

65 Marchetti P. New-onset diabetes after liver transplantation: from pathogenesis to management. Liver Transpl. 2005 Jun;11(6):612–20.

66 Shah T, Kasravi A, Huang E, Hayashi R, Young B, Cho YW, et al. Risk factors for development of new-onset diabetes mellitus after kidney transplantation. Transplantation. 2006 Dec;82(12):1673–6.

67 Mathew JT, Rao M, Job V, Ratnaswamy S, Jacob CK. Post-transplant hyperglycaemia: a study of risk factors. Nephrol Dial Transplant. 2003 Jan;18(1):164–71.

68 Everhart JE, Lombardero M, Lake JR, Wiesner RH, Zetterman RK, Hoofnagle JH. Weight change and obesity after liver transplantation: incidence and risk factors. Liver Transpl Surg. 1998 Jul;4(4):285–96.

69 Yau WP, Vathsala A, Lou HX, Chan E. Is a standard fixed dose of mycophenolate mofetil ideal for all patients? Nephrol Dial Transplant. 2007 Dec;22(12):3638–45.

70 Marterre WF, Hariharan S, First MR, Alexander JW. Gastric bypass in morbidly obese kidney transplant recipients. Clin Transplant. 1996 Oct;10(5):414–19.

71 Szomstein S, Rojas R, Rosenthal RJ. Outcomes of laparoscopic bariatric surgery after renal transplant. Obes Surg. 2010 Mar;20(3):383–5.

72 Rogers CC, Alloway RR, Alexander JW, Cardi M, Trofe J, Vinks AA. Pharmacokinetics of mycophenolic acid, tacrolimus and sirolimus after gastric bypass surgery in end-stage renal disease and transplant patients: a pilot study. Clin Transplant. 2008 May–Jun;22(3):281–91.

73 Seo S, Maganti K, Khehra M, Ramsamooj R, Tsodikov A, Bowlus C, et al. De novo nonalcoholic fatty liver disease after liver transplantation. Liver Transpl. 2007 Jun;13(6):844–7.

74 Duchini A, Brunson ME. Roux-en-Y gastric bypass for recurrent nonalcoholic steatohepatitis in liver transplant recipients with morbid obesity. Transplantation. 2001 Jul;72(1):156–9.

75 Giulianotti P, Gorodner V, Sbrana F, Tzvetanov I, Jeon H, Bianco F, et al. Robotic transabdominal kidney transplantation in a morbidly obese patient. Am J Transplant. 2010 Jun;10(6):1478–82.

76 Modi P, Rizvi J, Pal B, et al. Laparoscopic kidney transplantation: an initial experience. Am J Transplant. 2011;11(6):1320–4.

20 Critical Care Management of the Obese Patient after Bariatric Surgery

Scott E. Mimms and Samer G. Mattar

Indiana University, Indianapolis, IN, USA; Indiana University Health Bariatrics and Weight Loss, Indiana University Health North, Carmel, IN, USA

> **KEY POINTS**
> - Bariatric surgery has been performed with great success and with low mortality in well-established centers.
> - Patients who are male, older than 50 years, who are heavier (BMI > 60 kg/m2), and who have complications requiring reoperation will likely need intensive care and extended mechanical ventilation.
> - Survival of the morbidly obese patient hinges on early recognition and expedient treatment of postoperative complications.

INTRODUCTION

The National Institutes of Health (NIH), in cooperation with the North American Association for the study of Obesity (NAASO) and the Heart, Lung, and Blood Institute (NHLBI) Expert Panel, published a practical guide on the identification, evaluation, and treatment of overweight and obesity in adults [1]. The goal for treating obesity is to reduce excess body weight, prevent further weight gain, and improve the patient's overall health. Effective weight control involves multiple techniques and strategies including dietary therapy, physical activity, behavior therapy, and pharmacotherapy. Unfortunately, conservative medical treatment efforts have been largely unsuccessful in achieving and maintaining profound and durable results in morbidly obese patients.

Bariatric surgery is a collective term for surgical procedures that involve reducing the size of the gastric reservoir. These operations have yielded impressive results,

with approximately a 50% or more reduction in excess body weight by 18–24 months post operation [2]. Thus, it is not surprising that, in the USA, approximately 200 000 bariatric operations are performed each year, and these numbers are rapidly escalating. Although most patients have good outcomes, a certain proportion may develop postoperative complications.

BARIATRIC SURGERY AND CRITICAL CARE

Bariatric surgery has been performed with great success and with low mortality in well-established centers. Laparoscopic Roux-en-Y gastric bypass and laparoscopic adjustable gastric banding are the most commonly performed weight-reduction operations in the world. The sleeve gastrectomy is gaining increasing popularity, and the duodenal switch and biliopancreatic diversion continue to be performed, but with less frequency. Of particular distinction is the fact that successful clinical outcomes, regardless of which operation is offered, depend to a large extent on a detailed and comprehensive preoperative evaluation and optimization of the patient. Preoperative assessment and selection should be performed by a multidisciplinary team composed of clinicians who are dedicated to the management of the bariatric patient. It is especially helpful to include dedicated anesthesiologists in this team and seek their opinion early on in the patient's progress, to allow adequate assessment of the airway and the ability for thorough preparation. In a similar vein, dedicated

Critical Care Management of the Obese Patient, First Edition. Edited by Ali A. El Solh.
© 2012 John Wiley & Sons, Ltd. Published 2012 by John Wiley & Sons, Ltd.

pulmonologists, cardiologists, and endocrinologists should collaborate to optimize patients with a view to increasing physiological reserves and avoiding postoperative complications.

Currently, reported mortality for patients with a BMI < 50 is about 0.28% [3]. Most patients tolerate the operations well and, in most practices, are discharged within 2 days of surgery. In fact, the majority will not require admission to the intensive care unit (ICU) unless their hospital course is prolonged due to sustained postoperative sedation, or a postoperative complication such as an anastomotic leak, pulmonary embolism (PE), subphrenic abscess and/or systemic sepsis, or bowel obstruction. In aggregate, these major complications occur in less than 10% of patients [4]. The two most likely complications that would cause an ICU admission are an anastomotic leak and a PE, both of which may present with respiratory distress.

The ability to recognize risk factors for ICU admission has been of keen interest to many investigators. Clearly, open surgery is associated with increased trauma and an increased stress response when compared to minimally invasive techniques. In a randomized trial of open versus laparoscopic gastric bypass, 21% of patients who received open surgery required postoperative ICU care, whereas this incidence was only 7.6% in the laparoscopically treated group [5]. Helling et al. noted that patients who are male, older than 50 years, who are heavier (BMI > 60 kg/m²), and who have complications requiring reoperation will likely need intensive care and extended mechanical ventilation [6].

POSTOPERATIVE FLUID RESUSCITATION

Obese patients are in a chronically hypovolemic state, which manifests vividly in the perioperative period. Initiation of intravenous fluid administration preoperatively (typically 2 liters of resuscitative fluids administered in the preoperative area) is recommended. This is maintained through the postoperative period until euvolemia is achieved. The best measure for end resuscitation is the urine output, but consideration should also be given to the protracted effects on renal function of chronic diuretic or potentially nephrotoxic drug administration. An adequate goal in the postoperative patient should be an average of 30 cc of urine per hour, over a 2 hour period. If the urine output does not improve with initial resuscitation, an oliguria workup should be initi-

ated with measurement of serum electrolytes and a calculated fractional excretion of sodium (or urea). For patients with normal preoperative renal function, acute kidney insufficiency is most likely due to preoperative use of angiotensin-converting enzyme (ACE) inhibitors or nephrotoxic medications, the administration of toradol, or intraoperative hypotension causing acute tubular necrosis. For patients with preexisting kidney disease, simple fluid shifts may cause acute or chronic kidney insufficiency [7]. Improving renal function may require judicious fluid administration, diuresis, or both. Consultation with a nephrologist may be required for persistent oliguria or rising blood urea nitrogen and serum creatinine levels.

RESPIRATORY COMPLICATIONS POST BARIATRIC SURGERY

Because approximately 40% of bariatric surgery patients have obstructive sleep apnea, it is recommended that they are all screened and treated appropriately preoperatively [8,9]. Early recognition and treatment of occult sleep apnea may also dramatically reduce respiratory-related ICU stay, as demonstrated by Hallowell et al., with whom only 1 in 43 patients required such a level of postoperative care [10]. Patients with documented sleep apnea should be treated with continuous positive airway pressure (CPAP) as soon as they are extubated to maximize air exchange. Empirical CPAP may be instituted if patients are unable to complete preoperative testing or are suspected to have sleep apnea.

Prolonged respiratory failure after bariatric surgery is not common. In a series of 1067 gastric bypass patients, there were only 9 (0.6%) with respiratory failure [11]. Poulose et al. reported 7.3 cases of respiratory failure per 1000 bariatric patients, according to the 2002 Health Care Cost and Utilization Project National Inpatient Sample [12]. Patients with prolonged respiratory failure may benefit from early tracheostomy. Longer tracheostomy tubes with sharper angles may be necessary to accommodate for short and wide necks with substantial subcutaneous tissue [13,14]. There remains controversy whether percutaneous tracheostomy should be used in obese patients. Given the anatomy, both open and percutaneous techniques can be challenging. With either technique, it is advisable to have full extension of the neck and adequate lighting for the best exposure to

Table 20.1 Complications of bariatric surgery.

Early	Late
Anastomotic leak	Internal hernia
GI bleeding	Marginal ulcer
Mesenteric bleeding	Anastomotic stricture
Pulmonary embolism	Cholelithiasis
Myocardial infarction	Band slippage/prolapse
Aspiration	Band saline leak
Respiratory failure	Band erosion
Wound infection	Concentric dilatation
Rhabdomyolysis	Malnutrition
Thromboembolism	Contained leak/abscess
Obstruction	Gastric-gastric fistula

the trachea. Table 20.1 presents a list of potential complications post bariatric surgery.

GASTROINTESTINAL COMPLICATIONS POST BARIATRIC SURGERY

Gastrointestinal bleeding

Gastrointestinal (GI) bleeding occurs in approximately 1–2% of patients after Roux-en-Y gastric bypass, and usually occurs from one of the various staple lines [15]. In the early postoperative period (72 hours), significant bleeding is usually due to an intraoperative complication or anastomotic ischemia [16]. Peroral endoscopy should be avoided during this period, with a low threshold for early reoperation with intraoperative or laparoscopy-assisted endoscopy [17]. Transient obstruction from clot at the jejuno-jejunal anastomosis may increase risk of perforation at the gastro-jejunal anastomosis or gastric remnant. From 72 hours to 1 week, erosions and ulcerations occur at band sites or anastomosis (marginal ulcer). Endoscopy, including push enteroscopy to examine the Roux limb, is reasonable at this point, although it may be technically challenging. The gastric pouch and anastomotic staple lines are easily identified with upper endoscopy, and often so is the jejunojejunostomy, although this depends on the length of the Roux-en-Y limb [18]. Most surgeons make the Roux-en-Y limb between 75 and 150 cm. Bleeding can also occur from the gastric remnant staple line, but this is usually not accessible through standard endoscopy. Nonsteroidal antiinflammatory medications should be

avoided after undergoing Roux-en-Y bypass because their administration may result in staple-line bleeding or the formation of ulcers, which may also bleed. The bypassed stomach can be endoscoped with a pediatric colonoscope or some other type of enteroscope of adequate length to traverse the Roux limb [19]. Surgical intervention may be required if the site of bleeding cannot be identified. If this complication occurs remotely from the original operation, it can be managed by angiography. Endoscopy may also be performed through a surgically created gastrostomy into the excluded stomach. Ulcers may also be responsible for GI bleeding and may occur on the gastric or intestinal side of the gastro-jejunostomy. These ulcers are usually thought to be ischemic in nature; however, in most cases, the gastric pouch looks otherwise well perfused. Almost all of these patients will heal with a course of proton pump inhibition. Follow-up endoscopy may be performed to document resolution.

Anastomotic leak after bariatric surgery

Anastomotic leaks are the second most common cause of preventable death following gastric bypass surgery, after PE. The incidence ranges from 0.8 to 7% [20–30], with a mortality ranging from 6 to 17% [21,31]. In a series of 2675 patients, Thodiyil et al. [20] reported a leak rate of 1.7% and no deaths in the first 90 days after surgery. Minimizing mortality from anastomotic leaks is directly related to early recognition and treatment. Older, heavier male patients with multiple comorbidities, and patients undergoing revisional operations, have an increased risk for leaks. Poorly controlled diabetes, chronic steroid use, previous radiation, sepsis, infection, and hemodynamic compromise may also contribute to poor anastomotic healing. Although high ventilatory pressures and CPAP may cause gastric distention, neither has been shown to increase the rate of leaks [11].

Presenting symptoms may include respiratory distress and tachycardia, which can be mistaken for a PE. Failure of timely extubation or rapid respiratory decompensation should raise suspicion of intraabdominal pathology. Concurrent symptoms and findings, such as left shoulder pain, a perception of impending doom, an elevated white count, rising metabolic acidosis, or an isolated left pleural effusion on chest radiograph may help differentiate a leak from a PE. Upper GI contrast studies and computed tomography (CT) scans (Figure 20.1) can be helpful with confirming the

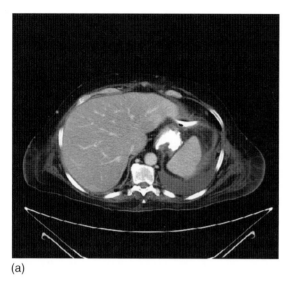 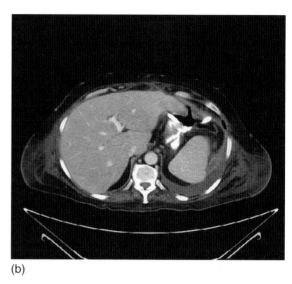

(a)   (b)

Figure 20.1 Computed tomography of the upper abdomen in a patient with an anastomotic leak. (a) Contrast filling of the gastric pouch with minimal extravasation of contrast adjacent to the drain. (b) More extravasation of contrast communicating to a pocket of air where the drain traverses.

diagnosis, but they lack sensitivity in the immediate postoperative period.

Failure to recognize an anastomotic leak, however, can result in rapid deterioration and death, and therefore the attending clinician should exercise a high level of suspicion. When a leak is suspected, it is highly recommended that aggressive and early surgical intervention be considered [13]. Surgical reexploration should not be deferred or postponed. Expedient diagnostic laparoscopy or laparotomy has the highest sensitivity, specificity, and accuracy for the definitive assessment of an anastomotic leak [32]. The majority of leaks after gastric bypass are radiologically contained (meaning they are not flowing freely within the peritoneal cavity), involve the gastroje-junostomy anastomosis or the gastric pouch staple line, and can be safely managed nonoperatively with bowel rest, intravenous fluids, antibiotics, and percutaneous drainage under image guidance [20]. Overall, early recognition and treatment is critical.

Cholelithiasis

The prevalence of gallstones 6 months following obesity surgery has been reported to be as high as 22% [33]. A reduction in the gallbladder emptying rate and a decrease in the gallbladder refilling rate contribute to gallbladder stasis and the formation of gallstones [34].

For these reasons, as well as the morbidity associated with pancreatitis in obese patients, some clinicians advocate performing prophylactic cholecystectomy in all patients at the time of bariatric surgical procedures. Most clinicians, however, resort to removing the gallbladder only in those who have gallstones at the time of surgery [35]. A dose of ursodiol 600 mg daily may provide prophylaxis against gallstone formation, although a strong evidence for this practice has not been validated in randomized trials.

Other complications

Obstruction and perforation of the excluded stomach are potentially fatal complications. If obstructed, the excluded stomach may dilate markedly and a perforation may occur, resulting in free intraperitoneal spillage. Gastro-gastric and gastrocutaneous fistulas may develop rarely, especially in cases with leakage of enteric contents, and usually require surgical repair.

WOUND INFECTION AND DEHISCENCE

Surgical-site infections may occur, usually within the first week. These may take the form of a port-site wound infection or, in an open case, an incisional wound infection.

The majority are treated with antibiotics. Occasionally the wound may need to be opened. The incidence of wound infection varies from 1 to 10%, according to the method: laparoscopic or open surgery, respectively. Fascial dehiscence may occur in up to 1% of trocar sites, and is managed with surgical repair. For large ventral hernias, which can occur in 15–20% of laparotomies, mesh repairs are common, as reapproximation usually fails and may be complicated by abdominal compartment syndrome [36].

THROMBOEMBOLIC DISEASE

Although standard of care dictates that bariatric surgeons use some form of prophylaxis to prevent thromboembolic disease, there is no consensus on any specific regimen for post bariatric surgery. The implementation of multiple-modality prophylaxis protocols that include early ambulation, intermittent pneumatic compression devices, and enoxaparin or heparin has been shown to achieve a low rate of postoperative venous thromboembolism [37]. Emphasis must be placed on proper timing of prophylaxis, with the initial dose of pharmacoprophylaxis given 1 to 2 hours preoperatively [13]. Additionally, early ambulation within 2 hours of surgery and every 2 hours thereafter during waking hours is commonly enforced if the patient is capable. An inferior vena cava filter, preferably of the retrievable type, may be placed prophylactically in patients with a prior history of PE, or those who have sustained venous thromboembolism while on anticoagulants. Signs of deep venous thrombosis (DVT) include asymmetrical swelling or edema, fever, and pain in the involved extremity. A duplex ultrasound of the affected extremity will confirm the diagnosis. A PE should be suspected if the stable and alert patient has dyspnea, chest pain, tachycardia, and fever, and if the ventilated patient has unexplained fever, electrocardiogram (EKG) changes, and poor arterial oxygenation. The gold standard for diagnosis of PE is pulmonary angiography and spiral CT pulmonary angiography. Both DVT and PE are treated with heparin anticoagulation. Massive PEs are treated with heparin anticoagulation, thrombolysis, or surgical embolectomy.

RHABDOMYOLYSIS

Postoperative rhabdomyolysis has been reported among morbidly obese patients following bariatric procedures and, especially, laparoscopic duodenal switch procedures, which have an associated incidence of 1.4% [38]. Affected patients present in the early postoperative period with muscle pain in the buttock, hip, or shoulder regions. Routine measurement of creatine kinase and serum creatinine levels, both prior to and following surgery, can aid detection. Treatment requires aggressive intravenous fluid administration and urine alkalinization.

NUTRITION

The postoperative diet for all types of bariatric operation should be started with water, ice chips, and clear, unsweetened beverages. Very small amounts (1 ounce or less) should be taken at first, but this can be increased, as tolerated by the patient [39]. The clear liquid diet for postoperative bariatric surgery patients varies from the regular clear liquid hospital diet in that carbonated, caffeinated, and sweetened beverages are not allowed.

Patients usually advance to a full liquid diet within 1 to 2 days. The full liquid diet should include liquids that contain protein, such as milk or protein supplements. Diet prescriptions vary among practitioners, and it should be noted that some practitioners prefer not to allow patients to use fruit juices on either the clear or the full liquid diet, due to the natural, or added, sugar concentration. However, milk has about the same amount of natural sugar as fruit juices and is considered an acceptable fluid for postsurgical patients, except for those patients who may develop lactose intolerance.

Puree or soft foods can be introduced around postoperative weeks 2 and 3. Many patients find it helpful to use baby foods at this point, rather than to attempt to puree solid foods with a blender at home. When soft foods are tolerated by the patient, advancement can be made to regular solid foods.

CONCLUSION

Bariatric surgery is increasingly being utilized to accomplish weight loss. Although generally effective and safe, outcomes can be improved and complications can be decreased.

The associated adverse events and true complications often necessitate frequent consultation with other specialties well versed in the care of post-bariatric surgery patients. Successful management of these patients involves communication with the bariatric surgeon, knowledge of postoperative anatomy, an understanding of the potential complications, and implementation of appropriate treatment.

BEST PRACTICE TIPS

1 All bariatric programs should institute a multidisciplinary team to provide optimal care to the obese patient before, during, and after bariatric surgery.

2 Aggressive resuscitation with intravenous fluids during surgery and close monitoring of urine output in the immediate postoperative period may prevent acute renal failure.

3 Patients with sleep apnea must receive CPAP immediately after surgery to prevent pulmonary complications.

4 Skilled endoscopists should be readily available for the diagnosis and treatment of suspected postoperative GI bleeding.

5 Expedient diagnostic laparoscopy or laparotomy has the highest sensitivity, specificity, and accuracy for the definitive assessment of an anastomotic leak. Surgical reexploration should not be deferred or postponed.

REFERENCES

1 The Practical Guide: Identification, Evaluation, and Treatment of Overweight and Obesity in Adults. National Institute of Health. Pub no 00–4084. Oct 2000. p. 39.

2 Balsiger BM, Murr MM, Poggio JL, Sarr MG. Bariatric surgery: surgery for weight control in patients with morbid obesity. Med Clin North Am. 2000;84:477–89.

3 Buchwald H, Estok R, Fahrbach K, Banel D, Sledge I. Trends in mortality in bariatric surgery: a systematic review and meta-analysis. Surgery. 2007 Oct;142(4):621–32, disc. 632–5.

4 Pories WG, Swanson MS, MacDonald KG, et al. Who would have thought it? An operation proves to be the most effective therapy for adult-onset diabetes mellitus. Ann Surg. 1995;222:339–50.

5 Nguyen NT, Goldman C, Rosenquist J, et al. Laparoscopic versus open gastric bypass: randomized study of outcomes, quality of life, and costs. Ann Surg. 2001;234:279–91.

6 Helling TS, Willoughby TL, Maxfield DM, Ryan P. Determinants of the need for intensive care and prolonged mechanical ventilation in patients undergoing bariatric surgery. Obes Surg. 2004 Sep;14(8):1036–41.

7 Thakar CV, Kharat V, Blanck S, Leonard AC. Acute kidney injury after gastric bypass surgery. Clin J Am Soc Nephrol. 2007 May;2(3):426–30. Epub 2007 Mar 14.

8 Byhahn C, Lischke V, Meninger D, et al. Peri-operative complications during percutaneous tracheostomy in obese patients. Anaesthesia. 2005;60:12–15.

9 Frey WC, Pilcher J. Obstructive sleep-related breathing disorders in patients evaluated for bariatric surgery. Obes Surg. 2003;13:676–83.

10 Hallowell PT, Jasper JJ, et al. Eliminating respiratory intensive care unit stay after gastric bypass surgery. Surgery. 2007 Oct;142(4):608–12,e1.

11 Livingston EH, Huerta S, Arthur D, et al. Male gender is a predictor for morbidity and age a predictor of mortality for patients undergoing bypass surgery. Ann Surg. 2002; 236:576–82.

12 Poulose BK, Griffen MR, Zhu Y, et al. National analysis of adverse patient safety events in bariatric surgery. Am Surg. 2005;71:406–13.

13 Pieracci FM, et al. Critical care of the bariatric patient. Crit Care Med. 2006;34(6):1796–804.

14 Davidson JE, Callery C. Care of the obesity surgery patient requiring immediate-level care or intensive care. Obesity Surgery. 2001;11:93–7.

15 Klein S, Wadden T, Sugerman HJ. AGA technical review on obesity. Gastroenterology. 2002;123:882–932.

16 Kaplan LM. Gastrointestinal management of the bariatric surgery patient. Gastroenterol Clin North Am. 2005;34: 105–125.

17 Huang CS, Farraye FA. Endoscopy in the bariatric surgical patient. Gastroenterol Clin North Am. 2005;34:151–66.

18 Huang CS, Forse RA, Jacobson BC, Farraye FA. Endoscopic findings and their clinical correlations in patients with symptoms after gastric bypass surgery. Gastrointest Endosc. 2003;58:859–66.

19 Park HK, Sinar DR, Sloss RR, Whitley TW, Silverman JF. Histologic and endoscopic studies before and after gastric bypass surgery. Arch Pathol Lab Med. 1986;110:1164–7.

20 Thodiyil PA, Mattar SG et al. Selective non-operative management of leaks after gastric bypass. Annals of Surgery Nov 2008;248(5):782–92.

21 Csendes A, Burdiles P, Burgos AM, et al. Conservative management of anastomotic leaks after 557 open gastric bypasses. Obes Surg. 2005;15:1252–6.

22 Fernandez AZ Jr, DeMaria EJ, Tichansky DS, et al. Experience with over 3,000 open and laparoscopic bariatric procedures: multivariate analysis of factors related to leak and resultant mortality. Surg Endosc. 2003;18:193–7.

23 Higa KD, Boone KB, Ho T. Complications of the laparoscopic Rouxen-Y gastric bypass: 1,040 patients – what have we learned? Obes Surg. 2000;10:509–13.

24 Schauer PR, Ikramuddin S, Gourash W, et al. Outcomes after laparoscopic Roux-en-Y gastric bypass for morbid obesity. Ann Surg. 2000;232:515–29.

25 Benotti PN, Wood GC, Rodriguez H, et al. Perioperative outcomes and risk factors in gastric surgery for morbid obesity: a 9-year experience. Surgery. 2006;139:340–6.

26 DeMaria EJ, Sugerman HJ, Kellum JM, et al. Results of 281 consecutive total laparoscopic Roux-en-Y gastric bypasses to treat morbid obesity. Ann Surg. 2002;235:640–5, disc. 645–7.

27 Shikora SA, Kim JJ, Tarnoff ME, et al. Laparoscopic Roux-en-Y gastric bypass: results and learning curve of a high-volume academic program. Arch Surg. 2005;140:362–7.

28 Mason EE, Renquist KE, Jiang D. Perioperative risks and safety of surgery for severe obesity. Am J Clin Nutr. 1992;55(Suppl 2):S573–6.

29 Hamilton EC, Sims TL, Hamilton TT, et al. Clinical predictors of leak after laparoscopic Roux-en-Y gastric bypass for morbid obesity. Surg Endosc. 2003;17:679–84.

30 Fernandez AZ Jr, Demaria EJ, Tichansky DS, et al. Multivariate analysis of risk factors for death following gastric bypass for treatment of morbid obesity. Ann Surg. 2004;239:698–702, disc. 702–3.

31 Carucci LR, Turner MA, Conklin RC, et al. Roux-en-Y gastric bypass surgery for morbid obesity: evaluation of postoperative extraluminal leaks with upper gastrointestinal series. Radiology. 2006;238:119–27.

32 Nguyen H, MD, et al. Bariatric surgery: the needs of the obese patient. Society of Critical Care Medicine August. 2009.

33 Weinsier RL, Wilson LJ, Lee J. Medically safe rate of weight loss for the treatment of obesity: a guideline based on risk of gallstone formation. Am J Med. 1995;98:115–17.

34 Al-Jiffry BO, Shaffer EA, Saccone GT, et al. Changes in gallbladder motility and gallstone formation following laparoscopic gastric banding for morbid obesity. Can J Gastroenterol. 2003;17:169–74.

35 Villegas L, Schneider B, Provost D, et al. Is routine cholecystectomy required during laparoscopic gastric bypass? Obes Surg. 2004;14:60–66.

36 Livingston EH. Complications of bariatric surgery. Surg Clin North Am 2005;85:853–68,vii.

37 Scholton DJ, Hoedema RM, Scholten SE. A comparison of two different prophylactic dose regimens of low molecular weight heparin in bariatric surgery. Obes Surg 2002;12:19–24.

38 Khurana RN, Baudendistel TE, Morgan EF, et al. Postoperative rhabdomyolysis following laparoscopic gastric bypass in the morbidly obese. Arch Surg. 2004;139:73–6.

39 Marcason W. What are the dietary guidelines following bariatric surgery? J Am Diet Assoc. 2004;104:487–8.

21 Nutritional Requirements of the Critically Ill Obese Patient

Bikram S. Bal,[1] Frederick C. Finelli,[2] and Timothy R. Koch[3]

[1]Section of Gastroenterology, [2]Department of Surgery, and [3]Department of Medicine, Washington Hospital Center and Georgetown University School of Medicine, Washington, DC, USA

KEY POINTS

- Optimal nutritional support of the critically ill obese patient is a considerable challenge.
- Critical illness in obese patients incites several paradoxical metabolic responses.
- Hypocaloric, high-protein nutritional support is recommended for critically ill obese patients.

INTRODUCTION

Medically complicated obesity is a rapidly spreading worldwide health problem reaching an epidemic magnitude. Over the past three decades, the prevalence of obesity has doubled in the USA [1]. Presently, about one third of Americans, roughly 100 million, are obese [1,2]. In the UK, the prevalence of obesity has multiplied three times over the past 15 years, and in Eastern Europe it has reached about 20% of the population [3,4]. Due to the briskly growing numbers of patients, physicians from all specialties are frequently encountering the unique challenges presented by these patients.

Obesity definitions in adults are based on body mass index (BMI), a ratio of weight (in kilograms) to height (in meters squared). BMI generally parallels body fat, although there are obvious limitations in using this method with patients at extremes of body composition. Table 21.1 outlines the National Institutes of Health (NIH) classification of obesity.

Obesity is associated with an increased risk for developing a number of chronic medical conditions and therefore obese individuals are at a higher risk for hospitalization and intensive care unit (ICU) admission. Multiple comorbidities also predispose these patients to medical and surgical catastrophes requiring intensive care [5]. Chronic medical conditions associated with obesity [6–10] are summarized in Table 21.2.

Nutritional support is a key component in managing critically ill patients, with early and aggressive feeding interventions shown to improve outcomes favorably. Like other aspects of care, feeding also becomes complicated in the presence of obesity.

Unfortunately, much controversy exists regarding the nutritional support of critically ill obese patients and there is no agreement among the various health care professionals about the best method to provide such support. This chapter will discuss the unique metabolic changes in critically ill obese patients and the challenges in providing them with nutritional support while in the ICU.

MICRONUTRIENT DEFICIENCIES IN THE MORBIDLY OBESE

Preoperative evaluation of patients with medically complicated obesity supports the notion that micronutrient malnutrition is a common finding in the morbidly obese.

A large percentage of patients were demonstrated to have micronutrient deficiencies in an Isreali study of preoperative obese patients [11]. Micronutrient deficiencies commonly reported were those of iron (35%), folic acid (24%), and vitamin B12 (3.6%); 39% of these patients had elevated parathyroid hormone levels, supporting the

Critical Care Management of the Obese Patient, First Edition. Edited by Ali A. El Solh.
© 2012 John Wiley & Sons, Ltd. Published 2012 by John Wiley & Sons, Ltd.

Table 21.1 National Institutes of Health classification of obesity. (Source: http://www.nhlbi.nih.gov/health/public/heart/obesity/lose_wt/bmi_dis.htm. Accessed April 14, 2011.)

Weight	BMI (kg/m²)	Associated health risk
Underweight	< 18.5	Low
Normal weight	18.5–24.9	Low
Overweight	25–29.9	Mild
Class I obesity	30–34.9	Moderate
Class II obesity	35–39.9	Severe
Class III obesity	≥ 40	Very severe

Table 21.2 Chronic medical conditions associated with obesity.

Organ system	Medical disorders
Cardiovascular	Congestive heart failure, hypertension, myocardial infarction, dyslipidemia
Respiratory	Hypoventilation (Pickwickian) syndrome, asthma, obstructive sleep apnea, respiratory failure
Gastrointestinal	Gastroesophageal reflux, nonalcoholic fatty liver disease (NAFLD), gastroparesis, gallstones, biliary tract disease, pancreatitis, hernias
Endocrine	Diabetes mellitus (type II), metabolic syndrome, infertility, polycystic ovarian syndrome, hypothyroidism
Neurological/psychological	Cerebral infarction, depression, disordered eating, idiopathic intracranial hypertension
Hematologic	Deep venous thrombosis (DVT), hypercoagulable state, chronic venous stasis
Musculoskeletal	Degenerative joint disease, chronic back pain
Immune system/infection	Pressure ulcers, skin-fold infections, poor wound healing, proinflammatory state
Increased cancer risk	Kidney, esophagus, pancreas, colon, breast, ovary, endometrial, prostate

presence of secondary hyperparathyroidism induced by vitamin D deficiency. The high percentage of patients with low folic acid and BMI > 50 kg/m² suggests that small-intestinal bacterial overgrowth is uncommon in super-obese patients, since elevated serum folate is an indirect indicator of small-intestinal bacterial overgrowth [12]. Similarly, a preoperative study from Switzerland showed that 57% of morbidly obese individuals had a micronutrient deficiency, most commonly vitamin D deficiency [13]. While subcutaneous and visceral adipose tissue does contain high concentrations of fat-soluble micronutrients [14], higher percentage body fat was associated with greater circulating concentrations of uncarboxylated prothrombin, indicative of lower hepatic utilization of vitamin K in both men and women. A high prevalence of vitamin A deficiency in obese, preoperative patients has also been described by investigators from Rio de Janeiro [15].

Of potential importance to morbidly obese individuals facing treatment in the ICU is the discovery that 15% of preoperative bariatric surgery patients have thiamine deficiency [16]. This has raised concern about precipitating Wernicke's syndrome while receiving parenteral nutrition [17]. A potential origin for development of a micronutrient deficiency is the intake of dietary supplements [18], a common practice among morbidly obese individuals.

METABOLIC RESPONSE TO CRITICAL ILLNESS IN OBESE PATIENTS

Critical illness incites a hypermetabolic inflammatory response directed at promoting acute survival, which affects macronutrient utilization throughout the body [19,20]. Obesity is a proinflammatory state and probably lowers the threshold at which these mechanisms become overwhelmed or exaggerated during a critical illness [21]. Compared with fasting nonobese, nonstressed subjects of normal weight, fasting obese, nonstressed subjects have increased levels of plasma substrates, including carbohydrates, amino acids, free fatty acids (FFAs), and so on. Under physiological stress, these endogenous substrates serve as fuel sources, with the metabolic responses being mediated by hormones including epinephrine, glucagon, cortisol, and growth hormone. The potential effect of physiological stress on this hormonal milieu is unknown in the obese patient [22].

Stress-induced hyperglycemia is a frequent complication of critical illness and obese patients are at a higher risk for this complication due to their high prevalence of diabetes and insulin resistance. Hyperglycemia may also be induced by the abovementioned phenomenon of excess circulating substrates in obese individuals.

Hyperglycemia is associated with a poor outcome and this may explain the reason for obese individuals being at greater risk than lean individuals for postoperative sepsis, bacteremia, and clinical sepsis after acute thermal injury [22,23]. Mortality has also been found to be higher in obese victims with blunt trauma [24]. Therefore, care should be taken to avoid iatrogenic hyperglycemia from overfeeding, as administration of excess glucose (calorie) loads can lead to increased lipogenesis, hepatic steatosis, and CO_2 production, which in turn increases the work of breathing [19,25].

Muscle protein catabolism is a hallmark feature of critical illness, regardless of an individual's BMI, with studies showing losses of up to 20% of skeletal muscle after 1 week in the ICU [26]. Contrary to general belief, acutely injured obese patients have a catabolic response to injury similar to that of normal-weight patients, which puts them at equal or greater risk for nutritional depletion. Obese persons have increased amounts of fat-free mass (FFM) over their height-matched lean counterparts, but are more likely to use this muscle mass as fuel during critical illness when fasted [20]. Despite having a relative abundance of serum FFAs and triglyceride-rich adipose stores, it appears obese individuals are ineffective at mobilizing or using these energy sources during critical illness [20,27]. The ultimate result is increased net protein oxidation and higher daily muscle mass degradation.

Based on their unique metabolism, hypocaloric and high-protein nutrition is a preferable approach in critically ill obese patients. It promotes endogenous fat oxidation and shifts obese patients away from utilization of FFM as the predominant fuel source. It also induces favorable changes in body composition [28,29]. Avoidance of overfeeding is also critical since excess caloric load is associated with increased protein turnover and fat storage [30].

INITIAL EVALUATION OF THE OBESE PATIENT

History

BMI does not correlate with nutritional status and obese patients often have micronutrient malnutrition as described above. History taking should be focused on identifying any preexisting nutritional risk factors. Specifically:
1 Any history of recent weight gain or weight loss should be obtained. Obese individuals in the process of losing weight follow food fads and often neglect essential nutrients.
2 Any risk factors predicting failure of enteral feeding should be investigated, including:
   a Changes in gastrointestinal function.

   b Prior abdominal surgeries with loss of bowel.
   c Prior bariatric or obesity surgery.
   d Mechanical limitations to feeding.

Physical examination

A thorough physical examination can be difficult and often limited in severely obese individuals. Physical examination that is pertinent to an individual's nutritional status and for determining nutritional needs should include:
1 Accurate determination of weight and height to calculate energy requirements.
2 Abdominal examination for previous surgeries and to asses bowel function.
3 Determination of volume status.
4 Identification of muscle wasting, which can suggest chronic protein-calorie malnutrition.
5 Examination of whole-body skin surface including skin folds to determine skin integrity and presence of wounds.
Postoperatively, all incision sites should be examined for healing as malnutrition is associated with poor healing of surgical sites.

DETERMINATION OF MACRONUTRIENT REQUIREMENTS IN THE OBESE PATIENT

Development of a nutrition care plan for critically ill obese patients can be both complex and challenging. The initial nutritional assessment should include evaluation for markers of protein status, such as a serum prealbumin level. However, the inherent variability of such markers' half-lives in relation to the ongoing metabolic stress while in the ICU should be kept in mind.

Determination of resting energy expenditure (REE) is an integral part of the nutrition assessment. This allows the clinician to minimize negative outcomes associated with underfeeding and overfeeding. Unfortunately, there is no consensus as to which prediction equation for REE is most accurate in hospitalized obese patients. Indirect calorimetry remains the "gold standard" method for measuring REE [31,32]. However, its use is limited by cost, availability of proper equipment and trained personnel, patient ventilatory status (an $FiO_2 > 60\%$ is generally excluded), and ability to use a handheld device in nonventilated patients [33].

There are various equations for the estimation of REE. However, most of these have fallen into disfavor and are not used clinically. Some of the equations commonly used today are summarized in Table 21.3: the Harris–Benedict equation (HBE) [34], the Mifflin–St

Table 21.3 Equations for the estimation of resting energy expenditure (REE).

Harris–Benedict equation (HBE)	For men: $kcal/d = 66.47 + 13.75(w) + 5(h) - 6.75(a)$
	For women: $kcal/d = 655.1 + 9.56(w) + 1.85(h) - 4.68(a)$
	Adjusted: $kcal/d = HBE \times (injury\ factor) \times (activity\ factor)$
Mifflin–St Jeor equation (MSJ)	For men: $kcal/d = 10(w) + 6.25(h) - 5(a) + 5$
	For women: $kcal/d = \frac{1}{4}10(w) + 6.25(h) - 5(a) - 161$
Ireton-Jones equation	Ventilator-dependent: $kcal/d = 1784 + 5(w) - 11(a) + 244\ (if\ men) + 239\ (if\ trauma) + 804\ (if\ burn)$
	Spontaneous breathing: $kcal/d = 629 - 11(a) + 25(w) - 609\ (if\ BMI > 27\ kg/m^2)$
Penn State equation	Harris–Benedict: $kcal/d = 0.85(HBE) + 175(T_{max}) + 33(Ve) - 6344$
	Mifflin: $kcal/d = 0.96(MSJ) + 167(T_{max}) + 31(Ve) - 6212$

a, age; h, height (in cm); T_{max}, maximum temperature (in centigrade) in a 24-hour period; Ve, minute ventilation; w, actual weight (in kg).

Jeor (MSJ) equation [35], the Ireton-Jones equation [36], and the Penn State equation [37].

While using predictive equations, determining how to use an obese patient's weight to avoid introducing bias into calculations is problematic and is a matter of much debate [38]. Using actual body weight (ABW) will likely overestimate caloric needs, because adipose tissue is felt to be less metabolically active than FFM [39,40]. However, using ideal body weight (IBW) will likely underestimate caloric needs because it does not appropriately reflect the increased amount of lean body mass present in the obese patient. This debate has led to the use of an adjusted body weight for determining the REE [41], which is:

adjusted body weight = [(ABW − IBW) − (0.25 to 0.5)] + IBW

However, the strategy of using an adjusted body weight is also thought to be flawed by some experts and hence has not been universally adopted [42].

Several recent studies have examined the usefulness of prediction equations for REE in obese patients. Anderegg et al. [43] compared five different prediction methods (MSJ, HBE, Ireton-Jones, and 21 or 25 kcal/kg/d) with indirect calorimetry measures. The HBE using adjusted body weight (25%) and a stress factor (1.2 for ward patients, 1.5 for ICU patients) most closely predicted REE within 10% of measured value, but only 50% of the time. Frankenfield et al. [45] noted that the Penn State equation (using HBE from adjusted weight) estimated REE with the least amount of bias across all age and BMI subgroups, with accuracy rates of 70 and 59%, respectively, in young (18–59 years) and elderly (> 60 years) obese patients.

Although no available equation reliably estimates REE, the Penn State equation and HBE have the strongest evidence supporting their use in the obese ICU patient population [43–47]. Port et al. [21] at the Boston University Medical Center have recommended using the Penn State method in ventilator-dependent obese patients, or HBE with ABW and a stress factor (of 1.1) if the patient is spontaneously breathing.

MACRONUTRITIONAL REGIMENS

There is debate regarding the appropriate nutritional regimen for the critically ill obese patient. The benefits of enteral versus parenteral nutrition are well established [48] and therefore enteral feeding is the preferred method when possible.

Enteral hypocaloric nutritional support in the critically ill obese patient is fast gaining momentum as the standard of care. The term "hypocaloric feeding" refers specifically to permissive underfeeding of a patient and is derived from the classical protein-sparing modified fast [49]. There is no standard method for hypocaloric feeding, but its use generally involves providing 30–70% of the estimated daily caloric needs in conjunction with a higher proportion of protein calories (intended to minimize glucose loads while sparing lean body mass from catabolism). Calorie-restricted nutrition markedly improves insulin sensitivity and glycemic control, in addition to preventing metabolic consequences of overfeeding such as hypercapnea, fluid retention, and hypertriglyceridemia.

In 1979, Greenberg and Jeejeebhoy [50] first introduced the notion of restricting energy intake during nutritional support in obese patients. During starvation, adaptive changes reduce energy requirements and allow fat stores to be used for energy while sparing muscle protein. Multiple studies since then have demonstrated positive outcomes in the ICU related to reduced caloric intake [28,51,52]. The landmark study in this regard was a well-designed retrospective trial by Dickerson et al. [28], which showed that hypocaloric enteral feeding in obese surgical patients was associated with improved nitrogen balance, shorter length of stay in the ICU, and decreased use of antibiotics.

The 2009 Consensus statement issued jointly by the Society of Critical Care Medicine (SCCM) and the American Society for Parenteral and Enteral Nutrition (ASPEN) endorsed hypocaloric feeding of critically ill obese patients with enteral feeds, with the goal of providing no more than 60–70% of target energy requirements or 11–14 kcal/kg ABW per day [42]. Based on nitrogen balance data from studies on hypocaloric feeding, the ASPEN/SCCM guidelines also recommend administration of protein in the range of at least 2.0 g/kg IBW per day for class I and II obese patients and at least 2.5 g/kg IBW per day for class III obesity.

Possible contraindications to the use of hypocaloric, high-protein, specialized nutritional support may include progressive renal insufficiency without renal replacement therapy and hepatic encephalopathy. Both conditions can be aggravated with higher protein intake as a way to compensate for the lower calories, in an effort to achieve protein anabolism. Other potential contraindications for hypocaloric, high-protein feeding are a history of diabetic ketoacidosis, hypoglycemia, age greater than 60 years, and severe immune system compromise [53].

DETERMINATION OF MICRONUTRIENT REQUIREMENTS IN THE OBESE PATIENT

Many laboratory analyses for micronutrients require hours to days to be completed. For those obese patients admitted to an ICU, consideration of a micronutrient deficiency may require considering a deficiency based on the patient's symptoms. As shown in Table 21.4, micronutrient deficiencies may induce a variety of neurological, cardiovascular, gastrointestinal, and visual symptoms, as well as the finding of anemia [54]. If there is a suspicion of a micronutrient deficiency, repletion therapy should be initiated while blood testing is pending. Since it is difficult to exclude malabsorptive disorders of the small intestine, if a micronutrient deficiency is suspected, parenteral replacement therapy should be started immediately. A typical daily intravenous infusion would include (mixed in 5% dextrose in aqueous solution): a standard injectable multivitamin formulation (several are commercially available) with a mixture of trace elements (such as Multitrace 5 concentrate), and both thiamine hydrochloride (100 mg/day) and folic acid (1 mg/day). Conditions such as acute psychosis and Wernicke's encephalopathy are medical emergencies and require supportive care with a minimum of 250 mg of thiamine hydrochloride given daily either intramuscularly or intra-

Table 21.4 Signs and symptoms suggesting a micronutrient deficiency.

Signs and symptoms	Laboratory blood testing
Tachycardia; respiratory distress; right ventricular dilation	Whole-blood thiamine
Peripheral edema	Selenium; plasma niacin; whole-blood thiamine
Blurred vision; loss of vision	Vitamin A; vitamin E; copper; whole-blood thiamine
Hallucinations; nystagmus; ataxia; aggressive behavior; confusion; ophthalmoplegia	Whole-blood thiamine
Numbness; muscle weakness; neuropathy; extremity pain; convulsions; exaggerated tendon reflexes	Vitamin B12, copper; whole blood thiamine; vitamin E; plasma niacin
Anemia	Ferritin; vitamin B12; folate; vitamin A; vitamin E; zinc; copper
Nausea; vomiting; constipation; abdominal pain; diarrhea	Whole-blood thiamine; plasma niacin
Dermititis-like skin disorder	Vitamin A; zinc; plasma niacin

venously (infused over 3–4 hours to reduce the risk of an anaphylactoid reaction), for at least 3–5 days [55].

NUTRITION AND ACUTE MEDICAL DISORDERS IN THE OBESE PATIENT

Sepsis

Hypocaloric enteral feeding is the preference in obese patients who have septic shock. Permissive underfeeding attenuates apoptosis, oxidant production, and cytokine release, thereby favoring cell survival and enhancing immune defense/repair systems [56]. Enteral feedings also aid in maintenance of the integrity of the gastrointestinal tract and prevention of transluminal bacterial translocation. However, there are no studies that support improved outcomes in septic patients who have received a hypocaloric diet.

Respiratory failure

Patients with chronic lung disease develop malnutrition as an adaptive mechanism to decrease the oxygen consumption and lower the work of breathing [57]. Sustained malnutrition alters host immune responses and contributes to poor outcomes. Studies support the notion that these patients should be fed immune-enhancing diets consisting of omega 3 fatty acid-supplemented formula [58]. Since fluid accumulation and pulmonary edema have been associated with poor outcomes for these patients, fluid-restricted nutrient formula [59] should be used (at 2 kcal/ml).

Diabetic ketoacidosis

Critically ill obese patients with diabetic ketoacidosis should undergo hypocaloric enteral nutrition for obvious reasons, as stated above. Hypocaloric feeding promotes euglycemia and improves outcomes by lowering infection rates [60]. However, the optimal duration of hypocaloric nutrition remains unclear.

Hepatic failure

Hepatic failure is associated with a high prevalence of malnutrition, which in turn is associated with compromised outcomes in this population. Due to the need for fluid restriction, it may be beneficial to choose nutrient-dense formulas (1.5–2.0 kcal/ml).

Despite conventional wisdom calling for protein restriction in hepatic failure, controlled trials have demonstrated that patients with hepatic failure not only require increased protein intake to maintain nitrogen balance, but commonly tolerate normal or increased protein intake without exacerbating encephalopathy [61]. Branched-chain amino acid formulas have been recommended for the prevention of encephalopathy. However, these formulas should be reserved for those patients who appear intolerant of adequate protein intake from standard formulas.

Thermal injury

There are no published studies examining the nutritional support of obese patients with major thermal injury. Major thermal injury is characterized by hypermetabolic responses. High exogenous calorie and nitrogen intake is required for wound healing as well as host resistance to infection in burn patients. Therefore, the maxim of hypocaloric feeding in critically ill obese patients should not be applied to obese patients with major thermal injury. Further studies are required to determine the optimal caloric and protein requirement in obese patients with major burns.

Acute renal failure

Acute renal failure is a catabolic state with increased skeletal muscle breakdown via the ubiquitin–proteasome proteolytic system [62–64]. Hemodialysis results in a loss of 6–12 g of amino acids, 2–3 g of peptides, and negligible amounts of protein per dialysis session [63]. Increasing protein to 2.0–2.5 g protein/kg will result in improved nitrogen balance in hospitalized patients with acute renal failure [65–67]. However, increasing protein intake beyond 1.5–1.6 g/kg may increase the rate of urea nitrogen appearance and increase the need for frequent dialysis. Protein and fluid restriction may be needed in patients who have not been initiated on dialysis. There are no calorie recommendations that are specific to acute renal failure in the critically ill obese patient to date.

CONCLUSION

Nutritional support in critically ill obese patients presents a unique set of challenges. Careful consideration must be given to energy and nutrient requirement calculations in this population, as prediction equations for REE are highly unreliable. Indirect calorimetry should always be the preferred method for measuring REE. When this is unavailable or impractical, the Penn State equation and/or the adjusted HBE have the strongest evidence to support their use. Adjusted body weight should be used in energy-expenditure calculations. Hypocaloric feedings with at least 2 g/kg IBW per day protein are probably the best approach to nutritional support in these patients, and are recommended by various major societies. Hypocaloric feedings promote protein anabolism and prevent complications of overfeeding such as hyperglycemia and fluid retention while promoting steady weight loss.

BEST PRACTICE TIPS

1 Nutritional support of critically ill obese patients should be rigorously evaluated.
2 BMI and nutritional status have no correlation and obese patients are often malnourished.
3 History and physical exam should be focused on determining preexisting nutritional risk factors, risk factors for failure of enteral feeding, and current nutritional status.
4 In the absence of indirect calorimetry, the Penn State equation and HBE should be used to calculate REE.
5 Consensus guidelines recommend enteral feeds with 11–14 kcal/kg ABW per day and protein intake of 2–2.5 g/kg IBW per day.

REFERENCES

1 Ogden CL, Carroll MD, Curtin LR, et al. Prevalence of over-weight and obesity in the United States, 1999–2004. JAMA. 2006;295:1549–1555.

2 United States Census Bureau. US and world population clocks: updated in real time.http://www.census.gov [Accessed 3 September 3, 2009].

3 Kopelman PG. Obesity as a medical problem. Nature. 2000;404:635–43.

4 Basdevant A. Obesity: epidemiology and public health. Ann Endocrinol (Paris). 2000;61:6–11.

5 Bercault N, Boulain T, Kuteifan K, et al. Obesity-related excess mortality in an adult intensive care unit: a risk adjusted matched cohort study. Crit Care Med. 2004;32:998–1003.

6 Must A, Spadano J, Coakley EH, et al. The disease burden associated with overweight and obesity. JAMA. 1999;282:1523–9.

7 Calle EE, Rodriguez C, Walker-Thurmond K, Thun MJ. Overweight, obesity, and mortality from cancer in a prospectively studied cohort of US adults. N Engl J Med. 2003;348:1625–38.

8 Friedenberg FK, Xanthopoulos M, Foster GD, et al. The association between gastroesophageal reflux disease and obesity. Am J Gastroenterol. 2008;103:2111.

9 Field AE, Coakley EH, Must A, et al. Impact of overweight on the risk of developing common chronic diseases during a 10-year period. Arch Intern Med. 2001;161:1581–6.

10 Fogarty AW, Glancy C, Jones S, et al. A prospective study of weight change and systemic inflammation over 9 y. Am J Clin Nutr. 2008;87:30–5.

11 Schweiger C, Weiss R, Berry E, et al. Nutritional deficiencies in bariatric surgery candidates. Obes Surg. 2010;20(2):193–7.

12 Camilo E, Zimmerman J, Mason JB, Golner B, Russell R, Selhub J, Rosenberg IH. Folate synthesized by bacteria in the human upper small intestine is assimilated by the host. Gastroenterology. 1996;110(4):991–8.

13 Gehrer S, Kern B, Peters T, et al. Fewer nutrient deficiencies after laparoscopic sleeve gastrectomy (LSG) than after laparoscopic Roux-Y-gastric bypass (LTYGB): a prospective study. Obes Surg. 2010;20(4):447–53.

14 Shea MK, Booth SL, Gundberg CM, et al. Adulthood obesity is positively associated with adipose tissue concentrations of vitamin K and inversely associated with circulating indicators of vitamin K status in men and women. J Nutr. 2010;140(5):1029–34.

15 Pereira S, Saboya C, Chaves G, et al. Class III obesity and its relationship with the nutritional status of vitamin A in pre- and postoperative gastric bypass. Obes Surg. 2009;19(6):738–44.

16 Carrodeguas L, Kaidar-Person O, Szomstein S, Antozzi P, Rosenthal R. Preoperative thiamine deficiency in obese populations undergoing laparoscopic bariatric surgery. Surg Obes Relat Dis. 2005;1(6):517–22.

17 Francini-Pesenti F, Brocadello F, et al. Wernicke's syndrome during parenteral feeding: not an unusual complication. Nutrition. 2009;25(2):142–6.

18 Sechi GP. Dietary supplements and the risk of Wernicke's encephalopathy. Clin Pharmacol Ther. 2010;88:164.

19 Mizock BA. Alterations in fuel metabolism in critical illness: hyperglycaemia. Best Pract Res Clin Endocrinol Metab. 2001;15:533–51.

20 Jeevanandam M, Young DH, Schiller WR. Obesity and the metabolic response to severe multiple trauma in man. J Clin Invest. 1991;87:262–9.

21 Port AM,"Apovian C. Metabolic support of the obese intensive care unit patient: a current prespective. Curr Opin Crit Care. 11:300–3.

22 Gottschlich MM, Mayes T, Khoury JC, et al. Significance of obesity on nutritional immunologic, hormonal, and clinical outcome parameters in burns. J Am Diet Assoc. 1993;93:1261–8.

23 Chandra RK. Nutrition and the immune system. Proc Nutr Soc. 1993;52:77–84.

24 Choban PS, Weireter LJ, Maynes C. Obesity and increased mortality in blunt trauma. J Trauma. 1991;31:1253–7.

25 Honiden S, McArdle JR. Obesity in the intensive care unit. Clin Chest Med. 2009;30:581–99.

26 Reid CL, Campbell IT, Little RA. Muscle wasting and energy balance in critical illness. Clin Nutr. 2004;23:273–80.

27 Schiffelers SL, Saris WH, van Baak MA. The effect of an increased free fatty acid concentration on thermogenesis and substrate oxidation in obese and lean men. Int J Obes Relat Metab Disord. 2001;25:33–8.

28 Dickerson RN, Boschert KJ, Kudsk KA. Hypocaloric enteral tube feeding in critically ill obese patients. Nutrition. 2002;18:241–6.

29 Dickerson RN. Hypocaloric feeding of obese patients in the intensive care unit. Curr Opin Nutr Metab Care. 2005;8:189–96.

30 Biolo G, Agostini F, Simunic B, et al. Positive energy balance is associated with accelerated muscle atrophy and increased erythrocyte glutathione turnover during 5 wk of bed rest. Am J Clin Nutr. 2008;88:950–8.

31 Makita K, Nunn JF, Royston B. Evaluation of metabolic measuring instruments for use in critically ill patients. Crit Care Med. 1990;18:638–44.

32 Epstein CD, Peerless JR, Martin JE, Malangoni MA. Comparison of methods of measurements of oxygen consumption in mechanically ventilated patients with multiple trauma: the Fick method versus indirect calorimetry. Crit Care Med. 2000;28:1363–9.

33 Wells JC, Fuller NJ. Precision and accuracy in a metabolic monitor for indirect calorimetry. Eur J Clin Nutr. 1998;52:536–40.

34 Harris JA, Benedict FG. A biometric study of basal metabolism in man. Publication 279. Washington, DC, Carnegie Institute of Washington. 1919.

35 Mifflin MD, St Jeor ST, Hill LA, et al. A new predictive equation for resting energy expenditure in healthy individuals. Am J Clin Nutr. 1990;51:241–7.

36 Ireton-Jones C, Jones JD. Improved equations for predicting energy expenditure in patients: the Ireton-Jones equations. Nutr Clin Pract. 2002;17:29–31.

37 Frankenfield DC, Coleman A, Alam S, Cooney RN. Analysis of estimation methods for resting metabolic rate in critically ill adults. JPEN. 2009;33:27–36.

38 Ireton-Jones C, Turner WW. Actual or ideal body weight: which should be used to predict energy expenditure? J Am Diet Assoc. 1991;91:193–5.

39 Ravussin E, Burnand B, Schutz Y, Jequier E. Twenty-four hour energy expenditure and resting metabolic rate in obese, moderately obese and control subjects. Am J Clin Nutr. 1982;35:566–73.

40 Zauner A, Schneeweiss B, Kneidinger N, et al. Weight adjusted resting energy is not constant in critically ill patients. Int Care Med. 2006;32:428–34.

41 Krenitsky J. Adjusted body weight, pro: evidence to support the use of adjusted body weight in calculating calorie requirements. Nutr Clin Pract. 2005;20:468–73.

42 McClave SA, Martindale RG, Vanek VW, et al. Guidelines for the provision and assessment of nutrition support therapy in the adult critically ill patient: Society of Critical Care Medicine (SCCM) and American Society for Parenteral and Enteral Nutrition (A.S.P.E.N.). JPEN. 2009:33(3)277–316.

43 Anderegg BA, Worrall C, Barbour E, et al. Comparison of resting energy expenditure prediction methods with measured resting energy expenditure in obese, hospitalized adults. JPEN. 2009;33:168–75.

44 Frankenfield DC, Rowe WA, Smith JS, et al. Validation of several established equations for resting metabolic rate in obese and nonobese people. J Am Diet Assoc. 2003;103:1152–9.

45 Alves V, da Rocha EE, Gonzalez MC, et al. Assessment of resting energy expenditure of obese patients: comparison of indirect calorimetry with formulae. Clin Nutr. 2009; 28:299–304.

46 Boullata J, Williams J, Cottrell F, et al. Accurate determination of energy needs in hospitalized patients. J Am Diet Assoc. 2007;107:393–401.

47 Hoher JA, Teixeira PJ, Hertx F, Moreira JS. A comparison between ventilation modes: how does activity level affect energy expenditure estimates? JPEN. 2008;32:176–83.

48 Kudsk KA, Croce MA, Fabian TC, et al. Enteral versus parenteral feeding: effects on septic morbidity after blunt and penetrating abdominal trauma. Ann Surg. 1992;215:503–11.

49 Palghi A, Reed JL, Greenburg I, et al. Multidisciplinary treatment of obesity with a protein-sparing modified fast: results in 668 outpatients. Am J Public Health. 1985;75:1190–4.

50 Greenberg GR, Jeejeebhoy KN. Intravenous protein-sparing therapy in patients with gastrointestinal disease. JPEN J Parenter Enter Nutr. 1979;3:427–32.

51 Krishnan JA, Parce PB, Martinez A. Caloric intake in medical ICU patients: consistency of care with guidelines and relationship to clinical outcomes. Nutr Clin Pract. 2004;19:645–6.

52 Choban PS, Burge JC, Scales D, Flancbaum L. Hypoenergetic nutrition support in hospitalized obese patients: a simplified method for clinical application. Am J Clin Nutr. 1997;66:546–50.

53 Liu KJ, Cho MJ, Atten MJ, et al. Hypocaloric parenteral nutrition support in elderly obese patients. Am Surg. 2000;66:394–99.

54 Koch TR, Finelli FC. Postoperative metabolic and nutritional complications of bariatric surgery. Gastroenterological Issues in the Obese Patient. Gastroenterol Clin North Am. 2010;39(1):109–24.

55 Thomson AD, Marshall EJ. The treatment of patients at risk of developing Wernicke's encephalopathy in the community. Alcohol Alcohol. 2006;41:159–67.

56 Heyland DK, Lukan JK, McClave SA. The role of nutritional support in sepsis. In Vincent JL, Carlet J, Opal S, editors. The Sepsis Text. Nowell, MA, Klumer Academic Publishers. 2002. pp. 479–90.

57 Henessey KA, Orr ME. Nutrition Support Nursing Core Curriculum in Respiratory Failure. 3 edn. Silver Spring, MD, ASPEN. 1996. p. 4.

58 Gadek J, DeMichele S, Karlstad M, et al. Effect of enteral feeding with eicosapentaenoic acid, gamma-linolenic acid, and antioxidants in patients with acute respiratory distress syndrome. Enteral Nutrition in ARDS Study Group. Crit Care Med. 1999;27:1409–20.

59 ASPEN Board of Directors and the Clinical Guidelines Task Force. Guidelines for the use of parenteral and enteral nutrition in adult and pediatric patients. JPEN. 2002 Jan–Feb;26(Suppl 1):1SA–138SA.

60 Pomposelli JJ, Baxter JK 3rd, Babineau TJ, et al. Early postoperative glucose control predicts nosocomial infection rate in diabetic patients. JPEN. 1998;22:77–81.

61 Kearns PJ, Young H, Garcia G, Blaschke T, O'Hanlon G, et al. Accelerated improvement of alcoholic liver disease with enteral nutrition. Gastroenterology. 1992;102:200–5.

62 Kinney JM. Calories: nitrogen: disease and injury relationships. In White PL, Nagy ME, editors. Total Parenteral Nutrition. Acton, MA, Publishing Sciences Group. 1974 pp. 81–91.

63 Kopple JD. Pathophysiology of protein-energy wasting in chronic renal failure. J Nutr. 1999;129(Suppl 1):247S–251S.

64 Mehrotra R, Kopple JD, Wolfson M. Metabolic acidosis in maintenance dialysis patients: clinical considerations. Kidney Int Supp. 2003 Dec;(88):S13–S25.

65 Scheinkestel CD, Kar L, Marshall K, Bailey M, Davies A, Nyulasi I, Tuxen DV. Prospective randomized trial to assess

caloric and protein needs of critically ill, anuric, ventilated patients requiring continuous renal replacement therapy. Nutrition. 2003;19(11–12):909–16.

66 Scheinkestel CD, Adams F, Mahony L, Bailey M, Davies AR, NyulasiI, Tuxen DV. Impact of increasing parenteral protein loads on amino acid levels and balance in critically ill anuric patients on continuous renal replacement therapy. Nutrition. 2003;19(9):733–40.

67 Bellomo R, Seacombe J, Daskalakis M, et al. A prospective comparative study of moderate versus high protein intake for critically ill patients with acute renal failure. Renal Failure. 1997;19:111–20.

Part VI Pharmacology

22 Drug Dosing in the Critically Ill Obese Patient

Brian L. Erstad

University of Arizona College of Pharmacy, Department of Pharmacy Practice & Science, Tucson, AZ, USA

KEY POINTS
- There is a paucity of information related to drug dosing in obesity, particularly in patients with more extreme forms of obesity.
- For weight-based dosing of drugs the ideal size descriptor would take into account height and body composition.
- The concept of dose proportionality is necessary to understand what size descriptor should be used for the weight-based dosing of drugs.

INTRODUCTION

Unfortunately, research related to drug dosing in overweight and obese patients has not kept pace with studies concerning the epidemiology and complications of obesity. This is particularly true for patients with severe or morbid obesity, which for the purposes of this chapter will be defined as an ideal body weight (IBW) at least twice the estimated normal value or a body mass index (BMI) of at least $40 \, \text{kg/m}^2$ [1]. The pivotal trials leading to drug approval typically include relatively few patients with extremes of weight relative to height. They usually focus on patients in non-intensive care unit (ICU) settings, and in some cases specifically exclude patients beyond a predefined weight. Furthermore, when the results of clinical trials are reported, patient weights are usually expressed in terms of summary statistics such as weight ± standard deviation (SD), rather than a more detailed breakdown of size descriptor information or body composition. This paucity of information extends to the official product information, where the term "weight" is often used without making clear whether it refers to actual body weight (ABW), which is usually the case, or some form of adjusted body weight (ABWadj).

Therefore, the clinician frequently must make dosing decisions with limited or no information on the clinical efficacy or toxicity, or the pharmacokinetics (how the body handles medications from absorption and distribution to elimination) or pharmacodynamics (the effects of the drug on the body), of medications in obese patients. The problem is compounded when using weight-based drug dosing in critically ill patients with rapidly fluctuating clinical conditions and organ dysfunction, which can alter drug disposition and effect.

ADVERSE DRUG EVENTS RELATED TO OBESITY

Lists of complications of obesity should include adverse drug events (ADEs) related to dosing. Whether a weight-based dosing ADE is preventable or nonpreventable depends on the specific situation and any change in classification that occurs over time as new knowledge is accrued. For example, in a life-threatening situation the clinician may not have access to a measured weight for weight-based dosing of a drug given intravenously (IV) by an infusion pump. If the weight estimate used by the clinician turned out to be wrong and the patient received an excessive dose of a medication, this should still be considered a nonpreventable ADE given the urgent nature of the situation and the clinician's best guess of the patient's weight. On the other hand, if a patient's weight was measured or recorded inaccurately and the clinician ignored warnings on the pump about the dose exceeding preprogrammed limits, a subsequent ADE due to an overdose should be considered a preventable ADE.

New technologies such as automated infusion devices (or smart pumps) and automated weight-based dosing

---

Critical Care Management of the Obese Patient, First Edition. Edited by Ali A. El Solh.

calculators have been shown to reduce the incidence of under- and overdosing of drugs and resultant medication errors when programmed and used appropriately [2,3]. However, for drugs administered by such devices using weight-based dosing regimens, the clinician is still faced with the difficult decision as to which weight to enter into the machine's software program when designing a dosing regimen for an obese patient.

SIZE DESCRIPTORS FOR DRUG DOSING

Weight-based dosing regimens are based on an assumed or proven relationship between patient weight and medication disposition such as clearance. Although patient weight is often the focus of discussions of drugs administered using weight-based dosing regimens, other factors such as height and body composition must be taken into account (Table 22.1). This point is readily illustrated using an example of three patients with the same disease state and all with an ABW of 80 kg and a height of 72 inches. Assume one patient has an ABW prior to admission of 65 kg and that the other 15 kg is related to fluid retention. Assume a second patient has an IBW of 70 kg and the other 10 kg is fat weight. Assume the third patient has relatively normal body composition with no excess fluid retention. All three patients have the same weight and height, but could have markedly different responses to weight-based drug dosing based on varying pharmacokinetic parameters such as volume of distribution (Vd) and clearance. At a minimum, a size descriptor should take into account age, gender, and height in addition to weight; depending on the medication, other factors such as race might need to be considered [4]. The ideal size descriptor would take into account these factors as well as body composition changes related to obesity. Furthermore, the descriptor would be robust for research purposes, yet practical for

Table 22.1 Changes in body composition during ICU stay that may affect drug disposition.

Lean vs Adipose Tissue Changes during More Prolonged Stays
  Loss of lean tissue
  Gain of adipose tissue
  Distribution of adipose tissue (e.g. subcutaneous vs visceral)

Gains or Losses of Total Body Water throughout Stay
  Distribution of retained fluid (e.g. intracellular vs extracellular, interstitial vs intravascular)

---

use in the clinical setting. While such a validated size descriptor currently does not exist (see Table 22.2) and may vary depending of the physicochemical characteristics of the medication, some interesting research is being performed on this subject.

Much current research is focused on the best size descriptor to use for renally cleared medications. In particular, it has been argued that lean body weight (LBW) is a better predictor of creatinine clearance than ABW [5] (Table 22.2). This is based on research of fat-free mass (FFM) measured by bioelectrical impedance and dual-energy X-ray absorptiometry. The resulting equations for males and females that take into account height and weight are based on FFM, but are assumed to apply to LBW, since LBW contains a relatively small amount of fat relative to total body weight [6]. Retrospective analyses have demonstrated that drug clearance is similar for subjects with similar and stable renal function regardless of height and weight when differences in body composition are adjusted by one LBW equation for males and another for females [7]. Further confirmation of this LBW correction factor was demonstrated in one of the uncommon studies that restricted enrollment to morbidly obese patients [8]. In this study, a variety of size descriptor equations were compared to creatinine clearance values measured by 24-hour urine collections. The Cockcroft–Gault equation adjusted for LBW was found to be the

Table 22.2 Weight descriptors commonly used in adult patients in the clinical setting.

Ideal body weight (IBW)
  IBW in kg for men = 50 kg + 2.3 kg for each inch in height over 60 inches
  IBW in kg for women = 45.5 kg + 2.3 kg for each inch in height over 60 inches

Adjusted body weight (ABWadj)
  ABWadj in kg = IBW + 0.4 (actual weight − IBW)

Lean body weight (LBW)
  LBW (men) = $(1.10 \times \text{weight in kg}) - 120 \times (\text{weight}^2 / (100 \times \text{height in m})^2)$
  LBW (women) = $(1.07 \times \text{weight in kg}) - 148 \times (\text{weight}^2 / (100 \times \text{height in m})^2)$

Body mass index (BMI)
  BMI = actual body weight (ABW) in kg divided by $(\text{height in m})^2$

Body surface area (BSA) in m²
  BSA = square root $((\text{height in cm} \times \text{ABW in kg}) / 3600)$

Various methods have been used for estimation – inclusion in this table should not be interpreted as support for a particular method.

best in terms of bias, accuracy, and clinical usefulness. The basic Cockcroft–Gault equation has the additional advantages that it is the most common equation used by investigators in preapproval drug studies and by clinicians to adjust drug doses for renal dysfunction. The positive results of these studies should be interpreted with a few caveats. First, the LBW estimates for males and females are based on specific equations and may not apply to estimates based on other equations. Second, IBW and LBW estimates are derived with different equations and should not be considered interchangeable. Finally, the research was restricted to adult patients. Other approaches have been used for children, since dosing predictions must take into account maturation as well as clearance [9].

ESTIMATES AND MEASUREMENT OF WEIGHT

A major source of drug-dosing variation and possibly medication errors is the initial determination of weight. Studies have shown substantial errors in weight estimations and measurements. In one study involving a medical/surgical ICU, 47% of weight estimates by medical and nursing staff were at least 10% different from measured values and 19% were at least 20% different [10]. Interestingly, height estimates were more accurate and were within 10% of measured values. In general, adult patients appear to be better at estimating their own weight compared to health care providers, although in one study 22% of patients did not estimate their own weight to within 5 kg [11]. The latter study was performed in an emergency department and presumes patients are able to communicate their weight, which is often not possible in the ICU setting. Similar to weight estimates, there are problems with weight measurements. In one study involving three tertiary care teaching hospitals only 65.7% of patients were weighed according to patient reports [12]. Of the weights in nursing records, 25.9% differed by at least 2.27 kg from values measured by research nurses. In addition to measurement errors, there is often intra- and inter-health professional inconsistency in the choice of weight being used for any given patient. Often estimates of weight are utilized, such as dry weight, which have no relationship to measured weight or weight estimated from other size descriptors such as height. The situation becomes more complicated with weight fluctuations during hospital stay due to fluid gains or losses, or alterations in lean-to-fat mass associated with prolonged immobilization. As much as possible and practical, the

Table 22.3 Estimates and measurements of size descriptors such as height and weight.

Strive for consistency and standardization within and between all health care professionals and staff involved in size-descriptor estimates and measurements. Examples include:
  Method of estimates including formulas and equations used for calculations.
  Instruments used for measurement and how utilized (e.g. clothes off or on for weight recordings).
  Recording and use of units of estimates and measurements (e.g. centimeters vs inches, pounds vs kilograms).
  Terminology related to size descriptors (e.g. ideal weight, adjusted weight).

Ensure proper communication and documentation of method (e.g. patient vs provider, estimate vs measurement) used to obtain estimates and measurements of size descriptors.

Have ongoing education with evaluation of all personnel involved in the determination and documentation of estimates and measurements.

Have periodic evaluation of compliance by area (e.g. ICU vs emergency department).

Ensure that age-appropriate instruments are available and have regularly scheduled calibration.

Use technology (e.g. automated infusion devices, dosing calculators) when available to reduce chance of medication errors.

---

way in which weight is estimated, measured, recorded, and utilized for drug dosing should be standardized to reduce variability that might lead to dosing errors. Some interesting research is being performed in the area of weight estimation, as exemplified by studies that demonstrate improvements in estimates with anthropometric measurements in adults and body-shape icons in children [13,14]. Consistency should be the theme, given the relative absence of evidence supporting any particular approach to dosing when weight changes over time (Table 22.3).

DRUG DISPOSITION IN OBESITY

Obesity may affect pharmacokinetics of medications, but these changes are difficult to elucidate in critically ill patients, who typically have substantial variability in parameters such as Vd and clearance. Therefore, information is often extrapolated from pharmacokinetic studies performed in non-ICU settings, but such extrapolation must be done with caution. For example, a critically ill patient may have gastrointestinal dysfunction that precludes adequate absorption despite high bioavailability of a drug in normal subjects. In general, the absorption of oral medications is not substantially diminished with increased body weight when due to adipose tissue. There are data to suggest that absorption of selected medications may be altered after bariatric surgery. In a systematic review of the literature, drug absorption of different medications was evaluated in patients who had undergone gastric or jejunoileal bypass, gastroplasty, or biliopancreatic diversion procedures [15]. Medications most likely to be affected were those that had bioavailability concerns such as poor absorption or enterohepatic recirculation even in normal-weight subjects. Examples of such medications were cyclosporine, phenytoin, rifampin, tacrolimus, and thyroxine.

There exists the potential for malabsorption of medications from parenteral (non-IV) routes of administration in obese patients. Unfortunately, there is a dearth of data concerning the absorption of drugs into the systemic circulation when given by subcutaneous (SC) or intramuscular (IM) routes in critically ill obese patients. This is not only true for newer drugs but also for drugs such as insulin where increased amounts of SC fat could delay absorption or result in variability in absorption between sites, depending on the distribution of the excess adipose tissue. Surprisingly few studies have been performed in obese patients with respect to SC absorption of drugs such as the rapid-acting insulin [16]. This is partially a function of the difficulties in conducting bioavailability studies in drugs with nonrenal routes of elimination, but is aggravated by the challenges of conducting studies in critically ill patients with factors to consider beyond weight. This is illustrated by the low-molecular-weight heparins (LMWHs) that are frequently administered by the SC route in critically ill patients. Studies with standard doses of this class of drug have demonstrated markedly reduced bioavailability as determined by factor Xa activity in patients with edema or in those receiving concomitant vasopressors [17,18]. Therefore, investigations into the independent effect of increasing body weight on bioavailability would need to control for these potential confounders.

The Vd is a constant that quantifies the volume in which the medication would be contained if the concentration throughout the body were the same as that in the measured fluid, which is usually plasma or serum. There are various forms of Vd depending on the time at which it is measured after administration of a medication. For example, the Vd of the central compartment is the volume of a theoretical compartment that reflects the initial rapid distribution of a drug when given by IV

bolus or rapid infusion. Other terms, such as Vd at steady state, are used to describe Vd after more time has elapsed with continued administration. The Vd of some drugs may be different in obese compared to normal-weight patients of the same height, age, and gender depending on the physicochemical properties of the drug such as degree of ionization and lipophilicity. For drugs that have a change in Vd associated with obesity, there are important implications for drug dosing. This is particularly the case for one-time IV bolus administration or infrequent, intermittent IV bolus administration, since the termination of drug effect in these cases is more likely to be the result of redistribution within the body and not clearance or actual elimination from the body.

In contrast to loading doses, which tend to be a function of Vd, maintenance doses are more a function of drug clearance. Although most medications are eliminated by the kidneys, some are eliminated by the liver and others through more unique pathways such as plasma esterases. As mentioned earlier, there is evidence to suggest that the clearance of drugs is similar in obese and normal-weight patients when adjusted by LBW and assuming other factors such as age, gender, and height are similar. This has mostly been supported by studies involving drugs that are eliminated by the kidneys. Since lean tissue accounts for the majority of metabolic processes in the body, it is expected that LBW would also normalize clearance of drugs by the liver, again assuming other factors are similar; however, the issue is complicated by the adverse effects of long-term obesity on liver function [19]. Similarly, although liver dysfunction may decrease albumin synthesis, there is no evidence to suggest clinically important alterations in the concentration of albumin or the binding properties of albumin due to obesity in the absence of comorbidities.

Most of the above information on Vd and clearance reflects drug administration by the IV route. There is less information on the disposition of drugs administered by other, less common routes (e.g. intrapleural, intraventricular) in patients with obesity. There has been some interesting data on epidural fat and drug disposition. Studies have demonstrated that the amount of epidural fat is not influenced by BMI or waist circumference [20,21]. These results seem to be supported by studies of local anesthetic dose requirements of women in labor. In one study, bupivacaine requirements in obese women were significantly reduced (p < 0.001), and they had a significantly higher level of block (p < 0.001) compared to nonobese women of similar height and age with similar pain scores [22]. Another study of intrathecal bupivacaine for cesarean delivery found that similar doses were needed in obese and nonobese women [23]. As a group, these studies demonstrate that the dose of drugs for regional anesthesia in obese patients should not be increased solely due to obesity and may need to be decreased to achieve similar effects to those noted in non-obese patients.

DRUG DOSING

Dose proportionality

Perhaps the single most important concept to appreciate when considering possible dose adjustments of drugs in obese patients is dose proportionality. This is most easy to appreciate when applied to drugs that have weight-based dosing recommendations (e.g. mg/kg). In order to justify the use of ABW for weight-based dosing in obese patients, the clinician must know that the pharmacokinetics and pharmacodynamics of a drug increase proportionally to weight (Table 22.4). For example, assume that a drug has a Vd of 5 l/kg and a clearance of 1 ml/kg/minute in

Table 22.4 Assessment of possible dose proportionality in studies with obese subjects.

Did the study involve a comparator group of normal-weight subjects with similar demographics (e.g. age, height, gender) and comorbidities to the obese subjects?

Did the values of pharmacokinetic parameters unadjusted for body weight (e.g. volume of distribution in ml and clearance in ml/minute) increase proportionally to weight in the obese versus the normal-weight subjects?

Were the values of pharmacokinetic parameters adjusted for ABW (e.g. volume of distribution in ml/kg and clearance in ml/minute/kg) similar in the obese and normal-weight subjects?

Did the values of pharmacokinetic parameters adjusted for IBW (e.g. volume of distribution in ml/kg and clearance in ml/minute/kg) increase proportionally to weight in the obese versus the normal-weight subjects?

Was the calculated half-life based on the pharmacokinetic parameters similar in the obese and normal-weight subjects?

When ABW was used in weight-based dosing protocols, were the therapeutic effects and dose-related adverse drug events similar in the obese and normal-weight subjects?

If the answer to all of these questions is yes, the data suggest that dose proportionality is present, although this does not necessarily mean that ABW should be used in weight-based dosing protocols.

relatively normal-weight patients. This would equate to a Vd of 400 l and a clearance of 80 ml/minute in an 80 kg patient. If these pharmacokinetic parameters increase proportionally to weight, a 160 kg obese patient with the same age, height, sex, and comorbidities as the 80 kg patient should have a Vd of 800 l and a clearance of 160 ml/minute. In this theoretical example, dose proportionality appears to be present with this drug, so ABW could be utilized when calculating mg/kg doses. This assumes no change in the pharmacodynamics of the drug in obesity with regards to either efficacy or adverse effects such as rate-related infusion reactions. Additionally, since Vd and clearance are independent parameters that may be affected in different ways by obesity, there is no reason to expect that because one of these parameters changes with increasing body weight, the other parameter will necessarily change in the same direction or to the same extent. These issues are compounded by the fact that for the majority of drugs used in the critical care setting there is inadequate research in obese and nonobese patients to assess for possible dose proportionality. Most of the pharmacokinetic studies that have investigated the issue of dose proportionality were conducted in non-critically ill patients, so the results must be extrapolated to the patient in the ICU.

Administration of boluses or single doses of drugs

One-time doses of drugs in the institutional setting are usually administered when a rapid effect is needed (e.g. acute pain, antimicrobials for sepsis), in which case the IV route is preferred. This would include loading doses of drugs that are given for rapid attainment of therapeutic concentrations. For a drug given as a bolus IV dose, the concentration immediately following injection is a function of the drug's Vd, not clearance. Depending on the physicochemical characteristics of a drug, the Vd may or may not change with increasing body weight. For many of the hydrophilic medications used in the ICU with an intermediate Vd, such as β-lactam antimicrobials, Vd increases with increasing obesity but the increase is not proportional to the increase in weight [24]. So, when loading doses of hydrophilic drugs are given, the dosing weight should be increased to account for distribution in the excess body weight. This correction factor is usually somewhere between 20 and 60% of the excess weight. Using a 40% correction factor, the adjusted weight in kg used for weight-based dosing would be equal to IBW + 0.4(ABW − IBW).

For a drug with small Vd, such as a drug with distribution limited to plasma volume, it is unlikely that its Vd would increase proportionally to the increase in excess weight, since plasma volume does not increase proportionally to excess weight [25]. For such a drug, the use of IBW or LBW (or at most ABWadj) would usually be safer when giving an obese patient a loading dose, although the decision must always be made with a risk/benefit assessment. For example, the nondepolarizing agent rocuronium has a relatively small Vd and one study performed in morbidly obese patients found that the duration of action based on twitch tension was 55 minutes when dosed by ABW, 22 minutes in morbidly obese patients dosed by IBW, and 25 minutes in normal-weight patients (p < 0.001 for ABW vs IBW plus normal weight) [26]. In light of these results, the authors recommended the use of IBW when giving single doses of rocuronium (e.g. for rapid sequence intubation) in order to avoid the delayed recovery noted with the use of ABW.

The difficulties with generalizations about weight and Vd are illustrated by the depolarizing neuromuscular blocking agent succinylcholine. As with rocuronium, succinylcholine has a small Vd, but its pharmacokinetics are complicated by very rapid clearance by plasma pseudo-cholinesterase [27]. In a study of succinylcholine in morbidly obese patients, there was no difference in the onset of maximum blockade between patients dosed on ABW, IBW, or LBW, but maximum block occurred in 100% of patients dosed on ABW compared to 93 and 99% for IBW and LBW, respectively [28]. Intubation conditions were evaluated as good to excellent for all patients dosed by ABW, but were poor for 33 and 27% of patients dosed by IBW and LBW, respectively. The time to 50% recovery of twitch response was 8.5 minutes for ABW compared to 5 and 7 minutes for IBW and LBW, respectively. Hence, the use of IBW would not provide for optimal intubating conditions in morbidly obese patients; furthermore, the rapid recovery from block with IBW would not prevent the occurrence of hypoxemia if laryngoscopy was delayed since desaturation occurs more rapidly in morbidly obese compared to normal-weight patients. These differences noted between neuromuscular blocking agents demonstrate important pharmacodynamic considerations beyond Vd when single doses of drugs are administered for rapid effect.

In general, more lipophilic drugs have larger volumes of distribution and would be expected to have at least some distribution into the excess adipose tissue associated with obesity. This would suggest that loading doses of such drugs should be based on ABW or ABWadj, but

this is not always the case. For example, digoxin has a large Vd, but the distribution is not significantly different between normal-weight and obese patients (937 ± 397 l versus 981 ± 301 l, respectively) [29]. In order to decrease the risk of dosing errors when prescribing boluses of drugs for obese patients in the absence of pertinent research, the clinician should consider factors other than drug distribution. For example, a series of smaller incremental doses titrated to clinical effect or blood concentration (if available) might obviate the need for conjectures about the size of a dose based on Vd and the risk of dose-related toxicities. An example of such an approach would be the use of IV opioids for acute, severe pain. The clinician could give a series of incremental doses titrated by a pain relief instrument rather than trying to estimate the one dose that would control a patient's pain while minimizing adverse effects such as respiratory depression. Further support for this specific approach with opioids is research that suggests that opioid requirements are not greater, and may even be less, in obese compared to normal-weight patients [30,31].

For a number of other drugs such as thrombolytics there is little information on how their efficacy or safety might change with alterations in body composition, so investigators often have an arbitrary upper dosing limit when weight-based dosing protocols are employed for calculating loading infusions [32,33]. Concerns with this approach include the assumption of dose proportionality with weight regardless of other factors such as height or body composition. Until more research is performed, arguments for or against this approach are based mostly on assumptions.

Administration of maintenance or multiple doses of drugs

Clearance is the pharmacokinetic parameter that is most applicable for determining dosing requirements of IV drugs over prolonged periods of time, as would occur with scheduled maintenance doses or continuous infusions. A number of antiarrhythmic and sedative drugs used in critically ill patients are cleared by the liver, so fatty infiltration associated with obesity has the potential to affect metabolic activity [34]. However, the majority of studies that have evaluated the pharmacokinetics of these agents in subjects with at least moderate degrees of obesity (e.g. weight at least 150% of IBW) have found no significant differences in clearance between obese and normal-weight subjects, although Vd changes were sometimes noted that would have implications for loading doses, drug half-life, and frequency of dosing [35–41]. This is not unexpected since liver clearance, as indicated by antipyrine clearance, is correlated with LBM [42]. One study of propofol anesthesia involving eight patients at least 170% of IBW found that clearance seemed to increase with body weight and there appeared to be no accumulation over time, but these results must be interpreted with caution given the small number of subjects and abbreviated infusions [43]. Since propofol accumulation likely occurs during sustained sedation, the use of IBW has been recommended for dosage titration [44].

Many of the shorter-acting drugs used in critically ill patients may have some portion metabolized by the liver, but also have alternative routes of breakdown or elimination that present challenges for the usual pharmacokinetic sampling and modeling techniques [45]. Examples include the nondepolarizing neuromuscular blocking agent cisatracurium, which is metabolized by Hofmann degradation, and vasoactive agents like epinephrine and norepinephrine, which are inactivated by enzymes such as catechol-*O*-methyltransferase (COMT) and monoamine oxidase (MAO), which are distributed throughout the body. Of the few such drugs that have been studied in subjects of various weights, clearance is either unrelated, or does not appear to increase in proportion, to body size [46–49]. Therefore, use of an IBW or LBW would appear to be most appropriate for weight-based dosing, particularly for those patients with more extreme forms of obesity. Table 22.5 provides suggested dosing regimens for commonly used drugs in the ICU when treating morbidly obese patients.

Table 22.5 Suggested weight for loading and maintenance doses of medications in moderately to severely obese patients.

Medication	Loading dose	Maintenance dose	Comment
Amiodarone	LBW	LBW or ABWadj	May need to give mini-loads for breakthrough arrhythmias
Aminoglycosides	ABWadj	ABWadj	Titrate to therapeutic concentrations
Argatroban	ABWadj	ABWadj	Duration of action may be prolonged with prolonged use
Benzodiazepines	ABWadj	ABWadj	Best to titrate with smaller doses to response
β-lactam antimicrobials	ABWadj	ABWadj	Higher end of dosing range if non-weight-based dosing
Cisatracurium	LBW	LBW or ABWadj	Titrate to effect; duration of action may be prolonged
Daptomycin	LBW	LBW	Higher end of dosing range if non-weight-based dosing
Dexmedetomide	LBW	ABWadj	May want to avoid load due to hypotension concerns
Digoxin	LBW	LBW	Lower end of dosing range if non-weight-based dosing
Fluconazole	ABWadj	ABWadj	Higher end of dosing range if non-weight-based dosing
Heparin, unfractionated	ABWadj	ABWadj	Titrate by coagulation studies
Lidocaine	ABWadj	LBW or ABWadj	Titrate to therapeutic concentrations and desired effect
Linezolid	ABWadj	ABWadj	Higher end of dosing range if non-weight-based
Low-molecular-weight heparins (LMWHs)	ABWadj	ABWadj	Anti-Xa monitoring may be warranted if available
Opioids	LBW	LBW	Best to titrate with smaller doses to response
Phenytoin	ABWadj	LBW	Titrate to therapeutic concentrations
Propofol	LBW	LBW or ABWadj	Titrate to effect; duration of action may be prolonged
Quinolone antimicrobials	ABWadj	ABWadj	Higher end of dosing range if non-weight-based dosing
Rocuronium (for intubation)	LBW		
Succinylcholine	ABW	NA	
Vancomycin	LBW	ABW	Titrate to therapeutic concentrations
Vecuronium	LBW	LBW	Titrate to desired effect

ABW, actual body weight; ABWadj, adjusted body weight; LBW, lean body weight (IBW (ideal body weight) is used as a surrogate of lean body weight since it is more familiar to clinicians and easy to calculate); NA, not applicable.

A number of recommendations in this table are based on relatively little data and primarily reflect the author's attempt to balance benefits versus risks in more severely obese patients; for example, some studies in less obese patients suggest that ABW is the preferred weight for some medications with weight-based dosing regimens, but adverse effect concerns (e.g. hypotension with loading doses) prompted a suggestion for use of a lower weight; individual patient issues must always be taken into account when making decisions regarding the most appropriate weight; medications should be titrated to clinical, laboratory, or blood concentration measurements depending on availability; see the text for a more in-depth discussion of dosing issues.

Most of the literature concerning the effects of obesity on clearance involves drugs that are primarily eliminated by the kidneys. In particular, the antimicrobial agents and anticoagulants have been most studied in patients of moderate to severe obesity (e.g. BMI > 35), although dosing recommendations for the latter category of drugs have been the most controversial due to the serious bleeding complications that may occur if excessive doses are used. This is of particular concern with therapeutic dosing, since substantially lower doses of heparin and LMWH are used for prophylaxis even with the dose increases over standard (approximately 30%, or use of weight-based dosing) typically recommended for the obese patient. Despite how long heparin has been used as an anticoagulant, virtually all of the data regarding dosing in more extreme forms of obesity is in the form of case reports and retrospective investigations. The data that are available suggest that use of ABW for therapeutic dosing of venous thromboembolism in such patients may lead to supratherapeutic activated partial thromboplastin times when using traditional unit/kg doses with or without protocols or nomograms [50]. The use of nomograms is unlikely to preclude this concern, since most were not derived from populations that had substantial numbers of patients of more extreme weight [51]. In the absence of further studies, use of an ABWadj would be the more conservative approach when initially dosing a morbidly obese patient, with subsequent adjustment based on laboratory and clinical monitoring.

The introduction of the LMWHs has added further confusion to anticoagulant dosing questions in patients undergoing treatment for venous thromboembolism. Available guidelines provide little guidance and simply refer to the need for dosage adjustments [52]. Enoxaparin has been the most studied LMWH in obese subjects and data from normal volunteer, small prospective, and large retrospective studies conclude there is no need for dosage adjustments in obese patients [53–55]. However, the smaller studies were unable to assess important clinical endpoints such as bleeding and the large retrospective studies often had small numbers of morbidly obese patients and did not control for factors such as height. Much of the debate concerns the weight at which ABW should no longer be used for weight-based dosing, since there is some data to suggest increased bleeding with substantially increased body weight [56]. The most aggressive recommendations came from one group, which recommends ABW for dosing LMWHs in conjunction with anti-Xa monitoring if the patient is more than 190 kg. If anti-Xa isn't available, the authors recommend

ABW with downward adjustment only for bleeding complications [57]. This is clearly not consistent with current clinical practice, as evidenced by the results of one large study in which 74% of patients above 100 kg received doses less than recommended [58]. The issue is further complicated by studies and recommendations that do not distinguish one LMWH from another, despite the varying pharmacokinetic and possibly therapeutic differences between them. Clearly more research is needed, along the lines of a prospective study that has found enoxaparin clearance to be best described by LBW, with recommendations for adjusting the interval as well as the dose in obese patients [59].

Dosing recommendations of antimicrobial agents in obesity have been less controversial than those concerning the LMWHs. This is likely due to the much larger therapeutic window for most antimicrobial agents and the uncommon use of weight-based dosing in adult patients. For the majority of antimicrobials an increased dose is usually needed in obese patients when intermittent IV doses are administered [60]. This is due to the increased Vd, and sometimes clearance, which is increased compared to nonobese patients, but not increased proportional to weight. The first evidence for this need for increased doses came from research involving normal-weight and morbidly obese patients with gram-negative rod infections who were given aminoglycosides [61–63]. These were some of the first studies that suggested the use of an ABWadj with correction factors to account for the influence of the excess weight on pharmacokinetic parameters.

Vancomycin is unique in that it is one of the few antimicrobials with sound pharmacokinetic data to suggest that clearance, using an equation that estimates FFM, is increased in proportion to body weight. The most applicable study was conducted prospectively and involved morbidly obese and normal-weight patients who were seriously ill [64]. The two groups were matched for important covariates (gender, age, IBW, and serum creatinine). The authors performed measures to ensure the accuracy of the pharmacokinetic parameters by determinations at steady state (≥5 estimated half-lives) with verification by follow-up concentration analysis. Creatinine clearance was estimated by the Salazar–Corcoran equation in the morbidly obese and by the Cockcroft–Gault equation in the normal-weight patients. The Salazar–Corcoran equation is one of the few equations designed to predict creatinine clearance and drug clearance in obese patients [65]. Mean creatinine clearance estimated by the Salazar–Corcoran equation was

209 ml/minute for the morbidly obese patients and the measured vancomycin clearance was 197 ml/minute. The results of this study have important implications for dosing vancomycin since they indicated that a dose of 30 mg/kg/day using ABW would be needed to achieve troughs of 5–10 mg/l. These troughs are much less than the currently recommended trough vancomycin concentrations of 15–20 mg/l for serious infections [66]. Hopefully, more studies using this type of methodology will be used to evaluate other antimicrobial agents in critically ill patients with more severe forms of obesity to help the clinician in making appropriate decisions regarding dosing.

BEST PRACTICE TIPS

1 Patients with the same weight and height could have markedly different responses to weight-based drug dosing based on varying pharmacokinetic parameters such as Vd and clearance.

2 As much as possible and practical, the way in which weight is estimated, measured, recorded, and utilized for drug dosing should be standardized to reduce variability that might lead to dosing errors.

3 The Cockcroft–Gault equation adjusted for LBW is the most accurate and useful method for estimating creatinine clearance in patients with more extreme forms of obesity.

4 Vd and clearance are independent pharmacokinetic parameters that do not necessarily change proportionally with increasing body weight.

5 A series of smaller incremental doses titrated to clinical effect or blood concentration (if available) might obviate the need for conjectures about dosing based on potential changes in pharmacokinetic parameters associated with obesity.

REFERENCES

1 Erstad BL. Dosing of medications in morbidly obese patients in the intensive care unit setting. Intensive Care Med. 2004;30:18–32.

2 Hennings S, Romero A, Erstad BL, Franke H, Theodorou AA. A comparison of automated infusion device technology to prevent medication errors in pediatric and adult intensive care unit patients. Hosp Pharm. 2010;45:464–71.

3 Ginzburg R, Barr WB, Harris M, Munshi S. Effect of a weight-based prescribing method within an electronic health record on prescribing errors. Am J Health-Syst Pharm. 2009; 66:2037–41.

4 Green B, Duffull SB. What is the best size descriptor to use for pharmacokinetic studies in the obese? Br J Clin Pharmacol. 2004;50:119–33.

5 Janmahasatian S, Duffull SB, Chagnac A, Kirkpatrick CM, Green B. Lean body mass normalizes the effect of obesity on renal function. Br J Clin Pharmacol. 2008;65:964–5.

6 Janmahasatian S, Duffull SB, Ash S, Ward LC, Byrne NM, Green B. Quantification of lean bodyweight. Clin Pharmacokinetic. 2005;44:1051–65.

7 Han PY, Duffull SB, Kirkpatrick CM, Green B. Dosing in obesity: A simple solution to a big problem. Clin Pharmacol Ther. 2007;82:505–8.

8 Demirovic JA, Pai AB, Pai MP. Estimation of creatinine clearance in morbidly obese patients. Am J Health-Syst Pharm. 2009;66:642–8.

9 Anderson BJ, Holford NH. Mechanistic basis of using body size and maturation to predict clearance in humans. Drug Metab Pharmacokinet. 2009;24:25–36.

10 Bloomfield R, Steel E, MacLennan G, Noble DW. Accuracy of weight and height estimation in an intensive care unit: Implications for clinical practice and research. Crit Care Med. 2006;34:2153–7.

11 Hall WL, Larkin GL, Trujillo MJ, Hinds JL, Delaney KA. Errors in weight estimation in the emergency department: Comparing performance by providers and patients. J Emerg Med. 2004;27:219–24.

12 Jensen GL, Friedmann JM, Henry DK, Skipper A, Beiler E, Porter C, et al. Noncompliance with body weight measurements in tertiary care teaching hospitals. J Parent Enter Nutr. 2003;27:89–90.

13 Lin BW, Yoshida D, Quinn J, Strehlow M. A better way to estimate adult patients' weights. Am J Emerg Med. 2009;27:1060–4.

14 Yamamoto LG, Inaba AS, Young LL, Anderson KM. Improving length-based weight estimates by adding a body habitus (obesity) icon. Am J Emerg Med. 2009;27:810–15.

15 Padwal R, Brocks D, Sharma AM. A systematic review of drug absorption following bariatric surgery and its theoretical implications. Obes Rev. 2010;11:41–50.

16 Barnett AH. How well do rapid-acting insulins work in obese individuals? Diab Obes Metab. 2006;8:388–95.

17 Haas CE, Nelsen JL, Raghavendran K, Mihalko W, Beres J, Ma Q, et al. Pharmacokinetics and pharmacodynamics of enoxaparin in multiple trauma patients. J Trauma. 2005;59:1336–44.

18 Dorffler-Melly J, de Jonge E, de Pont A, Meijers J, Vroom MB, Buller HR, et al. Bioavailability of subcutaneous low-molecular-weight heparin to patients on vasopressors. Lancet. 2002; 359:849–50.

19 Blouin RA, Warren GW. Pharmacokinetic considerations in obesity. J Pharm Sci. 1999;88:1–7.

20 Alicioglu B, Sarac A, Tokuc B. Does abdominal obesity cause increase in the amount of epidural fat? Eur Spine J. 208; 17:1324–8.

21 Wu HH, Schweitzer ME, Parker L. Is epidural fat associated with body habitus? J Comput Assist Tomogr. 2005;29:99–102.

22 Panni MK, Columb MO. Obese parturients have lower epidural local anaesthetic requirements for analgesia in labour. Br J Anaesth. 2006;96:106–10.

23 Lee Y, Balki M, Parkes R, Carvalho JC. Dose requirements of intrathecal bupivacaine for cesarean delivery is similar in obese and normal weight women. Rev Bras Anestesiol. 2009;59:674–83.

24 Falagos ME, Karageorgopoulos DE. Adjustment of dosing of antimicrobial agents for bodyweight in adults. Lancet. 2010;375:248–52.

25 Pearson TC, Guthrie DL, Simpson J, et al. Interpretation of measured red cell mass and plasma volume in adults: Ecpert panel on radionuclides of the International Council for Standardization in Haematology. Br J Haematol. 1995;89:748–56.

26 Leykin Y, Pellis T, Lucca M, Lomangino G, Marzano B, Gullo A. The pharmacodynamic effects of rocuronium when dosed according to real body weight or ideal body weight in morbidly obese patients. Anesth Analg. 2004;99:1086–9.

27 Roy JJ, Donati F, Boismenu D, Varin F. Concentration-effect relation of succinylcholine chloride during propofol anesthesia. Anesthesiol. 2002;97:1082–92.

28 Lemmens HJ, Brodsky JB. The dose of succinylcholine in morbid obesity. Anesth Analg. 2006;102:438–42.

29 Abernethy DR, Greenblatt DJ, Smith TW. Digoxin disposition in obesity: clinical pharmacokinetic investigation. Am Heart. J 1981;102:740–4.

30 Rand CSW, Kuldau JM, Yost RL. Obesity and post-operative pain. J Psychosom Res. 1999;29:43–8.

31 Bennett R, Baterhorst R, Graves DA, Foster TS, Griffen WO, Wright BD. Variation in postoperative analgesic requirements in the morbidly obese following gastric bypass surgery. Pharmacotherapy. 1982;2:50–3.

32 Hacke W, Kaste M, Fieschi C, et al. Intravenous thrombolysis with recombinant tissue plasminogen activator for acute hemispheric stroke. JAMA. 1995;274:1017–25.

33 The National Institute of Neurological Disorders and Stroke rt-PA Stroke Study Group. Tissue plasminogen activator for acute ischemic stroke. N Engl J Med. 1995;333:1581–7.

34 Blouin RA, Warren GW. Pharmacokinetic considerations in obesity. J Pharm Sci. 1999;88:1–7.

35 Abernethy DR, Greenblatt DJ. Lidocaine disposition in obesity. Am J Cardiol. 1984;53:1183–6.

36 Christoff PB, Conti DR, Naylor C, Jusko WJ. Procainamide disposition in obesity. Drug Intell Clin Pharm. 1983;17:516–22.

37 Cheymol G, Poirier JM, Carrupt PA, Testa B, Weissenburger J, Levron JC, et al. Pharmacokinetics of β-adrenoreceptor blockers in obese and normal volunteers. Br J Clin Pharmacol. 1997;43:563–70.

38 Cheymol G, Poirier JM, Barre J, Pradalier A, Dry J. Comparative pharmacokinetics of intravenous propranolol in obese and normal volunteers. J Clin Pharmacol. 1987;27:874–9.

39 Abernethy DR, Schwartz JB. Verapamil pharmacodynamics and disposition in obese hypertensive patients. J Cardiovasc Pharmacol. 1988;11:209–15.

40 Abernethy DR, Greenblatt DJ, Divoll M, Harmatz JS, Shader RI. Alterations in drug distribution and clearance in obesity. J Pharmacol Exp Ther. 1981;217:681–5.

41 Greenblatt DJ, Abernethy DR, Locniskar A, Harmatz JS, Limjuco RA, Shader RI. Effect of age, gender, and obesity on midazolam kinetics. Anesthesiology. 1984;61:27–35.

42 Nawaratne S, Brien JE, Seeman E, Fabiny R, Zalcberg J, Cosolo W, et al. Relationships among liver and kidney volumes, lean body mass and drug clearance. Br J Clin Pharmacol. 1998;46:447–52.

43 Servin F, Farinotti R, Haberer JP, Desmonts JM. Propofol infusion for maintenance of anesthesia in morbidly obese patients receiving nitrous oxide. Anesthesiology. 1993;78:657–65.

44 Barr J, Egan TD, Sandoval NF, Zomorodi K, Cohane C, Gambus PL, et al. Propofol dosing regimens for ICU sedation based upon an integrated pharmacokinetic-pharmacodynamic model. Anesthesiology. 2001;95:324–33.

45 Fisher DM. (Almost) everything you learned about pharmacokinetics was (somewhat) wrong? Anesth Analg. 1996;83:901–3.

46 Lam SW, Bauer SR, Cha SS, Oyen OJ. Lack of an effect of body mass on the hemodynamic response to arginine vasopressin during septic shock. Pharmacotherapy. 2008;28:591–9.

47 Leykin Y, Pellis T, Lucca M, Lomangino G, Marzano B, Gullo A. The effects of cisatracurium on morbidly obese women. Anesth Analg. 2004;99:1090–4.

48 MacGregor DA, Smith TE, Prielipp RC, Butterworth JF, James RL, Scuderi PE. Pharmacokinetics of dopamine in healthy male subjects. Anesthesiology. 2000;92:338–46.

49 Klem C, Dasta JF, Reilley TE, Flancbaum LJ. Variability of dobutamine pharmacokinetics in unstable critically ill patients. Crit Care Med. 1994;22:1926–32.

50 Myzienski AE, Lutz MF, Smythe MA. Unfractionated heparin dosing for venous thromboembolism in morbidly obese patients: case report and review of the literature. Pharmacotherapy. 2010;30:105e–12e.

51 Barletta JF, DeYoung JL, McAllen K, Baker R, Pendleton K. Limitations of a standardized weight-based nomogram for heparin dosing in patients with morbid obesity. Surg Obes Relat Dis. 2008;4:748–53.

52 Hirsh J, Bauer KA, Donati MB, Gould M, Samama MM, Weitz JI. Parenteral anticoagulants: American College of Chest Physicians Evidence-Based Clinical Practice Guidelines (8th edition). CHEST. 2008;133(6 Suppl):141S–59S.

53 Sanderlink GJ, Liboux AL, Jariwala N, Harding N, Ozoux ML, Shukla U, et al. The pharmacokinetics and pharmacodynamics of enoxaparin in obese volunteers. Clin Pharmacol Ther. 2002;72:308–18.

54 Bazinet A, Almanric K, Brunet C, Turcotte I, Martineau J, Caron S, et al. Dosage of enoxaparin among obese and renal impairment patients. Thromb Res. 2005;116:41–50.

55 Spinler SA, Inverso SM, Cohen M, Goodman SG, Stringer KA, Antman EM for the ESSENCE and TIMI 11B Investigators. Am Heart J. 20003;146:33–41.

56 Spinler SA, Ou FS, Roe MT, Gibler WB, Ohman EM, Pollack CV, et al. Weight-based dosing of enoxaparin in obese patients with non-ST segment elevation acute coronary syndromes: Results from the CRUSADE initiative. Pharmacotherapy. 2009;29:631–8.

57 Nutescu EA, Spinler SA, Wittkowsky A, Dager WE. Low-molecular-weight heparins in renal impairment and obesity: Available evidence and clinical practice recommendations across medical and surgical settings. Ann Pharmacother. 2010;43:1165–72.

58 Barba R, Marco J, Martin-Alvarez H, Rondon P, Fernandez-Capitain C, Garcia-Bragado F, et al. The influence of extreme body weight on clinical outcome of patients with venous thromboembolism: findings from a prospective registry (RIETE). J Thromb Haemost. 2005;3:356–62.

59 Green B, Duffull SB. Development of a dosing strategy for enoxaparin in obese patients. Br J Clin Pharmacol. 2003; 56:96–103.

60 Wurtz R, Itokazu G, Rodvold K. Antimicrobial dosing in obese patients. Clin Infect Dis. 1997;25:112–18.

61 Blouin RA, Mann HJ, Griffen WO, Bauer LA, Record KE. Tobramycin pharmacokinetics in morbidly obese patients. Clin Pharmacol Ther. 1979;26:508–12.

62 Bauer LA, Blouin RA, Griffen WO, Record KE, Bell RM. Amikacin pharmacokinetics in morbidly obese patients. Am J Hosp Pharm. 1980;37:519–22.

63 Bauer LA, Edwards WA, Dellinger EP, Simonowitz DA. Influence of weight on aminoglycoside pharmacokinetics in normal weight and morbidly obese patients. Eur J Clin Pharmacol. 1983;24:643–7.

64 Bauer LA, Black DJ, Lill JS. Vancomycin dosing in morbidly obese patients. Eur J Clin Pharmacol. 1998;54:621–5.

65 Salazar DE, Corcoran GB. Predicting creatinine clearance and renal drug clearance in obese patients from estimated fat-free body mass. Am J Med. 1988;34:1053–60.

66 Rybak M, Lomaestro B, Rotschafer JC, Moellering R, Craig W, Billeter M, et al. Therapeutic monitoring of vancomyin in adult patients: a consensus review of the American Society of Health-System Pharmacists, the Infectious Diseases Society of America, and the Society of Infectious Diseases Pharmacists. Am J Health-Syst Pharm. 2009;66:82–98.

Part VII Prognosis and Ethics

23 Prognosis and Outcome of the Critically Ill Obese Patient

Yasser Sakr,[1] Mohamed Zeiden,[2] and Juliana Marques[1]

[1]Department of Anaesthesiology and Intensive Care, Friedrich Schiller University Hospital, Jena, Germany
[2]Department of Anaesthesiology and Intensive Care, Theodor Bilharz Institute, Cairo, Egypt

KEY POINTS

- Obese patients are at increased risk of organ dysfunction in the intensive care unit and consume more resources than nonobese patients.
- Obesity does not seem to be associated with a greater risk of death in the intensive care unit.
- In some subgroups of critically ill patients, obesity may be associated with improved survival.

INTRODUCTION

Overweight and obese adults are at increased risk of morbidity and mortality from many acute and chronic medical conditions [1]. In a collaborative analysis of data from 900 000 adults in 57 prospective studies [2], the overall mortality was lowest at a body mass index (BMI) of about 22.5–25 kg/m². Above this range, each 5 kg/m² increase in BMI was associated with about a 30% higher all-cause mortality. Management of obese patients, particularly in the intensive care unit (ICU), is often demanding and complications are common [3]. However, despite a greater prevalence of comorbid conditions and an increased liability to develop physiological derangements, which may impair the ability of obese patients to compensate for the stress of critical illness, an independent effect of obesity on outcome from critical illness has never been conclusively demonstrated. Studies have given conflicting results as to whether obesity increases the risk of death in critically ill patients or not [4].

In this chapter, we review the current evidence about the possible effects of obesity on outcome from critical illness in terms of morbidity and mortality.

RELATIONSHIP BETWEEN OBESITY AND MORBIDITY IN THE ICU

Obesity and organ dysfunction

Cardiovascular system

Although resting cardiac output is increased, obese patients have impaired left ventricular contractility and a depressed ejection fraction (EF), both at rest and with exercise [5]. The left ventricular chamber dilates to accommodate the increased venous return and, in turn, develops an eccentric type of hypertrophy [6]. The left atrium also enlarges in obese individuals due to increased blood volume and venous return. Later, other factors, like left ventricular hypertrophy and diastolic dysfunction, may also be responsible for increased left atrial size and could lead to an increased propensity to develop pulmonary edema during high cardiac output states or conditions of fluid loading in critical illness [7]. Various cardiac tissues, like the sinus node, atrioventricular node, right bundle branch, and the myocardium near the atrioventricular ring, are replaced by fat cells in obese individuals and this can occasionally cause conduction defects like sinoatrial block, bundle branch block, and, rarely, atrioventricular block [8].

Despite the above mentioned cardiovascular morbidity in relation to obesity, results from a meta-analysis showed that being overweight or obese was associated with lower all-cause and cardiovascular mortality rates in patients with congestive heart failure and was not associated with increased mortality in any of the included studies [9]. Mortality rates were, however, higher among underweight patients, probably due to the presence of low protein and energy intake in these patients [10]. Patients who have decompensated heart failure may also lose weight because of extensive caloric demands associated with the increased work of breathing.

Respiratory system

Total body fat and central adiposity are inversely proportional to lung function [11]. This may be the result of several mechanisms: obesity causes restriction of normal ventilatory patterns because of reduced chest-wall compliance [12] and may increase airway collapsibility and interfere with the function of the inspiratory and expiratory muscles that maintain airway caliber, thus contributing to serious ventilation and perfusion mismatch with a greater incidence of basal atelectasis, leading to hypoxemia [13]. Obese patients may also be prone to severe chest trauma, rib fractures, and pulmonary contusions [14]. Nonetheless, BMI values less than 22.5 kg/m² were also associated with diminished forced expiratory volume in 1 second (FEV1) in elderly critically ill patients [11].

Several studies have shown increased duration of mechanical ventilation in obese and severely obese patients [15–17]. An increase in the risk of aspiration and subsequent ventilator-associated pneumonia was also reported in severely obese patients [18]. In addition, difficult intubation occurs more frequently in obese patients, and postextubation stridor is common [19]. In a cohort study of critically ill patients at risk for acute respiratory distress syndrome (ARDS), there was a strong association between increasing BMI and the risk of developing ARDS [20]. However, a subgroup analysis demonstrated that obese patients had higher peak inspiratory (PIP) and positive end-expiratory (PEEP) pressures than nonobese patients, suggesting that the initial ventilatory strategy varies by weight and may contribute to the development of ARDS in obese patients [20]. In another study, severely obese patients with acute lung injury (ALI) had increased morbidity, as measured by duration of mechanical ventilation and length of stay (LOS), and were more likely to require care in a rehabilitation facility or skilled nursing facility (SNF) after hospital discharge [21]. However, other investigators reported that, after risk adjustment, overweight and obese patients with ALI had outcomes similar to those of patients with normal BMI [15]. Beneficial effects of lower tidal volume ventilation for patients with ALI were also reported in overweight and obese patients in this study [15].

Renal system

The formation of uremic toxins may be dependent on body composition, with the mass of metabolically active organs being mainly responsible [22]. In patients with low BMI, the relative organ mass and formation of uremic toxins are high, but the distribution volume and "buffer" potential for water-soluble and lipid-soluble toxins are low. In a recent study, obesity was reported to be an independent risk factor for developing acute kidney injury (AKI) [23]. However, the authors found that patients with AKI who were moderately obese had a better prognosis than those who were of normal or below-normal weight. A cohort study of 1346 primarily African American subjects receiving maintenance hemodialysis [24] demonstrated that for each one-unit increase in BMI the relative risk of dying was reduced by 4% per year. Underweight patients had a 60% higher mortality rate than the normal-BMI cohort.

Liver

Nonalcoholic fatty liver disease (NAFLD) is an increasingly recognized cause of liver-related morbidity and mortality. The majority of cases of NAFLD occur in patients who are obese or present other components of the metabolic syndrome (hypertension, dyslipidaemia, diabetes) [25]. NAFLD comprises a morphological spectrum of liver lesions ranging from simple triglyceride accumulation in hepatocytes (hepatic steatosis) to inflammatory and hepatocellular ballooning injury (nonalcoholic steatohepatitis, NASH), eventually leading to fibrosis and cirrhosis [26]. The possible impact of these lesions on outcome from critical illness has not been reported.

Infectious complications

Obese patients may be at a higher risk of developing infections, particularly surgical-site infections [27], including those related to cardiac surgery [17,28,29]. In a large prospective observational study of critically ill surgical patients [30], there was an increased risk of catheter-related infections and of other blood-stream infections in obese patients. In another study, obese patients had a more than two-fold increase in the risk of acquiring a bloodstream, urinary tract, or respiratory infection, or of being admitted to the ICU [31]. Recently, the observational European Sepsis Occurrence in Acutely ill Patients (SOAP) study reported no relationship between BMI and sepsis, severe sepsis, or septic shock as reason for admission to the ICU [4]. Another study found no association between obesity and outcome in patients with septic shock [32]. However, low BMI has been reported to be associated with a worse outcome in patients with infections [33]. This could be attributed to the state of malnutrition that is often present in underweight patients.

Thromboembolic complications

Obesity has been reported to be the single most important risk factor for development of recurrent thromboembolic disease [34]. Obesity may be associated with both arterial and idiopathic venous thrombotic events [34]. The risk of pulmonary embolism (PE) was also reported to be higher in patients with the obesity hypoventilation syndrome or sleep apnea [34].

Resource utilization

Staff caring for the obese ICU patient should be aware of the potential effects of personal prejudice against the obese, who may have insecurities about body image. In one survey of patients undergoing gastric bypass, 55% felt they had been treated disrespectfully by health care providers because of their weight [35]. Skin integrity can be particularly problematic in obese patients. Multiple skinfolds can lead to the buildup of moisture, posing a threat to skin integrity. Limited mobility, difficulty in nurse-assisted turning, and decreased vascularity within adipose tissue all contribute to an increased risk of decubitus ulceration [36]. Turning patients, particularly those with very high BMIs, can present a risk for injury to the patient and staff members, but these risks can be minimized with proper training, staffing, and equipment [37]. Obesity is, therefore, associated with higher nursing requirements in the intensive care setting.

Several studies have also shown a strong association between obesity and prolonged ICU and hospital LOS [13,41,43]. This has been attributed to the greater dependence of obese patients on mechanical ventilation or the increased risk of acquiring infection [4]. Prolonged ICU and hospital LOS have also been reported among underweight patients [4]. However, the increase in resource utilization, as evident from prolonged hospitalization and increased nursing requirements, was not associated with worse outcomes in critically ill obese patients [4].

RELATIONSHIP BETWEEN OBESITY AND MORTALITY IN THE ICU

Several studies have reported increased mortality in obese critically ill patients [38–40]. However, this observation cannot be considered as a cause–effect

relationship. Since obesity is associated with increased comorbidity, a confounding effect cannot be excluded. Indeed, three recent metaanalyses [38–40] could not demonstrate any association between obesity and mortality in critically ill adults. Yet, two of these metaanalyses [39,40] reported a trend towards improved outcome in overweight and obese patients when compared to those with normal BMI, a phenomenon known as the obesity survival paradox [41]. Several potential mechanisms have been proposed to elucidate why the "overweight or obese" might do better. Although the association is likely not causative, being overweight or obese may be a marker of improved general health status. Adipose tissue helps provide reserves of energy and lipid-soluble nutrients that are beneficial during the highly catabolic states of critical illness. Furthermore, adipose tissue could be considered an active metabolic and endocrine organ since hormones secreted by fat cells (leptin and interleukin-10) have immune effects that might reduce the inflammatory response and improve survival during severe illness [42]. For instance, leptin levels are positively correlated to BMI, and clinical studies in humans have also reported higher leptin levels in survivors of severe sepsis and septic shock than in nonsurvivors. However, these endocrine effects and the precise immunomodulation that they induce have not yet been fully elucidated. In a recent metaanalysis, the possible association between obesity and favorable outcome, in terms of survival benefit, was not confirmed [38]. One potential explanation is the use of a BMI cutoff of 30kg/m^2. This may have introduced heterogeneity into the case mix of the two groups by including morbidly obese and underweight patients with no, or low, survival benefit.

An association between underweight BMI and poor outcome has also been reported. In a retrospective analysis of 1488 patients with ALI [33], being overweight or obese was associated with a lower risk of death, while a lower BMI was associated with a higher risk. Likewise, an increased mortality rate in underweight patients but not in overweight, obese, or severely obese patients was observed [43]. In a retrospective review [44] of the Study to Understand Prognoses and Preferences for Outcomes and Risks of Treatment (SUPPORT), a low BMI, but not a high BMI, was a significant and independent predictor of mortality. A metaanalysis including 23 studies demonstrated that the risk of mortality was only increased in underweight (i.e. cachectic) patients [40]. Whether this observation was due to diminished metabolic reserves or a confounding effect of possible associated comorbidities, or not, is a matter of speculation.

OBESITY AND OUTCOME IN SOME SPECIFIC ICU POPULATIONS

General surgical ICU patients

In surgical ICU patients, ICU and hospital mortality rates were increased in morbidly obese, critically ill surgical patients when compared with patients with a normal BMI [45]. Morbid obesity was also an independent risk factor for death in these patients [45]. However, the reference group included underweight and obese patients, limiting the interpretation of these data. In critically ill trauma patients, obese patients were 7.1 times more likely to die than nonobese patients after controlling for age, diabetes, gender, obesity, chronic obstructive pulmonary disease (COPD), and injury severity score [31]. Further studies are needed to clarify whether obesity is deleterious in this population or not and to assess the possible differences in outcome between various surgical interventions according to the degree of obesity.

Patients undergoing cardiac surgery

Several complications have been related to obesity in patients undergoing cardiac surgery. Sternal infections are common in obese and morbidly obese patients [28,46]. Although alterations in pulmonary function may theoretically lead to more respiratory-related complications, Yap et al. [17] did not find any increase in the occurrence of pneumonia, reintubation, or prolonged ventilation in obese patients after cardiac surgery. However, in a cohort study of 10 590 patients after cardiac surgery, Engel et al. [46] demonstrated that being underweight was associated with prolonged mechanical ventilation. The risk of postoperative renal failure has also been reported to be higher in obese patients undergoing cardiac surgery [29]. It is possible that the higher prevalence of hypertension and diabetes in obese patients may be associated with compromised preoperative renal function, which is exacerbated by the inflammatory response to cardiopulmonary bypass (CPB) and cardiac surgery. Obesity was also reported to be an independent risk factor for new episodes of atrial fibrillation following cardiac surgery [47]. The risk of postoperative bleeding was shown to be inversely correlated to BMI [28]. Underweight patients may experience relatively increased hemodilution caused by the priming volume of the CPB circuit. This may exacerbate CPB-related coagulopathy,

leading to increased rates of postoperative bleeding in these patients.

In patients undergoing cardiac surgery, underweight status was an independent predictor for worse outcome; however, obesity did not affect the risk of perioperative death [28,46].

Trauma patients

Obese blunt-trauma patients sustain different injuries than lean patients. In particular, obese patients suffer fewer and less severe head injuries and more thoracic and extremity injuries [14]. In a retrospective analysis of 242 severely injured blunt-trauma patients, obese patients had similar demographics, mechanisms of injury, and injury patterns but higher mortality than their nonobese counterparts [48]. Multiple organ failure occurs more often as a complication in obese patients and is twice as often the cause of death in this population [49]. Brown et al. reported that although obese patients with traumatic brain injury had higher morbidity and mortality than lean patients with similar head injuries, the poor outcome appeared to be related to age, admission hypotension, and associated injuries [14]. In contrast, several studies in patients with traumatic injuries [40,50] found an association between obesity and increased risk of death in these patients. The obesity survival paradox has not been reported in this population.

Patients undergoing organ transplantation

Morbid obesity is increasingly observed in patients being evaluated for heart transplantation and represents a relative contraindication. In patients who underwent heart transplantation, morbidly obese patients experienced higher rates of pretransplant diabetes and prolonged waiting times before transplantation [51]. However, there were no significant differences in postoperative complications including rejection, major and minor infections, and survival between the obese and nonobese patients after a mean follow-up of 4 years. On the other hand, in patients who underwent lung transplantation, obesity and being underweight were independent risk factors for postoperative mortality [52]. Similarly, in patients undergoing orthotopic liver transplantation, underweight patients were more likely to die from hemorrhagic complications and cerebrovascular accidents [53], but severely obese patients had a higher number of infectious complications and cancer events leading to death. In patients undergoing renal transplantation, obesity seems to influence delayed graft failure, graft survival, and patient survival [54]. A BMI of $\geq 35 \, kg/m^2$ is significant for greater post-transplant complications, especially new-onset transplant diabetes mellitus, wound complications, and weight gain [54].

Patients undergoing weight-reduction surgery

The type and frequency of complications from weight-reduction surgery vary depending on whether the surgery is performed laparoscopically or as an open procedure. A review of approximately 3500 patients who underwent laparoscopic gastric bypass surgery found that laparoscopic procedures were associated with fewer iatrogenic splenectomies, wound infections, incisional hernias, and overall mortality compared with open surgical procedures [55]. However, with laparoscopic procedures there appears to be an increase in both early and late bowel obstruction, gastrointestinal hemorrhage, and stomal stenosis. Pneumonia, PE, and anastomotic leak occur with equal frequency in both procedures, with PE and anastomotic leak accounting for a significant proportion of postoperative deaths; PE accounted for half the deaths in open and laparoscopic procedures [55].

CONCLUSION

Obesity is associated with significant morbidity and mortality in the general population. However, in critically ill patients, obesity does not seem to be associated with a greater risk of death, despite an increased prevalence of comorbid conditions and increased liability to develop physiological derangements that may impair the ability of these patients to compensate for the stress of critical illness. Nevertheless, obese patients are at increased risk of organ dysfunction in the ICU and consume more resources than nonobese patients. Underweight patients are at risk of considerable morbidity and decreased survival in the ICU and require special attention from health care providers. In some subgroups of critically ill patients, obesity may be associated with improved survival, a phenomenon known as the obesity survival paradox. Obesity should not be regarded, therefore, as a barrier to health care.

> **BEST PRACTICE TIPS**
>
> 1 Underweight rather than obese patients are at an increased risk of death in the ICU.
> 2 Although obesity is associated with an increased risk of organ dysfunction in the ICU and obese patients consume more resources than nonobese patients, obesity per se should not be considered as a barrier to health care.
> 3 Management of postoperative critically ill obese patients should include early mobilization and appropriate treatment of complications.
> 4 The association between obesity and outcome from critical illness is always confounded by other factors, including age, comorbidities, case mix, and associated injuries.

REFERENCES

1 National Task Force on the Prevention and Treatment of Obesity. Overweight, obesity, and health risk. Arch Intern Med. 2000;160:898–904.

2 Whitlock G, Lewington S, Sherliker P et al. Body-mass index and cause-specific mortality in 900 000 adults: collaborative analyses of 57 prospective studies. Lancet. 2009;373:1083–96.

3 Joffe A, Wood K. Obesity in critical care. Curr Opin Anaesthesiol 2007;20:113–18.

4 Sakr Y, Madl C, Filipescu D, et al. Obesity is associated with increased morbidity but not mortality in critically ill patients. Intensive Care Med. 2008;34:1999–2009.

5 Nakajima T, Fujioka S, Tokunaga K, et al. Noninvasive study of left ventricular performance in obese patients: influence of duration of obesity. Circulation. 1985;71:481–6.

6 Kaltman AJ, Goldring RM. Role of circulatory congestion in the cardiorespiratory failure of obesity. Am J Med. 1976;60:645–53.

7 Ku CS, Lin SL, Wang DJ, Chang SK, Lee WJ. Left ventricular filling in young normotensive obese adults. Am J Cardiol. 1994;73:613–15.

8 Balsaver AM, Morales AR, Whitehouse FW. Fat infiltration of myocardium as a cause of cardiac conduction defect. Am J Cardiol. 1967;19:261–5.

9 Oreopoulos A, Padwal R, Kalantar-Zadeh K, et al. Body mass index and mortality in heart failure: a meta-analysis. Am Heart. J 2008;156:13–22.

10 Anker SD, Rauchhaus M. Insights into the pathogenesis of chronic heart failure: immune activation and cachexia. Curr Opin Cardiol. 1999;14:211–16.

11 Wannamethee SG, Shaper AG, Whincup PH. Body fat distribution, body composition, and respiratory function in elderly men. Am J Clin Nutr. 2005;82:996–1003.

12 Stadler DL, McEvoy RD, Sprecher KE, et al. Abdominal compression increases upper airway collapsibility during sleep in obese male obstructive sleep apnea patients. Sleep. 2009;32:1579–87.

13 Vgontzas AN, Tan TL, Bixler EO, et al. Sleep apnea and sleep disruption in obese patients. Arch Intern Med. 1994;154:1705–11.

14 Brown CV, Rhee P, Neville AL, et al. Obesity and traumatic brain injury. J Trauma. 2006;61:572–6.

15 O'Brien JM Jr, Welsh CH, Fish RH, Ancukiewicz M, Kramer AM. Excess body weight is not independently associated with outcome in mechanically ventilated patients with acute lung injury. Ann Intern Med. 2004;140:338–45.

16 El Solh A, Sikka P, Bozkanat E, Jaafar W, Davies J. Morbid obesity in the medical ICU. Chest. 2001;120:1989–97.

17 Yap CH, Mohajeri M, Yii M. Obesity and early complications after cardiac surgery. Med J Aust. 2007;186:350–4.

18 Vaughan RW, Conahan TJ III. Part I: cardiopulmonary consequences of morbid obesity. Life Sci. 1980;26:2119–27.

19 Erginel S, Ucgun I, Yildirim H, Metintas M, Parspour S. High body mass index and long duration of intubation increase post-extubation stridor in patients with mechanical ventilation. Tohoku J Exp Med. 2005;207:125–32.

20 Gong MN, Bajwa EK, Thompson BT, Christiani DC. Body mass index is associated with the development of acute respiratory distress syndrome. Thorax. 2010;65:44–50.

21 Morris AE, Stapleton RD, Rubenfeld GD, et al. The association between body mass index and clinical outcomes in acute lung injury. Chest. 2007;131:342–8.

22 Marik P, Varon J. The obese patient in the ICU. Chest. 1998;113:492–8.

23 Druml W, Metnitz B, Schaden E, Bauer P, Metnitz PG. Impact of body mass on incidence and prognosis of acute kidney injury requiring renal replacement therapy. Intensive Care Med. 2010;36:1221–8.

24 Fleischmann E, Teal N, Dudley J, et al. Influence of excess weight on mortality and hospital stay in 1346 hemodialysis patients. Kidney Int. 1999;55:1560–7.

25 Qureshi K, Abrams GA. Metabolic liver disease of obesity and role of adipose tissue in the pathogenesis of nonalcoholic fatty liver disease. World J Gastroenterol. 2007;13:3540–53.

26 Brunt EM. Nonalcoholic steatohepatitis (NASH): further expansion of this clinical entity? Liver. 1999;19:263–4.

27 Falagas ME, Athanasoulia AP, Peppas G, Karageorgopoulos DE. Effect of body mass index on the outcome of infections: a systematic review. Obes Rev. 2009;10:280–9.

28 Rahmanian PB, Adams DH, Castillo JG, et al. Impact of body mass index on early outcome and late survival in patients undergoing coronary artery bypass grafting or valve surgery or both. Am J Cardiol. 2007;100:1702–8.

29 Tolpin DA, Collard CD, Lee VV, Elayda MA, Pan W. Obesity is associated with increased morbidity after coronary artery bypass graft surgery in patients with renal insufficiency. J Thorac Cardiovasc Surg. 2009;138:873–9.

30 Dossett LA, Dageforde LA, Swenson BR, et al. Obesity and site-specific nosocomial infection risk in the intensive care unit. Surg Infect (Larchmt). 2009;10:137–42.

31 Bochicchio GV, Joshi M, Bochicchio K, et al. Impact of obesity in the critically ill trauma patient: a prospective study. J Am Coll Surg. 2006;203:533–8.

32 Wurzinger B, Dunser MW, Wohlmuth C, et al. The association between body-mass index and patient outcome in septic shock: a retrospective cohort study. Wien Klin Wochenschr. 2010;122:31–6.

33 O'Brien JM Jr, Phillips GS, Ali NA, et al. Body mass index is independently associated with hospital mortality in mechanically ventilated adults with acute lung injury. Crit Care Med. 2006;34:738–44.

34 Goldhaber SZ, Grodstein F, Stampfer MJ, et al. A prospective study of risk factors for pulmonary embolism in women. JAMA. 1997;277:642–5.

35 Rand CS, Macgregor AM. Morbidly obese patients' perceptions of social discrimination before and after surgery for obesity. South Med J. 1990;83:1390–5.

36 El Solh AA. Clinical approach to the critically ill, morbidly obese patient. Am J Respir Crit Care Med. 2004;169:557–61.

37 Hurst S, Blanco K, Boyle D, Douglass L, Wikas A. Bariatric implications of critical care nursing. Dimens Crit Care Nurs. 2004;23:76–83.

38 Akinnusi ME, Pineda LA, El Solh AA. Effect of obesity on intensive care morbidity and mortality: a meta-analysis. Crit Care Med. 2008;36:151–8.

39 Hogue CW, Jr., Stearns JD, Colantuoni E, et al. The impact of obesity on outcomes after critical illness: a meta-analysis. Intensive Care Med. 2009;35:1152–70.

40 Oliveros H, Villamor E. Obesity and mortality in critically ill adults: a systematic review and meta-analysis. Obesity (Silver Spring). 2008;16:515–21.

41 Romero-Corral A, Montori VM, Somers VK, et al. Association of bodyweight with total mortality and with cardiovascular events in coronary artery disease: a systematic review of cohort studies. Lancet. 2006;368:666–78.

42 Hauner H. Adipose tissue inflammation: are small or large fat cells to blame? Diabetologia. 2010;53:223–5.

43 Tremblay A, Bandi V. Impact of body mass index on outcomes following critical care. Chest. 2003;123:1202–7.

44 Galanos AN, Pieper CF, Kussin PS, et al. Relationship of body mass index to subsequent mortality among seriously ill hospitalized patients. SUPPORT Investigators. The Study to Understand Prognoses and Preferences for Outcome and Risks of Treatments. Crit Care Med. 1997;25:1962–8.

45 Nasraway SA, Jr., Albert M, Donnelly AM, et al. Morbid obesity is an independent determinant of death among surgical critically ill patients. Crit Care Med. 2006;34:964–70.

46 Engel AM, McDonough S, Smith JM. Does an obese body mass index affect hospital outcomes after coronary artery bypass graft surgery? Ann Thorac Surg. 2009;88:1793–800.

47 Filardo G, Hamilton C, Hamman B, Hebeler RF Jr, Grayburn PA. Relation of obesity to atrial fibrillation after isolated coronary artery bypass grafting. Am J Cardiol. 2009; 103:663–6.

48 Neville AL, Brown CV, Weng J, Demetriades D, Velmahos GC. Obesity is an independent risk factor of mortality in severely injured blunt trauma patients. Arch Surg. 2004;139:983–7.

49 Ciesla DJ, Moore EE, Johnson JL, et al. Obesity increases risk of organ failure after severe trauma. J Am Coll Surg. 2006;203:539–45.

50 Brown CV, Velmahos GC. The consequences of obesity on trauma, emergency surgery, and surgical critical care. World J Emerg Surg. 2006;1:27.

51 Macha M, Molina EJ, Franco M, et al. Pre-transplant obesity in heart transplantation: are there predictors of worse outcomes? Scand Cardiovasc. J 2009;43:304–10.

52 Lederer DJ, Wilt JS, D'Ovidio F, et al. Obesity and underweight are associated with an increased risk of death after lung transplantation. Am J Respir Crit Care Med. 2009;180:887–95.

53 Dick AA, Spitzer AL, Seifert CF, et al. Liver transplantation at the extremes of the body mass index. Liver Transpl. 2009;15:968–77.

54 Kent PS. Issues of obesity in kidney transplantation. J Ren Nutr. 2007;17:107–13.

55 Podnos YD, Jimenez JC, Wilson SE, Stevens CM, Nguyen NT. Complications after laparoscopic gastric bypass: a review of 3464 cases. Arch Surg. 2003;138:957–61.

24 Ethical Considerations in the Critically Ill Obese Patient

Mark D. Siegel

Pulmonary & Critical Care Section, Department of Internal Medicine, Yale School of Medicine, New Haven, CT, USA

KEY POINTS

- Obese patients are at risk for bias and unfair discrimination traditionally recognized in other marginalized groups.
- Increased resources may be required to care for obese patients, but outcomes appear to rival those of normal-weight individuals.
- Carefully selected obese individuals offer important opportunities to expand the pool of organ donors.

INTRODUCTION

Critical care demands expertise in medical ethics. Every day, ethically charged problems arise in the intensive care setting when it comes to subjects related to end-of-life decisions and triage. Obesity introduces special ethical challenges [1]. Physicians must afford obese patients access to the same high-quality care given to normal-weight individuals, while institutions are challenged to provide resources, such as larger beds and sufficient staffing [1,2].

The management of obese patients introduces intellectual challenges. The extent to which data from studies in general populations should inform treatment decisions in obese patients is unknown. Concerns about bias and undue pessimism raise troubling questions about the quality of care given to obese patients [3–8]. The ethics of caring for obese patients is receiving increasing attention, but relatively little has focused on the critically ill. This chapter will explore the ethics of caring for obese patients in the intensive care unit (ICU), emphasizing issues related to prognostication, triage, end-of-life decision making, and organ donation.

ETHICAL PRINCIPLES AND OBESITY

Four ethical principles are commonly cited to guide medical practice: respect for patient autonomy, beneficence, nonmaleficence, and justice [9]. Autonomy denotes the patient's right to refuse unwanted care and choose among treatment options. Beneficence refers to a physician's duty to help patients and nonmaleficence to the duty to minimize harm. Justice refers to the obligation to ensure fair access to care. Obesity should not impact the spirit of these principles, but it may affect their application.

Autonomy

Respect for autonomy requires two elements. First, patients need the capacity to weigh the burdens and benefits of treatment options. Second, they need information to make informed decisions. Most critically ill patients lack decisional capacity because of cognitive impairment, sedation, or delirium, leading family members to serve as surrogate decision makers [10].

By itself, obesity should not impact autonomy rights. However, the relative paucity of data specifically focused on outcomes in obese patients challenges autonomous decision making. The extent to which data from studies in general populations should be extrapolated to obese individuals is unknown. Similarly, the relationship between weight and prognosis in critical care is uncertain, posing a special challenge to families trying to balance the burdens and therapies of treatment options. Such uncertainty is pervasive in critical care, however, and not unique to obese patients.

Critical Care Management of the Obese Patient, First Edition. Edited by Ali A. El Solh.
© 2012 John Wiley & Sons, Ltd. Published 2012 by John Wiley & Sons, Ltd.

Beneficence and nonmaleficence

Beneficence and nonmaleficence require physicians to use their skills to help patients and minimize harm. Obese patients sometimes receive suboptimal care compared to normal-weight individuals. For example, excessive tidal volumes are often chosen, risking ventilator-induced lung injury [11]. Physicians should know how weight impacts critical illness. Safe intubation requires special skill [12]. Dose adjustments may be needed for medicines such as heparin, which are dosed by weight [13]. Additional resources may be required for obese patients to get physical therapy [14]. Ultimately, intensivists must ensure that obese patients have access to the same safe, effective care given to normal-weight individuals.

Justice

Justice requires that all patients get a fair opportunity to receive medical care. Justice becomes paramount during triage, for example when there are not enough ICU beds to meet demand. Intensivists may be challenged to choose between competing patients, potentially subjecting some to inferior care [15–17]. Ethically sound triage systems must promote equity (fairness) and utility (benefit), recognizing that a balance may have to be struck between the two [18]. Well-considered systems generally seek to maximize benefit to the population while ensuring fair opportunity to those seeking care [15,16,19]. It is never appropriate to discriminate by race, ethnicity, gender, sexual orientation, or ability to pay [15,16,20].

It would generally be considered inappropriate to discriminate because of obesity unless a convincing argument can be made that it is relevant to triage. Two caveats must be emphasized. First, data suggesting a relationship between obesity, outcomes, and resource use are tenuous. Second, triaging on the basis of obesity could marginalize a population already subject to bias.

OBESITY AND DISCRIMINATION

"Discrimination" is a charged word with two distinct meanings, one essential to good care and the other ethically dubious [21]. Discrimination acknowledges relevant distinctions between obese and nonobese patients, for example related to presentation, pathophysiology, and treatment needs. Excess weight is a risk factor for respiratory failure from H1N1 influenza [22] and obese patients may require larger beds and special approaches to mechanical ventilation [1,23]. Many assumed differences between obese and nonobese patients are unfounded,

however. Early work suggested that obese patients had worse outcomes [24], but more recent studies show outcomes that are comparable if not better [2,25].

Unfair discrimination could compromise care. "Anti-fat bias" is pervasive in the general and medical communities [1,3,5,7,26]. From 1994–1995 to 2004–2006, the prevalence of obese individuals reporting discrimination increased from 7.3 to 12.2% [26]. A survey of college students showed that bias against the obese was as strong as that against homosexuals and Muslims [3]. Anti-fat bias is often unrecognized and rarely discussed publicly [5,7,26,27]. The common perception that obese patients are responsible for their condition may foster a sense that bias is socially acceptable. No federal laws protect obese individuals from discrimination in any domain, including health care [26].

Physicians and nurses may harbor negative attitudes towards obese patients, including beliefs that they are lazy, worthless, and noncompliant [5]. One survey showed that physicians had less respect for patients with a higher body mass index (BMI) [4]. Similar attitudes have been demonstrated in nurses and nursing students [28]. Medical students report that attendings, residents, and students commonly direct derogatory comments against obese patients, particularly on surgery and obstetrics-gynecology services [29].

Bias may lead to health care inequities. A hypothetical study demonstrated that lay individuals used weight to choose among patients competing for dialysis machines [6]. Obese patients commonly cite prejudice against them by professionals and nonprofessionals [4,5,28,30]. Patients report insults by physicians or nurses, leading them to avoid health care visits [30]. Physicians appear to spend less time with obese patients and believe obese patients are less likely to follow their advice [31]. Whether bias impacts ICU care is unknown.

Respect for patients is a core physician value and it is important to be mindful of the potential for bias against obese patients [4]. To this end, the National Association to Advance Fat Acceptance (NAAFA) has produced the "Declaration of Health Rights for Fat People" [32]. Highlights include 1) a right to nondiscrimination on the basis of weight, 2) a right to quality medical care, including adequate physical accommodations, equipment, and testing facilities, and 3) freedom from ridicule, coercion, and harassment from caregivers.

OBESITY AND OUTCOMES

The literature on prognosis in obese patients is mixed. Some studies suggest worse outcomes, including increased mortality, morbidity, and resource utilization [24,33]. Others show no effect or even a favorable impact

[8,11,34,35]. A metaanalysis found no impact on mortality but did document increased length of stay and duration of mechanical ventilation [2]. A protective effect on mortality was suggested after morbidly obese patients were excluded. A more recent metaanalysis showed lower hospital mortality, although length of stay and duration of mechanical ventilation were unaffected [25]. The authors noted a critical lack of information pertaining to long-term outcomes. A recent retrospective study focusing on morbidly obese patients found no increase in mortality with higher BMI quartiles, but ICU admission, hospital length of stay, and need for mechanical ventilation and tracheotomy were increased [35].

Several factors contribute to uncertainty about the relationship between obesity and outcomes. Severity-of-illness scores generally do not specifically account for obesity [33]. The effects of obesity and related comorbidities are difficult to distinguish [34]. Studies use a variety of thresholds to denote excess weight. Some studies analyse weight as a dichotomous variable and some as a continuous variable [33]. The relationship between weight and outcome is almost certainly nonlinear, complicating statistics [8]. A paucity of data makes it particularly difficult to draw conclusions at the extremes of weight, for example in the super obese. Finally, recorded weight may be unreliable, particularly if fluid resuscitation is not considered [8].

The most commonly used variable, BMI, fails to distinguish adipose from muscle tissue, and the impact of ethnicity, which impacts thresholds for diagnosing obesity, is not always considered [27]. BMI fails to account for fat distribution. Measuring sagittal anteroposterior diameter may be better than BMI at identifying central obesity and predicting poor outcomes [36]. Further work is necessary to validate this approach.

Obesity can influence how physicians prognosticate. In one study, intensivists were asked to predict outcomes in patients whose clinical features varied by several factors, including BMI [37]. Higher mortality was predicted in those with increased BMI. Given uncertainty about the relationship between BMI and survival, this observation suggests undue pessimism among some physicians and the potential to undermine treatment decisions.

SPECIFIC ETHICS CHALLENGES

End-of-life decision making

Most ICU deaths in the USA follow decisions to forgo life support, usually after meetings with patients' families [10,38]. Family meetings should foster decisions that support the patient's wishes. Key elements include reviewing the patient's clinical course, prognosticating, discussing the patient's preferences, and making decisions. Multiple meetings may be needed to discern the patient's clinical trajectory and foster consensus.

Families commonly experience anxiety and depression during their loved one's course, complicating decision making [39]. Support for families should include access to information as well as emotional and spiritual counseling, if requested [40]. Family members need prognostic estimates, even if uncertain [41]. Many but not all families want physicians to participate in decision making [42].

By itself, obesity should not influence decision making, beyond recognizing factors relevant to the patient's course. Families should know that obesity, particularly when severe, may increase duration of mechanical ventilation and length of stay, and impose additional challenges during recovery. The uncertain relationship between obesity and outcome should be acknowledged; however, it would be inappropriate to forgo life support on the basis of obesity alone.

Triage and rationing

The pressure to ration ICU resources is growing, particularly as the population ages and the prevalence of critical illness increases [43]. Triage forces physicians to choose some patients over others, recognizing that those who fail to gain access may fare relatively poorly.

Several approaches can be used to guide triage, which vary to the extent that factors such as age, comorbidities, and severity of illness are considered [15–17,19,44]. The American Thoracic Society has suggested an egalitarian approach, advocating a first come, first serve approach to all patients with some chance of survival [16]. Other approaches seek to maximize utility by considering factors such as prognosis and age [15,17,44].

A controversial approach to triage employs reciprocity or desert, which considers past actions and behaviors [6,19]. In practice, this approach could punish patients considered responsible for their conditions; for example, obese patients might receive lower priority based on the belief that they precipitated their illnesses by excess eating [6]. Popular sentiment may support this approach. In one study, lay individuals were asked to consider a hypothetical scenario involving patients competing for dialysis [6]. Normal-weight patients were favored against those who were overweight. Such an approach to triage is morally problematic and would almost certainly expose obese patients to inferior treatment [20].

To ensure justice, triage systems must explicitly avoid bias. It would generally be inappropriate to consider weight during triage barring incontrovertible evidence of inferior outcomes or unsustainable resource use. Considering weight-related comorbidities could indirectly discriminate against obese patients. For this reason, it is essential to guard against marginalization of the obese, as with any vulnerable population.

Organ transplant

Transplantable organs are in scarce supply: each year in the USA, only one fifth of patients on the kidney waiting list receive transplants [18]. An ethical approach to distributing organs demands a balance between equity and utility [18]. Equity requires that all those seeking transplant be given the opportunity to be considered; utility requires an approach that maximizes health benefits to the population.

Concern about poor outcomes has traditionally excluded obese patients, but it is becoming increasingly common to offer them transplant [45,46]. Data comparing outcomes in obese and normal-weight patients are mixed. Some studies suggest obesity worsens outcomes [18,47–50], while others do not [51–53]. Obese patients may have more perioperative morbidity, particularly wound complications [46]. Erratic drug absorption may complicate immunosuppression [46]. One group reported that obese patients had delayed improvement in quality of life after liver [54] but not kidney transplant [55].

Moderate obesity should not, by itself, exclude patients from transplantation [46]. Unfortunately, obese patients spend more time on waiting lists and are less likely to be transplanted than those with normal weight [56,57]. Legitimate risk/benefit concerns may explain some of this disparity, but the possibility of bias is difficult to exclude. Additional work is needed to determine the degree to which obesity should influence transplant decisions.

Live organ donation

Cadaveric organs are in scarce supply and live donation plays a crucial role in helping to meet the need for transplantable organs. Key ethical principles govern live donation. First, an individual's decision to donate must be made freely, respecting autonomy. Second, the likelihood of successful transplant must be maximized, promoting beneficence. Third, risk to the donor must be minimized, ensuring nonmaleficence.

Careful selection is essential to protect the donor. Among kidney donors, perioperative and one-year mortality is negligible, the result of diligent attention to selection and technique [58]. Individuals with significant underlying diseases, such as diabetes and hypertension, are generally excluded, both to ensure acceptable organs for transplant and to protect the potential donor from complications [59]. Obese individuals are often excluded from donation due to comorbidities and weight-related risks [60–65].

The shortage of organs provides a compelling argument to expand the donor pool to include traditionally excluded individuals, including those with obesity [62,64–67]. The willingness to consider obese donors varies by center; 52% exclude potential kidney donors with a BMI > 35 kg/m^2 and 10% exclude those with a BMI > 30 kg/m^2 [65]. Estimates of the prevalence of obese kidney donors range from 13 to 23% [58,64]. Appropriately selected obese donors appear to tolerate nephrectomy well. Minor wound-related complications may be increased, but major morbidity and short-term mortality appear comparable to normal-weight individuals.

Obese kidney donors may be subject to long-term complications. Obesity is associated with hypertension, diabetes, and microalbuminuria, although the connection to past donation is uncertain [61,66,68]. Obese donors may be unable to compensate fully for lost renal function [62]. Hyperfiltration in the remaining kidney, the result of nephrectomy, could predispose donors to chronic kidney disease [66].

Obese candidates for kidney donation must be thoroughly evaluated for comorbidities, including microalbuminuria, impaired glucose tolerance, hypertension, hyperlipidemia, cardiovascular disease, sleep apnea, and liver disease [59]. Uncertainties about long-term complications must be discussed with donor candidates [61,64]. Consensus guidelines recommend 1) excluding candidates with a BMI > 35 kg/m^2, especially in the setting of comorbidities, 2) encouraging obese candidates to lose weight before donating and advising against donation if they have associated comorbidities, 3) informing obese patients of acute and long-term risks, especially in the presence of comorbid conditions, and 4) providing healthy lifestyle education [59]. Long-term follow up is required for all renal donors, but assumes special importance in obese individuals given the predisposition to chronic kidney disease [61].

Preliminary work suggests that liver donation is feasible in carefully selected obese individuals [67,69]. Obese donor candidates have traditionally been excluded due to concerns about complications as well as the potential for obesity-related steatosis and nonalcoholic fatty liver disease (NAFLD) [69,70]. Compared to nephrectomy, liver-donation surgery is more complicated and risky [60]. However, carefully selected donors appear to have outcomes similar to normal-weight individuals, except for some increased risk for wound infections [69]. Preliminary work suggests that the obese donor does not negatively impact recipient outcomes [71]. Weight loss, dietary modifications, exercise, and medication may reverse steatosis, making donation possible [72]. Additional data on long-term outcomes is needed to better understand how to balance the risks and benefits of liver donation from obese individuals.

CONCLUSION

Sophistication in medical ethics is essential to good critical care. The core values of medical ethics – respect for autonomy, beneficence, nonmaleficence, and justice – should not be affected by obesity. However, caring for obese patients introduces special considerations, including uncertainty about prognosis, special challenges to providing optimal care, and concerns about bias. More research is needed to better understand how obesity impacts outcomes and treatments. Commitment to ethical duties provides an important safeguard to ensure that obese patients receive the same outstanding care all patients deserve.

BEST PRACTICE TIPS

1 In isolation, obesity is irrelevant to triage considerations.
2 Clinicians must be familiar with the ways obesity affects important aspects of critical care such as intubation and choosing mechanical ventilation settings.
3 Institutions should ensure that adequate resources, such as appropriately sized beds, are available to manage obese patients.
4 Obese kidney donors require careful follow up, especially in view of a higher risk of chronic kidney disease compared to normal-weight donors.
5 Special care should be taken to ensure that obese patients are not subject to unfair bias in the delivery of health care.

REFERENCES

1 Reynolds LR, Rosenthal MS. Are we providing ethical care for the severely obese? South Med J. 2010;103:498–9.
2 Akinnusi ME, Pineda LA, El Solh AA. Effect of obesity on intensive care morbidity and mortality: a meta-analysis. Crit Care Med. 2008;36:151–8.
3 Latner JD, O'Brien KS, Durso LE, et al. Weighing obesity stigma: the relative strength of different forms of bias. Int J Obes (Lond). 2008;32:1145–52.
4 Huizinga MM, Cooper LA, Bleich SN, et al. Physician respect for patients with obesity. J Gen Intern Med. 2009;24:1236–9.
5 Puhl RM, Heuer CA. The stigma of obesity: a review and update. Obesity (Silver Spring). 2009;17:941–64.
6 Furnham A, Loganathan N, McClelland A. Allocating scarce medical resources to the overweight. J Clin Ethic. 2010;21:346–56.
7 Puhl RM, Heuer CA. Obesity stigma: Important considerations for public health. Am J Public Health. 2010;100:1019–28.
8 O'Brien JM Jr, Phillips GS, Ali NA, et al. Body mass index is independently associated with hospital mortality in mechanically ventilated adults with acute lung injury. Crit Care Med. 2006;34:738–44.
9 Beauchamp TL, Childress JF. Principles of Biomedical Ethics. 6 edn. New York, Oxford University Press. 2009.
10 Berger JT, DeRenzo EG, Schwartz J. Surrogate decision making: reconciling ethical theory and clinical practice. Ann Intern Med. 2008;149:48–53.
11 Anzueto A, Frutos-Vivar F, Esteban A, et al. Influence of body mass index on outcome of the mechanically ventilated patients. Thorax. 2011;66:66–73.
12 Frat JP, Gissot V, Ragot S, et al. Impact of obesity in mechanically ventilated patients: a prospective study. Intensive Care Med. 2008;34:1991–8.
13 Riney JN, Hollands JM, Smith JR, et al. Identifying optimal initial infusion rates for unfractionated heparin in morbidly obese patients. Ann Pharmacother. 2010;44:1141–51.
14 Needham DM, Korupolu R, Zanni JM, et al. Early physical medicine and rehabilitation for patients with acute respiratory failure: a quality improvement project. Arch Phys Med Rehab. 2010;91:536–42.
15 Anonymous. Consensus statement on the triage of critically ill patients. Society of Critical Care Medicine Ethics Committee. JAMA. 1994;271:1200–3.
16 Anonymous. American Thoracic Society. Fair allocation of intensive care unit resources. Am J Respir Crit Care Med. 1997;156:1282–301.
17 Sprung CL, Zimmerman JL, Christian MD, et al. Recommendations for intensive care unit and hospital preparations for an influenza epidemic or mass disaster: summary report of the European Society of Intensive Care Medicine's task force for intensive care unit triage during an influenza epidemic or mass disaster. Intensive Care Med. 2010;36:428–43.
18 Courtney AE, Maxwell AP. The challenge of doing what is right in renal transplantation: balancing equity and utility. Nephron Clin Pract. 2009;111(1):62–7.
19 Persad G, Wertheimer A, Emanuel EJ. Principles for allocation of scarce medical interventions. Lancet. 2009;373:423–31.
20 Council on Ethical Judicial Affairs, American Medical Association. Ethical considerations in the allocation of organs and other scarce medical resources among patients. Arch Intern Med. 1995;155:29–40.

21 http://dictionary.reference.com/browse/discrimination [accessed April 10, 2011].

22 Estenssoro E, Rios FG, Apezteguia C, et al. Pandemic 2009 Influenza A in Argentina: a study of 337 patients on mechanical ventilation. Am J Respir Crit Care Med. 2010;182:41–8.

23 Pelosi P, Croci M, Ravagnan I, et al. The effects of body mass on lung volumes, respiratory mechanics, and gas exchange during general anesthesia. Anesth Analg. 1998;87:654–60.

24 El Solh A, Sikka P, Bozkanat E, et al. Morbid obesity in the medical ICU. Chest. 2001;120:1989–97.

25 Hogue CW Jr, Stearns JD, Colantuoni E, et al. The impact of obesity on outcomes after critical illness: a meta-analysis. Intensive Care Med. 2009;35:1152–70.

26 Andreyeva T, Puhl RM, Brownell KD. Changes in perceived weight discrimination among Americans, 1995–1996 through 2004–2006. Obesity (Silver Spring). 2008;16:1129–34.

27 Anand SS. Obesity: the emerging cost of economic prosperity. CMAJ. 2006;175:1081–2.

28 Poon MY, Tarrant M. Obesity: attitudes of undergraduate student nurses and registered nurses. J Clin Nurs. 2009;18:2355–65.

29 Wear D, Aultman JM, Varley JD, et al. Making fun of patients: Medical students' perceptions and use of derogatory and cynical humor in clinical settings. Acad Med. 2006;81:454–62.

30 Hansson LM, Naslund E, Rasmussen F. Perceived discrimination among men and women with normal weight and obesity: a population-based study from Sweden. Scand J Public Health. 2010;38:587–96.

31 Hebl MR, Xu J. Weighing the care: Physicians' reactions to the size of a patient. Int J Obes Relat Metab Disord. 2001;25:1246–52.

32 Meletiche L. Declaration of health rights for fat people. Available at: http://www.grandstyle.com/declaration.htm [accessed April 10, 2011].

33 Goulenok C, Monchi M, Chiche JD, et al. Influence of overweight on ICU mortality: a prospective study. Chest. 2004;125:1441–5.

34 Slynkova K, Mannino DM, Martin GS, et al. The role of body mass index and diabetes in the development of acute organ failure and subsequent mortality in an observational cohort. Crit Care. 2006;10:R137.

35 Westerly BD, Dabbagh O. Morbidity and mortality characteristics of morbidly obese patients admitted to hospital and intensive care units. J Crit Care. 2011;26:180–5.

36 Paolini JB, Mancini J, Genestal M, et al. Predictive value of abdominal obesity vs. body mass index for determining risk of intensive care unit mortality. Crit Care Med. 2010;38:1308–14.

37 O'Brien JM Jr, Aberegg SK, Ali NA, et al. Results from the national sepsis practice survey: predictions about mortality and morbidity and recommendations for limitation of care orders. Crit Care. 2009;13:R96.

38 Curtis JR, White DB. Practical guidance for evidence-based ICU family conferences. Chest. 2008;134:835–43.

39 Pochard F, Azoulay E, Chevret S, et al. Symptoms of anxiety and depression in family members of intensive care unit patients: ethical hypothesis regarding decision-making capacity. Critical Care Medicine. 2001;29:1893–7.

40 Lautrette A, Darmon M, Megarbane B, et al. A communication strategy and brochure for relatives of patients dying in the ICU. New Engl J Med. 2007;356:469–78.

41 Evans LR, Boyd EA, Malvar G, et al. Surrogate decision-makers' perspectives on discussing prognosis in the face of uncertainty. Am J Respir Crit Care Med. 2009;179:48–53.

42 Johnson SK, Bautista CA, Hong SY, et al. An empirical study of surrogates' preferred level of control over value-laden life support decisions in intensive care units. Am J Respir Crit Care Med. 2011;183:915–21.

43 Sinuff T, Kahnamoui K, Cook DJ, et al. Rationing critical care beds: a systematic review. Crit Care Med. 2004;32:1588–97.

44 White DB, Katz MH, Luce JM, et al. Who should receive life support during a public health emergency? Using ethical principles to improve allocation decisions. Ann Intern Med. 2009;150:132–8.

45 Thuluvath PJ, Guidinger MK, Fung JJ, et al. Liver transplantation in the United States, 1999–2008. Am J Transplant. 2010;10:1003–19.

46 Potluri K, Hou S. Obesity in kidney transplant recipients and candidates. Am J Kidney Dis. 2010;56:143–56.

47 Chang SH, Coates PT, McDonald SP. Effects of body mass index at transplant on outcomes of kidney transplantation. Transplantation. 2007;84:981–7.

48 Hillingso JG, Wettergren A, Hyoudo M, et al. Obesity increases mortality in liver transplantation: the Danish experience. Transpl Int. 2005;18:1231–5.

49 Lederer DJ, Wilt JS, D'Ovidio F, et al. Obesity and underweight are associated with an increased risk of death after lung transplantation. Am J Respir Crit Care Med. 2009;180:887–95.

50 Russo MJ, Hong KN, Davies RR, et al. The effect of body mass index on survival following heart transplantation: do outcomes support consensus guidelines? Ann Surg. 2010;251:144–52.

51 Mehta R, Shah G, Leggat JE, et al. Impact of recipient obesity on living donor kidney transplant outcomes: a single-center experience. Transplant Proc. 2007;39:1421–3.

52 Macha M, Molina EJ, Franco M, et al. Pre-transplant obesity in heart transplantation: are there predictors of worse outcomes? Scand Cardiovasc J. 2009;43:304–10.

53 Leonard J, Heimbach JK, Malinchoc M, et al. The impact of obesity on long-term outcomes in liver transplant recipients-results of the NIDDK liver transplant database. Am J Transplant. 2008;8:667–72.

54 Zaydfudim V, Feurer ID, Moore DE, et al. The negative effect of pretransplant overweight and obesity on the rate of improvement in physical quality of life after liver transplantation. Surgery. 2009;146:174–80.

55 Zaydfudim V, Feurer ID, Moore DR, et al. Pre-transplant overweight and obesity do not affect physical quality of

life after kidney transplantation. J Am Coll Surg. 2010;210:336–44.

56 Segev DL, Thompson RE, Locke JE, et al. Prolonged waiting times for liver transplantation in obese patients. Ann Surg. 2008;248:863–70.

57 Segev DL, Simpkins CE, Thompson RE, et al. Obesity impacts access to kidney transplantation. J Am Soc Nephrol. 2008;19:349–55.

58 Segev DL, Muzaale AD, Caffo BS, et al. Perioperative mortality and long-term survival following live kidney donation. JAMA. 2010;303:959–66.

59 Anonymous. A report of the amsterdam forum on the care of the live kidney donor: data and medical guidelines. Transplantation. 2005;79(6 Suppl):S53–66.

60 Charlton M. Obesity in potential living donors: success with simplicity. Liver Transpl. 2004;10:726–7.

61 Heimbach JK, Taler SJ, Prieto M, et al. Obesity in living kidney donors: clinical characteristics and outcomes in the era of laparoscopic donor nephrectomy. Am J Transplant. 2005;5:1057–64.

62 Davis CL. Living kidney donors: current state of affairs. Adv Chronic Kidney Dis. 2009;16:242–9.

63 Reese PP, Feldman HI, Asch DA, et al. Short-term outcomes for obese live kidney donors and their recipients. Transplantation. 2009;88:662–71.

64 Reese PP, Feldman HI, McBride MA, et al. Substantial variation in the acceptance of medically complex live kidney donors across us renal transplant centers. Am J Transplant. 2008;8:2062–70.

65 Mandelbrot DA, Pavlakis M, Danovitch GM, et al. The medical evaluation of living kidney donors: a survey of US transplant centers. Am J Transplant. 2007;7:2333–43.

66 Nogueira JM, Weir MR, Jacobs S, et al. A study of renal outcomes in obese living kidney donors. Transplantation. 2010;90:993–9.

67 Tisone G, Manzia TM, Zazza S, et al. Marginal donors in liver transplantation. Transplant Proc. 2004;36:525–6.

68 Ibrahim HN, Foley R, Tan L, et al. Long-term consequences of kidney donation. New Engl J Med. 2009;360:459–69.

69 Moss J, Lapointe-Rudow D, Renz JF, et al. Select utilization of obese donors in living donor liver transplantation: implications for the donor pool. Am J Transplant. 2005;5:2974–81.

70 Lee JY, Kim KM, Lee SG, et al. Prevalence and risk factors of non-alcoholic fatty liver disease in potential living liver donors in Korea: a review of 589 consecutive liver biopsies in a single center. J Hepatol. 2007;47:239–44.

71 Yoo HY, Molmenti E, Thuluvath PJ. The effect of donor body mass index on primary graft nonfunction, retransplantation rate, and early graft and patient survival after liver transplantation. Liver Transpl. 2003;9:72–8.

72 Hwang S, Lee SG, Jang SJ, et al. The effect of donor weight reduction on hepatic steatosis for living donor liver transplantation. Liver Transpl. 2004;10:721–5.

Multiple Choice Questions

CHAPTER 1

1) Which of the following hemodynamic changes is not typically associated with obesity in the absence of systemic hypertension?
   a. Increased circulating blood volume.
   b. Increased cardiac output.
   c. Reduced systemic vascular resistance.
   d. None of the above.

2) In normotensive morbidly obese persons, which type of LV hypertrophy is most commonly encountered?
   a. Concentric LV hypertrophy.
   b. Eccentric LV hypertrophy.
   c. Eccentric–concentric LV hypertrophy.
   d. Asymmetric septal hypertrophy.

3) Which of the following statements is/are true concerning LV function in class III obesity?
   a. LV diastolic function is often impaired.
   b. LV diastolic function is usually normal.
   c. LV systolic function is usually normal.
   d. LV systolic function is usually reduced.
   e. a and c are correct.
   f. b and d are correct.

CHAPTER 2

1) Which of the following statements are true?
   a. In supine position, FRC approaches RV.
   b. Only ERV is reduced in obesity.
   c. In RT position, lung volume improves.
   d. Total respiratory compliance is unchanged in obesity.
   e. a and c are correct.
   f. b and d are correct.

2) Which of the following statements are false?
   a. Lung function improves with weight loss.
   b. Recruitment maneuver every 10 minutes improves oxygenation.
   c. Morbidly obese patients who undergo laparoscopic gastric bypass or gastric banding improve their spirometry 12 months after surgery.
   d. The prophylactic use of BiPAP System 12/4 (but not 8/4) during the first 24 hours postoperatively does not reduced pulmonary dysfunction after gastroplasty.

3) Which of the following statements are true?
   a. DLC improves with weight loss.
   b. An increased DLCO in obese patients is probably related to increased pulmonary blood volume and flow.
   c. In RT the alveolar/arterial oxygen difference was significantly increased in gastric surgery.
   d. Morbid obesity is associated with low arterial pressure of oxygen (PaO_2) and a decrease in alveolar/arterial oxygen partial pressure difference.
   e. a and c are correct.
   f. b and d are correct.

CHAPTER 3

1) Which of the following mechanisms predisposes obese patients to gastroesophageal reflux disease?
   a. Reduced lower esophageal sphincter relaxation.
   b. Raised intraabdominal pressure.
   c. Reduced gastric capacity.
   d. Reduced local acid environment.

2) Which of the following metabolic disturbances contribute to the development of nonalcoholic fatty liver disease?
   a. Increased hepatic fatty acid uptake.
   b. Reduced de novo hepatic fatty acid synthesis.
   c. Increased hepatic fatty acid oxidation.
   d. Increased hepatic fatty acid VLDL export.

3) Which of the following statements is true with regards to the gut microbiology in obesity?
   a. Gut bacteria colonization remains stable throughout life.
   b. Gut bacteria increase the energy yield from ingested food and can thus contribute to weight gain.
   c. Bacteroidete numbers decrease and Firmicute numbers increase in obese subjects in all published trials.
   d. Manipulation of the gut flora may be used therapeutically to promote weight loss.
   e. a and c are true.
   f. b and d are true.

CHAPTER 4

1) Which of the following hormonal alterations is not typical of overweight and obesity in men?
   a. Hyperinsulinemia.
   b. Increased TSH and T3.
   c. Increased testosterone levels.
   d. Decreased ghrelin.

2) Leptin is a polypeptide hormone secreted by which of the following?
   a. Pituitary.
   b. F-cells of the pancreatic islets of Langerhans.
   c. Stomach.
   d. Adipose tissue.

3) Which of the following is true?
   a. GH secretion is only dependent on the interaction between GHRH and somatostatin.
   b. The altered somatotroph function of obesity is functional and can be reversed in different situations.
   c. Ghrelin is a new nonnatural GHS.
   d. In obesity, FFA levels are decreased.
   e. a and c are true.
   f. b and d are true.

CHAPTER 5

1) How should kidney function in obese ICU patients be evaluated?
   a. By equations such as the Cockcroft–Gault or MDRD.
   b. By serum creatinine concentration.
   c. By serum urea or BUN concentration.
   d. By measured urinary creatinine clearance.

2) What is the consensus definition for acute kidney injury (AKI)?
   a. An increase of serum creatinine above 2 mg/dl within 48 hours.
   b. An increase of serum creatinine $\geq 25\%$ within 48 hours.
   c. An increase of serum creatinine by 0.3 mg/dl within 48 hours, or an increase by 100–200% above baseline within 7 days.
   d. Urine output < 0.3 ml/kg per hour for 3 hours or more.

3) Which mechanism is least likely to play a role in the untoward effects of obesity on kidney function?
   a. Hyperfiltration.
   b. Hypotension.
   c. Glomerulosclerosis.
   d. Intraabdominal hypertension.

CHAPTER 6

1) Linking daily spontaneous awakening trials with daily spontaneous breathing trials is NOT associated with which of the following?
   a. Decreased morbidity and mortality.
   b. Reduced exposure to sedative medication.
   c. Increased rate of self-extubation, though not reintubation rates.
   d. Increased risk of PTSD and neuropsychological dysfunction.

2) Obesity affects pharmacokinetics and pharmacodynamics of sedative agents due to which of the following?
   a. Decrease in lean body mass of obese patients.
   b. Decrease in the glomerular filtration rate in obese patients.
   c. Increase in the cardiac output of obese patients.
   d. Increased protein binding in obese patients.

3) Which of the following is true with regards to dexmedetomidine?
   a. It is a selective GABA receptor agonist which produces analgesia and sedation without respiratory depression.
   b. It should have its dose adjusted for renal dysfunction.
   c. It improves delirium outcomes.
   d. It is associated with tachycardia.
   e. a and c are true.
   f. b and d are true.

CHAPTER 7

1) Which of the following patient characteristics is not potentially associated with difficult laryngoscopy?
   a. Mallampati score of III or IV.
   b. Neck circumference > 40 cm.
   c. Edentulous.
   d. Limited mouth opening.
   e. Prior head and neck radiation.

2) Which of the following patient characteristics is not associated with a greater likelihood of difficult mask ventilation?
   a. Male gender.
   b. Age > 55.
   c. Presence of a beard.
   d. Edentulous.
   e. Prominent incisors.

3) Which of the following medications would be appropriately dosed based on TBW?
   a. Succinylcholine.
   b. Rocuronium.
   c. Vecuronium.
   d. Remifentanil.
   e. Fentanyl.

CHAPTER 8

1) Which of the following is not true for use of mechanical ventilation in an obese patient?
   a. Attempts should be made to use optimal PEEP.
   b. Tidal volume should be calculated based on actual body weight.
   c. Patient should be placed in reverse Trendelenburg position.
   d. Recruitment maneuvers are not routinely recommended.

2) Which of the following is true for outcomes in obese patients with hypoxic respiratory failure when compared to normal-weight patients?
   a. Obese patients have increased mortality.
   b. Both groups have similar likelihood of being discharged to a skilled nursing facility.
   c. Obese patients have an increase in duration of mechanical ventilation.
   d. Postextubation respiratory failure can be safely treated with noninvasive ventilation.

3) Which of the following statements is not true?
   a. FRC is decreased in obese patients.
   b. Spirometry usually demonstrates an obstructive defect in obese patients.
   c. OHS increases the likelihood of respiratory failure in obese patients.
   d. Total respiratory system compliance is decreased in obese patients.
   e. a and c are not true.
   f. b and d are not true.

CHAPTER 9

1) In ALI patients requiring mechanical ventilation, tidal volume should be calculated based on which of the following factors?
   a. Height.
   b. Age.
   c. Gender.
   d. Weight.
   e. a and c.
   f. b and d.

2) Which of the following statements describing the relationship between obesity and ALI/ARDS is true? I. Obesity has been associated with increased incidence of ARDS. II. Obesity has been associated with higher mortality in ALI.
   a. I.
   b. II.
   c. I and II.
   d. Neither I nor II.

3) Which of the following therapies for ALI improves respiratory physiology in healthy obese patients?
  a. Low tidal volumes.
  b. Prone positioning.
  c. Low plateau pressures.
  d. High PEEP.
  e. a and c.
  f. b and d.

CHAPTER 10

1) Obese patients are believed to be prone to enhanced systemic reaction to infection due to which of the following?
  a. Secretion of IL-1, IL-6, and TNF-α from adipocytes.
  b. Secretion of adipokines, including leptin and resistin.
  c. Elevated MCP-1.
  d. All of the above.

2) Which of the following is a false statement regarding the cutaneous physiology of healing in obese critically ill patients?
  a. Intraoperative subcutaneous oxygen partial pressure at the incision site is lower in obese patients than in nonobese patients.
  b. The "decisive period" when, if tissue oxygenation is low, an SSI may develop occurs 3 hours prior to the skin incision.
  c. A low tissue oxygen partial pressure correlates with reduced oxidative neutrophil activity.
  d. Ischemic tissue necrosis may result from the relative hypoperfusion of subcutaneous fat in obese patients, second to an increase in fat cell size without an increase in circulatory flow rate.

3) Key management strategies for infectious complications in critically ill obese patients include all of the following except which?
  a. Proper skin cleansing prior to CVC insertion is best accomplished with chlorhexidine, instead of povidone-iodine solutions.
  b. Obese surgical patients should ideally be maintained in a hyperglycemic, normothermic state pre-, intra-, and postoperatively.
  c. Daily assessment of every catheter in place in an obese patient should be performed to determine which ones can be discontinued, in an attempt to decrease infectious complications.
  d. Ventilator tidal volumes should be calculated based on ideal body weight to decrease risk of alveolar overdistension, barotrauma, and possibly pneumonia.

CHAPTER 11

1) Which of the following are not in the Atlanta Criteria for Pancreatitis Severity?
  a. Abdominal pain of at least 8/10 in severity.
  b. Cardiovascular shock with a systolic blood pressure (SBP) <90 mm Hg.
  c. Renal failure serum creatinine >2 mg/dl.
  d. GI bleeding >500 ml in 24 hours.

2) Which of the following would not be a worrisome sign in a bariatric surgery postoperative patient?
  a. Heart rate >120.
  b. Temperature >102 °F (39 °C).
  c. Patient experiencing anxiety as anesthesia wears off.
  d. Patient appearing systemically ill.

3) Which of the following bladder pressures most clearly indicates the need for surgical decompression when IAH and end-organ damage is suspected?
  a. 5 mm Hg.
  b. 12 mm Hg.
  c. 18 mm Hg.
  d. 25 mm Hg.

CHAPTER 12

1) Which of the following is the most common metabolic complication in critically ill obese patients besides hyperglycemia?
  a. Pituitary disease.
  b. Primary hypothyroidism.
  c. Cushing's syndrome.
  d. Hyperprolactinemia.

2) What glucose level must not be exceeded in the critically ill obese patient?
  a. 150 mg/dl.
  b. 160 mg/dl.
  c. 180 mg/dl.
  d. 200 mg/dl.

3) Which of the following conditions has been identified as an important risk factor for the development of adrenal insufficiency in ICU patients?
  a. Low HDL.
  b. High LDL.
  c. Low VLDL.
  d. High HDL.

CHAPTER 13

1) When treating the critically ill obese patient for PE, how should you dose UFH?
   a. On ideal body weight.
   b. On actual body weight.
   c. On actual body weight adjusted for extracellular water.
   d. With twice the initial bolus as you would for the nonobese patient.

2) When LMWHs are used to treat PE and DVT in the obese, which of the following best predicts antifactor Xa clearance?
   a. Body mass index.
   b. Ideal body weight.
   c. Total body weight.
   d. Height of the patient.

3) Which technique is used to improve the diagnostic accuracy for DVT and PE in the obese patient?
   a. Electronic filters with tissue harmonic imaging during compression ultrasonography.
   b. Increasing the kVp to 140 when CTPA scanning is done.
   c. Slowing the gantry rotation time when CTPA is done.
   d. Allowing a longer duration for data collection when V/Q scanning is done.
   e. All of the above.

CHAPTER 14

1) What is the best position to optimize diaphragmatic excursion in the extremely obese critically ill patient?
   a. Supine.
   b. Reverse Trendelenberg at a 30–45° angle.
   c. Head-of-bed elevation at 30° with the knees flexed.
   d. Prone.

2) What is the risk of pressure ulcer development in patients with a BMI ≥40 when compared with patients of normal size?
   a. No difference in risk.
   b. 1.5 times greater.
   c. 3 times greater.
   d. 4.5 times greater.

3) What unique challenges are posed by the extremely obese patient?
   a. Assessment and monitoring.
   b. Specialized equipment.
   c. Understanding of the pathophysiology of obesity.
   d. All of the above.

CHAPTER 15

1) Cardiac index is cardiac output indexed to body surface area (in formula: cardiac index = cardiac output/body surface area in m^2). In obese patients, cardiac output is increased. Which of the following is true concerning the cardiac index in obese patients compared with nonobese patients?
   a. It is increased.
   b. It is similar.
   c. It is decreased.
   d. It is unpredictable.

2) Which of the following is true concerning cardiac output measurement by means of uncalibrated blood pressure pulse contour (or waveform) analysis in the obese patient?
   a. It is reliable.
   b. It is unreliable. It is invalidated by pre-assumptions regarding vessel compliance (derived from nonobese individuals).
   c. It is unreliable, as stated in b), but can be used for trending in cardiac output in time.
   d. It is unreliable. Blood pressure waveform analysis in obese patients cannot be used at all.

3) What is the least preferred location for central venous catheterization in obese patients?
   a. Subclavian vein.
   b. Internal jugular vein.
   c. Femoral vein.
   d. Brachial vein.

CHAPTER 16

1) What is the maximum available weight limit for a multidetector CT scan?
   a. 250 kg/550 lb.
   b. 270 kg/600 lb.
   c. 310 kg/680 lb.
   d. 320 kg/700 lb.

2) What is th most commonly performed radiological examination in the critically ill obese patient?
   a. Abdominal CT.
   b. Chest radiograph.
   c. Head MRI.
   d. Upper GI contrast examination.

3) What is the common imaging finding of ACS?
   a. Bowel wall thickening.
   b. Hemoperitoneum.
   c. Increasing abdominal girth.
   d. All of the above.

CHAPTER 17

1) Which of these statements is true regarding the postoperative analgesia management of the obese patient?
   a. Intramuscular injection of analgesic drugs is an efficient and reliable method to deliver narcotics to these patients.
   b. Nonsteroidal antiinflammatory drugs should be avoided in the obese patient.
   c. Epidural anesthesia provides better postoperative analgesia as compared to parenteral opioids.
   d. The patient's body weight has a significant effect on morphine PCA dosing rate requirements.
   e. a and c are true.
   f. b and d are true.

2) Which of the following statements is not true?
   a. ACE inhibitor should be the first-line agent in the treatment of hypertension in the obese patient.
   b. Postoperatively, unfractionated heparin and LMWH are equally effective in preventing DVT in the obese patient.
   c. Obese patients are less prone to decubitus ulcer formation, due to a thicker adipose tissue layer.
   d. Adequate postoperative analgesia decreases the risk of cardiac and pulmonary complications.

3) Which of the following is true with respect to the obese patient with OSA?
   a. NPPV should be started in the recovery room when the patient is fully awake.
   b. OSA does not increase the risk of tachybradyarrhythmia.
   c. OSA is characterized by recurrent episodes of upper airway obstruction during sleep, due to a lack of neuromuscular ventilatory effort.
   d. OSA is a risk factor for respiratory compromise in the postoperative period.

CHAPTER 18

1) The Advance Trauma Life Support (ATLS) guidelines recommend that when assessing the obese trauma patient, the trauma team should first assess which of the following?
   a. BMI.
   b. Airway, breathing, and circulation.
   c. The most obvious and severe injury.
   d. Neurological status.

2) During the resuscitation of the obese trauma patient, which of the following is true?
   a. Pulse oximetry is not always accurate in the obese patient, since excess adipose tissue can create a barrier for the penetration of the light sensor.
   b. Vital signs may be erroneously elevated if the blood pressure cuff is too small. To obtain an accurate measurement, the cuff should be ≥40% of the patient's arm circumference.
   c. The reliability of a 12-lead EKG can be affected by inaccurate lead positioning due to indistinct landmarks and inconsistent voltages.
   d. All of the above.
   e. None of the above.

3) Regarding the impact of obesity on trauma, which of the following is true?
   a. There is a consensus within the published literature that obesity in trauma patients is associated with increased mortality
   b. Obesity is associated with increased risk of pelvic fractures.
   c. Compared to nonobese trauma patients, obese trauma patients require a longer period of mechanical ventilation.
   d. All of the above.
   e. None of the above.

CHAPTER 19

1) BMI becomes a relative contraindication for organ transplantation at what level?
   a. 30–35.
   b. 36–40.
   c. 41–45.
   d. ≥46.

2) Which immunosuppression agent should be avoided perioperatively in the obese patient due to concerns about wound complications?
   a. Tacrolimus.
   b. Prednisone.
   c. Sirolimus.
   d. Mycophenolatemoetil.

3) Which risk factor is most associated with coronary heart disease after kidney transplant?
   a. New-onset diabetes mellitus.
   b. Hypertension.
   c. Hyperlipidemia.

CHAPTER 20

1) Which of the following statements is true?
   a. Bariatric surgery is associated with a high mortality rate.
   b. Approximately 30% of patients who have bariatric surgery are admitted to the ICU.
   c. Patients who are female, older than 60 years, heavier (BMI > 60 kg/m²), and who have complications of any kind will most likely need intensive care.
   d. Preoperative assessment and selection should be performed by a multidisciplinary team composed of clinicians who are dedicated to the management of the bariatric patient.

2) Which of the following is not true when caring for obese patients after bariatric surgery?
   a. Because obese patients have more reserve from excess adipose tissue, they should receive fewer calories than calculated from ideal body weight.
   b. Patients with documented sleep apnea should be treated with continuous positive airway pressure (CPAP) as soon as they are extubated to maximize air exchange.
   c. Failure to recognize an anastomotic leak can result in rapid deterioration and death, and therefore the attending clinician should exercise a high level of suspicion.
   d. Central venous pressure readings in obese patients may be falsely elevated due to high thoracic pressures from the weight of the chest and abdomen. Therefore, the assessment of the patient should not be limited to any single value, but rather should look at trends and physiological responses.

3) Which of the following signs or symptoms may help to distinguish an anastomotic leak from PE?
   a. Tachycardia.
   b. Respiratory distress.
   c. Left shoulder pain.
   d. Hemodynamic compromise.

CHAPTER 21

1) What is the most reliable method for measuring REE in a critically ill obese patient?
   a. Harris–Benedict equation (HBE).
   b. Indirect calorimetry.
   c. Ireton-Jones equation.
   d. Penn State equation.

2) The 2009 Consensus guidelines by the Society of Critical Care Medicine and the American Society for Parenteral and Enteral Nutrition recommend which of the following nutritional regimens for a critically ill obese patient?
   a. Normal calorie and normal protein parenteral feeding.
   b. High-calorie and high-protein enteral feeding.
   c. Low-calorie and high-protein enteral feeding.
   d. Low-calorie and high-protein parenteral feeding.

3) Which of the following critically ill obese patients is better suited to receiving parenteral nutrition?
   a. Patient with prior history of extensive small-intestinal resection for Crohn's disease.
   b. Patient with stress-induced hyperglycemia.
   c. Patient with urosepsis.
   d. Patient with prolonged respiratory failure.

CHAPTER 22

1) Which of the following weights is most predictive of creatinine clearance in morbidly obese patients?
   a. Actual.
   b. Ideal.
   c. Lean.
   d. Adjusted.

2) Increased body weight relative to height due to obesity is most likely to affect which pharmacokinetic parameter of a lipophilic drug that is cleared by the liver?
   a. Absorption.
   b. Vd.
   c. Clearance.
   d. Protein binding.

3) Which of the following characteristics of a drug is most consistent with the concept of dose proportionality when a group of obese subjects who average 120 kg is compared to a group of normal-weight subjects who average 60 kg, assuming age, height, gender, and comorbidities are similar between the two groups?
   a. Clearance is 100 ml/minute in the obese and 50 ml/minute in the normal-weight subjects.
   b. Clearance is 100 ml/minute in the obese and 100 ml/minute in the normal-weight subjects.
   c. Half-life in hours is much greater in the obese compared to the normal-weight subjects.
   d. Vd in liters is similar in the obese compared to the normal-weight subjects.

CHAPTER 23

1) Obesity in the ICU is associated with all of the following, except which?
   a. Increased risk of organ dysfunction.
   b. Increased risk of infectious complications.
   c. Prolonged ICU and hospital length of stay.
   d. Increased mortality rates.

2) The obesity survival paradox could be explained by all of the following, except which?
   a. Obesity may be a marker of improved general health status.
   b. Adipose tissue may help in providing reserves of energy and lipid-soluble nutrients
   c. Hormones secreted by fat cells have immune effects that might reduce the inflammatory response and improve survival.
   d. Obese patients usually have fewer comorbidities on admission to the ICU.

3) Complications of nonlaparoscopic weight-reduction operations include all of the following, except which?
   a. Higher rates of wound infections.
   b. Higher rates of incisional hernias.
   c. Lower rates of gastrointestinal hemorrhage.
   d. Higher rates of early and late bowel obstruction.

CHAPTER 24

1) Which of the following is true of kidney donation in obese individuals?
   a. The long-term risk of chronic kidney disease should dissuade obese individuals from donation.
   b. Transplantation outcomes from obese donors fail to justify the risk.
   c. Carefully selected obese donors provide an opportunity to expand the donor pool.
   d. Effective management of diabetes and hypertension creates important opportunities for obese individuals to donate kidneys.

2) Which of the following is true?
   a. The AMA condones triage on the basis of conditions brought on by patient behavior, including obesity.
   b. Anti-fat bias has been demonstrated in health care professionals, including physicians and nurses.
   c. To avoid discrimination, weight should not be taken into account when managing obese patients.
   d. Worse survival in obese patients may have to be considered when discussing the burdens and benefits of mechanical ventilation.

3) Which of the following characterizes prognosis in obese patients who are critically ill?
   a. Available metaanalyses suggest that survival in obese patients rivals that of normal-weight individuals.
   b. Length of stay is unaffected by obesity.
   c. BMI is an effective way to describe multiple patterns of fat distribution, which appear to have an equivalent impact on comorbidities.
   d. Paradoxically, obese patients have more ventilator-free days than normal-weight controls.

Answers to Multiple Choice Questions

Chapter 1

1. d
2. b
3. e

Chapter 2

1. e
2. d
3. f

Chapter 3

1. b
2. a
3. f

Chapter 4

1. c
2. d
3. b

Chapter 5

1. d
2. c
3. b

Chapter 6

1. d
2. c
3. c

Chapter 7

1. c
2. e
3. a

Chapter 8

1. b
2. c
3. b

Chapter 9

1. f
2. a
3. f

Chapter 10

1. d
2. b
3. b

Chapter 11

1. a
2. c
3. d

Chapter 12

1. b
2. c
3. a

Chapter 13

1. b
2. c
3. e

Chapter 14

1. b
2. c
3. d

Chapter 15

1. b
2. c
3. c

Chapter 16

1. c
2. b
3. d

Chapter 17

1. c
2. c
3. d

Chapter 18

1. b
2. d
3. e

Chapter 19

1. c
2. c
3. a

Chapter 20

1. d
2. a
3. c

Chapter 21

1. b
2. c
3. a

Chapter 22

1. c
2. b
3. a

Chapter 23

1. d
2. d
3. d

Chapter 24

1. c
2. b
3. a

Index

Critical Care Management of the Obese Patient, First Edition. Edited by Ali A. El Solh.
© 2012 John Wiley & Sons, Ltd. Published 2012 by John Wiley & Sons, Ltd.